The NEW
GLUCOSE
Revolution for
DIABETES

To stay up to date with the latest research on carbohydrates, the GI, and your health, and the latest books in the series, check out the free online monthly newsletter *GI News*, produced by Dr. Jennie Brand-Miller's GI Group at the University of Sydney: http://ginews.blogspot.com.

The NEW GLUCOSE Revolution for DIABETES

The Definitive Guide to Managing Diabetes and Prediabetes Using THE GLYCEMIC INDEX

Jennie Brand-Miller, PhD
Kaye Foster-Powell, M Nutr & Diet
Stephen Colagiuri, MD
Alan W. Barclay, B Sci, Grad Dip Dietetics

Da Capo

LIFE LONG

A MEMBER OF THE PERSEUS BOOKS GROUP

Copyright © 2007 by Jennie Brand-Miller, Kaye Foster-Powell, Dr. Stephen Colagiuri, Alan Barclay

Designed by Pauline Neuwirth, Neuwirth & Associates, Inc.
Set in 11.5 point Fairfield LH by the Perseus Books Group

Cataloging-in-Publication data for this book is available from the Library of Congress.

ISBN: 978-1-56924-307-7

Published by Da Capo Press
A Member of the Perseus Books Group
www.dacapopress.com
Note: The information in this book is true and complete to the best of our knowledge. This book is intended only as an informative guide for those wishing to know more about health issues. In no way is this book intended to replace, countermand, or conflict with the advice given to you by your own physician. The ultimate decision concerning care should be made between you and your doctor. We strongly recommend you follow his or her advice. Information in this book is general and is offered with no guarantees on the part of the authors or Da Capo Press. The authors and publisher disclaim all liability in connection with the use of this book. The names and identifying details of people associated with events described in this book have been changed. Any similarity to actual persons is coincidental.

Da Capo Press books are available at special discounts for bulk purchases in the U.S. by corporations, institutions, and other organizations. For more information, please contact the Special Markets Department at the Perseus Books Group, 2300 Chestnut Street, Suite 200, Philadelphia, PA, 19103, or call (800) 810-4145, ext. 5000, or e-mail special.markets@perseusbooks.com.

10 9 8 7 6

*This book is for all the people who live
with diabetes and have so openly shared
their experiences with us.*

■

Contents

The NEW

GLUCOSE
Revolution for
DIABETES

Introduction

Diabetes has been around for thousands of years, and was once relatively rare. Its literal meaning is "to pass through"—referring to the passing of liquids through the body. The ancient Egyptians recommended that those suffering from "the passing of too much urine" eat a diet of fruit, grain and sweet beer. The Greeks, who mistakenly thought it was a weakness of the kidneys, prescribed exercise, "preferably on horseback."

Diabetes is no longer rare. In fact, it is one of the fastest-growing diseases in the world. About 246 million people in the world have diabetes, and that number is expected to reach 380 million by the year 2025. It can cause heart disease, blindness and kidney failure, and can lead to amputation. It can be a killer.

In the United States, diabetes and prediabetes affect 62 million adults. Every day nearly 300 people, including children, are being diagnosed with diabetes. And for every person diagnosed there's someone else who is undiagnosed. Millions of dollars are being spent by governments in treating, managing and preventing the epidemic, but the way to stem the tide really begins with us as individuals.

Living in the United States and Canada offers us immense potential for good health, but many people are uninformed about or confused by what's involved in a healthy lifestyle. Living well with diabetes doesn't mean being on a "diet." It means eating nutritious foods—and not eating whatever happens to be in front of you. It means making smarter food choices. And making the effort to move more.

In the last decade, research has yielded overwhelming evidence that lifestyle changes such as maintaining a healthy eating plan and increasing exercise can make a real difference in our risk of developing diabetes and in the quality of our health if we already have it. It's never too late to make a difference. There is the potential to turn back the clock.

HOW TO USE THIS BOOK

There are many types of diabetes and many different approaches to managing it. As the title says, this book is a diet and lifestyle guide to living well with diabetes or prediabetes, and there are many ways to do that. Our aim is to translate the current scientific evidence about managing and preventing diabetes into an accessible, practical resource, giving you the information to use so that you can discover what works best for you.

Whether you have **prediabetes**, **type 1 diabetes**, **type 2 diabetes** or **gestational diabetes**, this book has something for you.

The book sets out clearly and simply what you need to eat and do to:

- Reduce your risk of developing diabetes
- Improve your cardiovascular health
- Keep your **blood glucose levels (BGLs)**, **blood pressure** and blood fats under control, and
- Maintain a healthy body.

Part 1: Understanding diabetes, prediabetes and the metabolic syndrome will spell out the differences between the various types of diabetes, tell you how they are diagnosed and explain key aspects of their management.

In Part 2: What you can do, you'll learn the five fundamental steps to take to maintain a healthy lifestyle.

Part 3: Living with diabetes and prediabetes consists of sections on each type of diabetes and includes daily food guides, sample menu plans, recipes, a chart for converting from imperial to metric measurements (for Canadian readers) and the answers to frequently asked questions.

We have also included comprehensive GI tables to help you make smart food choices, and a detailed glossary to help demystify common medical terms and inform you so you can take control of your diabetes.

Diabetes is a complex condition, and there are aspects of its management—such as blood glucose monitoring, medications and **insulin**—which are not covered in detail. Nor do we cover management of diabetes **complications** (we hope this book will mean you never get them). The information in this handbook is not intended to take the place of individual consultation with your doctor or diabetes health professionals.

We hope that this book will help you to manage your diabetes successfully or turn back the clock with prediabetes. On the pages you will find anecdotes, comments and stories from people with diabetes whom we've spoken with throughout the years. We hope these inspire you, although keep in mind that what works for one person may not work for another. At the very least, we hope you might find familiarity with some of them and realize that you are not alone in your experience of managing diabetes.

We wish you success in preventing or managing diabetes.

ALAN BARCLAY
JENNIE BRAND-MILLER
STEPHEN COLAGIURI
KAYE FOSTER-POWELL
Sydney, January 2007

PART 1

Understanding Diabetes, Prediabetes and the Metabolic Syndrome

· 1 ·

Understanding Diabetes

FELIX

BACK IN LATE 2003, at age 41, although my general health appeared okay, I began to notice that my weight was inexplicably starting to drop, and I was starting to drink a lot of water and felt the need to urinate a lot. By early 2004 things had worsened considerably. Basically, I began to feel very unwell. Dizzy, extreme lethargy, blurry vision . . . and the weight loss continued. Although I realized that something was clearly wrong with my health and I was worried, I was extremely reluctant to visit my doctor! In the end, urged by family, I did, and the blood tests that followed showed a very high blood glucose level of 414. Yes, I had type 2 diabetes.

$\mathcal{D}$**iabetes mellitus is** a chronic condition. In simple terms, this means that your **blood glucose** (sometimes called blood sugar) is too high. There is no cure. It can be successfully managed, but it will never go away. It changes your life, so it's not surprising that anger and denial are really common reactions to a diagnosis of diabetes.

In fact, the range of feelings many people experience when first diagnosed are not dissimilar to those of grieving. In a way, a diagnosis of diabetes represents the loss of your healthy whole self. Your initial reaction may be "not me" denial or "why me?" anger. You may even try bargaining, perhaps with the "Almighty." You may experience a period of depression. Hopefully, finally will come acceptance that you have diabetes, that life will be different, but you can manage it successfully, and life will go on.

Whatever your reaction to the diagnosis, your feelings are perfectly natural. You are not alone. If it is any consolation, the pain you are feeling now may help you manage your health positively in the years to come. Having diabetes need not stop you from enjoying life to the full and achieving whatever you want from life.

According to research from the *Diabetes Information Jigsaw*, "depression greatly reduces the ability of people with diabetes to manage their condition, which can result in poorer management of blood glucose levels and difficulty in sticking to exercise, diet and treatment programs." The most important thing you can do is take control of the things in your life you can change and get informed about your body and what is happening to it. Knowing what you need to do to manage diabetes will allow you to live well and lessen the impact of this disease.

To understand why diet and lifestyle are so important in managing diabetes successfully, it is useful to know about how your body normally handles the nutrients in the food you eat, and how (and why) disturbances to its **metabolism** can affect your overall health.

BLOOD GLUCOSE AND INSULIN

Your body is incredibly complex, and is delicately tuned to deliver peak performance. You really are what you eat. "Metabolism" is the term that describes the processes (a complex series of biochemical reactions) that direct **energy** from the food you eat into fueling normal growth, development and physical activity; or into storage, such as **fat**.

Your body needs protein to build and maintain tissues, good fats to function and thrive, and **carbohydrates** as an energy source. It is important to understand carbohydrate's role. When you eat carbohydrate foods such as bread, cereals and fruit, your body converts them into a **sugar** called **glucose**. It is this glucose that is absorbed from your intestine and becomes the fuel that circulates in your bloodstream.

Glucose is a universal fuel for your body cells, the primary fuel source for the brain, red blood cells and a growing fetus, and the main source of energy during strenuous exercise.

In a healthy person, when glucose levels in the blood rise after a meal, the **beta cells** in the **pancreas** get the message to secrete a **hormone** called insulin. Insulin drives glucose out of the blood and into the cells. Once inside the cells, glucose is channeled into various pathways—to be used as an immediate source of energy, or converted to **glycogen** (a storage form of glucose) or to fat. **Insulin has been likened to the key that opens the cell door to let the glucose inside.**

Sometimes glucose builds up in the blood. There are two reasons for this. Either the pancreas can't produce enough insulin on demand (some or all of the keys are missing) or the cells do not respond to the insulin in the blood the way they should (the locks are malfunctioning).

"Insulin deficiency" is when the pancreas does not produce enough insulin to reduce blood glucose levels; "insulin resistance" is when the insulin can't do its job properly. Both these conditions lead to glucose accumulating in the bloodstream and to high blood glucose levels. Depending on how high the levels of glucose are, the condition is classified as:

- Diabetes, or
- Prediabetes (see chapter 2).

How active you are and how much you weigh have a very important effect on your metabolism, especially on the way your body handles carbohydrates. Being overweight or obese is a very common cause of insulin resistance, and losing a little weight is a powerful way of reducing insulin resistance. Exercise and improving your physical strength are also good ways of reducing insulin resistance.

TYPES OF DIABETES

There are three main kinds of diabetes, and although many of the symptoms are the same, the causes are very different.

Type 1 diabetes

Type 1 diabetes is an **autoimmune disease** and is one of the most common childhood diseases. Rates are increasing throughout the world, and no one knows exactly why. Certain environmental triggers have been proposed as possible contributors.

About 10 percent of people with diabetes have type 1. In this type of diabetes, the pancreas does not produce any insulin, so you need insulin injections. Maintaining a balanced blood glucose level (BGL) requires regulating your food intake, your insulin dose and your exercise.

Formerly called juvenile diabetes or insulin-dependent diabetes, type 1 diabetes is usually first diagnosed in children, teenagers or young adults. At the moment, half of all people with type 1 diabetes are diagnosed before the age of 16. Within this group there are two peaks in the age of onset: the major peak at 10–12 years and a smaller one at 5–6 years. For some reason, type 1 diabetes is more commonly diagnosed in the winter months.

The risk of someone developing type 1 diabetes if no one in the family has it is around 1 in 200. If there is a family history, the chances of developing it are much higher: about 1 in 17 if you have a brother or sister under the age of 30 who has it, and about 1 in 3 if your identical twin has it. Children whose mothers have type 1 diabetes have about a 1 in 75 chance of developing the condition; children whose fathers have it have a much higher chance—1 in 16.

Where you live also seems to affect your chances of developing the disease. Children in Finland have the greatest risk (37 per 100,000), whereas children in Fiji have a very low chance (1 per 1 million). Overall, boys and girls have the same degree of risk.

In chapters 30–34 we look at managing type 1 diabetes.

Type 2 diabetes

Eighty-five to ninety percent of people with diabetes have type 2 diabetes. Usually, type 2 diabetes develops after the age of 40. With our society's increasing trend to physical inactivity and **obesity**, however, this type of diabetes is being found in younger and younger people, and in some indigenous populations, even in children less than 10 years old. Overeating, being overweight and not exercising enough are important factors (what we call lifestyle factors) that can lead to this type of diabetes, especially in a family where someone already has diabetes.

WORLDWIDE, OVER THE last twenty years the total number of people with diabetes has risen from 30 million to 230 million. Similarly, data collected in the United States confirms the rising rate of diabetes among children—around 39,000 teenagers between the ages of twelve and nineteen may have type 2 diabetes, and 2.8 million may have prediabetes.

Most children with type 2 diabetes are being diagnosed in ethnic groups that already have a high susceptibility: African Americans, Latinos, Pacific Islanders, subcontinental Indians, and Asians. This link with ethnicity reflects a genetic susceptibility, as does a strong family history of type 2 diabetes. For example, we know it's highly likely that a child with type 2 will have at least one parent or grandparent with type 2 diabetes.

People get type 2 diabetes because their insulin is not working properly (insulin resistance, when the locks are malfunctioning). For a long time the body will struggle to make extra insulin to overcome the problem, but eventually people with type 2 diabetes develop a shortage of insulin (the keys get lost). The aim of treatment is to help people with type 2 diabetes make the best use of the insulin they have and make it last as long as possible. Pills or insulin injections may be necessary.

Being diagnosed with type 2 diabetes can be a shock. However, if current estimates are anything to go by, you shouldn't feel that you have been singled out. There are around 246 million people with diabetes worldwide; this number is expected to reach 380 million, or 7 percent of the adult population, by 2025. A recent Canadian study found that the rate of diabetes among people 20–50 years old has increased almost 100 percent in the last ten years—and it's still on the rise.Right now in America there are nearly 21 million people with diabetes—almost 10 percent of the population. Makes it sound pretty common, doesn't it?

In fact, scientists are predicting that 1 out of every 3 people born in the United States during the year 2000 will develop type 2 diabetes.

The cost of having type 2 diabetes to you as an individual and our community as a whole is enormous. The American Diabetes Association in 2002 found that total healthcare cost for people with type 2 diabetes who had no complications was over $13,000 for each person, each year. One out of every $10 spent on health care in the United States goes toward diabetes The total annual healthcare cost for diabetes and its complications is $92 billion—10% of the money spent on health care in the United States. The real challenge will be to fund and develop medical and public health programs that will help people manage their condition and prevent its complications.

The other scary thought is that for every person with diagnosed diabetes, there is someone else walking around with the condition who doesn't know it. In fact, many people have type 2 diabetes for several years before it is picked up—often during a routine medical exam, or after a major event like a heart attack or stroke. Regular health checks and screening by your doctor are a good idea after the age of 45, particularly if you have a close relative with the condition.

Why did you get it?

We know that the number of people with type 2 diabetes is increasing dramatically. Why? Mostly, it's a combination of unlucky genetics, increasing rates of overweight and obesity, and other lifestyle factors, particularly decreasing levels of physical activity. People from certain ethnic backgrounds and age groups are at greatest risk. Also, many people who develop type 2 diabetes have had **impaired glucose tolerance** or **impaired fasting glucose** (both are early signs of imminent diabetes) for many years.

Insulin resistance, which occurs without your even knowing it, is thought to be an underlying cause of type 2 diabetes. With insulin resistance, your muscle and liver cells are not good at taking up glucose from the blood, unless there's a truckload of insulin around. This makes the beta cells in your pancreas work overtime to produce extra insulin so that your muscle cells get enough glucose for making energy. Once your beta cells are unable to produce enough insulin to overcome the resistance, you get high blood glucose levels . . . and along with that, the diagnosis of diabetes.

IMPAIRED GLUCOSE TOLERANCE and impaired fasting glucose are often referred to as prediabetes. They are conditions in which blood glucose levels are higher than normal, but not high enough for a diagnosis of diabetes. People with prediabetes are at increased risk of developing diabetes, heart disease and stroke.

Coming to terms with prediabetes ("impaired glucose tolerance" and "impaired fasting glucose").

- **Prediabetes** is a term used to describe people who are at increased risk of developing diabetes.
- **Impaired fasting glucose** is a condition in which the fasting blood glucose level is elevated (110–125 mg/dL [6.1–7.0 mmol/L]) after an overnight fast, but is not high enough to be classified as diabetes.
- **Impaired glucose tolerance** is a condition in which the blood glucose level (BGL) is elevated (greater than 140 mg/dL [7.8 mmol/L]) 2 hours after an oral glucose tolerance test, but is not high enough to be classified as diabetes (that is, less than 200 mg/dL [11.1 mmol/L]).

Many factors are being identified as contributing to this failure of the beta cells, and it is believed to be at least partially genetically preprogrammed. This is why type 2 diabetes is more common among certain groups: African Americans, Hispanic Americans, Native Americans Aboriginal Australians or Torres Strait Islanders, Maoris, Pacific Islanders, Southeast Asians and Asian Indians. People from an Anglo-Celtic background, on the other hand, appear to be less susceptible.

■

**Genetics may load the cannon,
but human behavior pulls the trigger.**

Frank Vinicor,
United States Centers for Disease Control and Prevention

■

However, genes alone do not account for the increasing diabetes rates. Environmental factors such as reduced activity and a high-calorie diet have led to increased rates of overweight and obesity. Not surprisingly, around 80 percent of all people with type 2 diabetes are either overweight or obese.

Overweight is not only one of the underlying causes of type 2 diabetes. It also increases the risk of developing high blood pressure, high LDL ("bad") **cholesterol** and **triglycerides**, and as a result of all these things, it also dramatically increases your risk of developing **atherosclerosis** (hardening and narrowing of the **arteries**) or blocked arteries. In addition to these factors, more and more women are developing a condition called **polycystic ovarian syndrome** (PCOS), which is also thought to be due to insulin resistance.

Occasionally there are other causes of diabetes. There are some medical disorders that cause secondary diabetes, such as pancreatitis (inflammation of the pancreas) and acromegaly (due to excessive growth hormone production).

A number of medications also increase the risk of type 2 diabetes— the most important of these are the glucocorticoids or "steroids" that are often used by people with severe asthma or arthritis. People who need to take certain antipsychotic drugs for mental disorders, or anti-HIV drugs for AIDS, may also increase their risk of developing type 2 diabetes.

Did You Know?

THE RISK OF dying from a heart attack increases 2–3 times if you have diabetes.

In chapters 24, 25, 26 and 27 we look at managing type 2 diabetes.

Gestational diabetes

Gestational diabetes is the type of diabetes that women can develop during pregnancy. In any pregnancy, insulin resistance develops naturally as a pregnant woman's insulin needs are 2–3 times her normal needs. If a woman is overweight during pregnancy, it's worse. If a woman's body cannot produce enough insulin to overcome the insulin resistance, her blood glucose levels increase above normal.

In most women, when the baby is born, her blood glucose returns to normal and the gestational diabetes disappears. However, the risk of these women developing permanent diabetes later in life is very high, and they are strongly encouraged to eat well, watch their weight and exercise regularly to reduce their chance of developing it. They should also have regular blood checks for diabetes, because it can develop "silently."

In the United States, about 5 percent of pregnant women, or 1 in every 20, develops gestational diabetes. The number of women developing gestational diabetes is increasing, and again it is more common in women of certain groups (Asian Americans, African Americans, Hispanics, and Native Americans, for example). It is also more likely in women over 30, with multiple pregnancies, in overweight women and in those who have a family history of diabetes or previous gestational diabetes.

If gestational diabetes is not detected and treated properly it places the baby at risk of growing too big in the womb, which can make the birth difficult. Also, the baby is at increased risk of other complications and is more likely to be overweight as a child and develop other health problems (e.g., high blood pressure, heart disease and diabetes). That is why the American College of Obstetricians and Gynecologists recommends that women should be tested for gestational diabetes at 24–28 weeks of every pregnancy.

In chapters 28 and 29 we look at managing gestational diabetes.

DIAGNOSING DIABETES

The main symptoms of diabetes are:

- Increased thirst
- Tiredness
- Blurred vision
- Leg cramps
- Increased urine output
- Always feeling hungry
- Itching, skin infections, cuts that won't heal, and
- Unexplained weight loss.

However, the majority of people (except those with type 1), especially early in the development of diabetes, have no obvious symptoms at all.

Diabetes is diagnosed by a blood test. If your doctor suspects diabetes, either because of symptoms (listed above) or because you are in one of the high-risk groups (listed below), they will arrange for you to have a blood test to measure your blood glucose level (BGL). This is best done after fasting overnight (no food between dinner and the test the following morning).

Are You at Risk of Having Undiagnosed Diabetes?

IF YOU CAN say yes to any of the following questions, you should be having annual checks of your blood glucose levels. This is the only way to find out if you have undiagnosed diabetes. Your doctor can arrange this.

- Are you over 55?
- Do you have a family history of diabetes?
- Are you overweight or obese?
- Do you have high blood pressure?
- Did you have diabetes during pregnancy (gestational diabetes)?
- Are you an African American, Hispanic American, Native American, Pacific Islander, Southeast Asian or Asian Indian?

If there are questions in this list that you don't know the answer to, make an appointment with your doctor for a checkup.

If the result is very high and you have symptoms, that is all that is needed to make the diagnosis.

If it is moderately high, the test should be repeated to make sure of the diagnosis.

If the result is a little bit higher than normal, you will need to have an oral glucose tolerance test to make the diagnosis. This involves fasting overnight, then having a blood test to measure the fasting blood glucose, then drinking a sweet drink with 75 grams of glucose, and then measuring the blood glucose again 2 hours later.

The end result of these tests is that you might have diabetes, or your tests could be normal, or you could have prediabetes.

Diagnosing and treating diabetes (or prediabetes) early is an important way to prevent complications.

For every person who is known to have type 2 diabetes, there is another who has it but does not know it. Having diabetes and not knowing about it is like walking along with a hole in your wallet. About 1 in 4 people already have signs of permanent damage from diabetes by the time it is diagnosed. This is because they have had diabetes for a long time without knowing it and their high blood glucose levels have been quietly causing problems.

·2·

Understanding Prediabetes

SUSIE

WHEN I WAS diagnosed with prediabetes, I didn't know where to start or how to begin to plan my meals. I did know that I really had to lose some weight, as I was 200 pounds. In 3 months I managed to lose just over 13 pounds. I found it useful having an actual program, as it took a lot of the thinking out of planning meals. I didn't feel like I was on a "diet" as such because I felt as though I was always eating. It took a little getting used to at first because I'm not a veggie person at all, but I found that using balsamic vinegar with salads helped. And I did modify my dinner entrées by having gravy—I don't like dry food or veggies, but I ate them. And I did do much more exercise.

If **you have** prediabetes (the term used to describe impaired glucose tolerance and/or impaired fasting glucose), it means that you have blood glucose levels somewhere between normal and diabetes.

It's diagnosed by either a fasting blood glucose test or an oral glucose tolerance test.

Studies around the world show that there are twice as many people with prediabetes as with diabetes—in fact, it is currently estimated that there are about 300 million people worldwide with prediabetes. So it is a major public health problem that's only going to get worse unless something is done.

Left untreated, prediabetes can develop into type 2 diabetes. It also puts you at risk of some of the complications associated with diabetes, such as heart attack and stroke. That's why as well as making lifestyle changes to deal with prediabetes, you could also benefit from advice on how to prevent heart disease and stroke.

The good news is that there is very strong evidence that you can prevent, or at the very least delay, getting type 2 diabetes—and all of its complications. In fact, several large studies have shown that 3 out of 5 people with prediabetes can prevent the development of type 2 diabetes—very good odds indeed.

Be Well, Know Your BGL
(Blood Glucose Level)

Normal ranges for:

Fasting glucose	< 100 mg/dL (< 5.6 mmol/L)
Nonfasting glucose	< 140 mg/dL (< 7.9 mmol/L)
Glycated hemoglobin	4.0–6.0 percent

RISK FACTORS FOR DEVELOPING PREDIABETES

If there's type 2 diabetes in your family you probably already know that you have an increased chance of getting it too. But genetics alone doesn't account for the current diabetes/prediabetes epidemic. Instead, it's what researchers call our "diabetogenic environment"— the food we eat and our sedentary lifestyle. The most obvious trigger is that we're all getting heavier, and carrying extra body fat goes hand in hand with prediabetes and type 2 diabetes. People who are overweight, particularly around their middle, have up to three times more chance of developing type 2 diabetes than people who are in the healthy weight range.

Risk factors you cannot change

- A family history of diabetes
- Your ethnic background (people of Asian, Indian, African, Pacific Island, Hispanic and Native American background have a greater risk)
- Having polycystic ovarian syndrome (PCOS)
- Having diabetes in pregnancy or giving birth to a big baby (more than 9 pounds)
- Having heart disease, angina, or having had a heart attack, and
- Having familial hypercholesterolemia (an inherited condition that leads to higher than normal LDL cholesterol and potentially a heart attack early in life).

Risk factors you can do something about

- Smoking
- Being sedentary
- Having high blood pressure
- Having high triglycerides
- Having low **HDL** (good) **cholesterol**
- Having high total **LDL cholesterol**, and
- Being overweight, especially if that weight is around your middle.

Of course not every overweight person is going to develop prediabetes or type 2 diabetes (many don't), but the underlying metabolic problem in prediabetes and type 2 diabetes—that is, insulin resistance—is exacerbated by being overweight.

As we explain in chapter 1, insulin resistance means your body cells are resistant to the action of insulin (plenty of keys but the locks are malfunctioning). They don't let glucose in as easily as normal, so the blood glucose level (BGL) tends to rise. To compensate, the pancreas makes more and more insulin. This eventually moves the glucose into the cells, but the blood insulin levels stay high. Having high insulin levels all the time spells trouble.

Being overweight makes this situation worse because the excess fat "blocks" the action of the insulin, putting added pressure on the body's ability to maintain optimal blood glucose levels.

WHAT'S THE BEST WAY OF PREVENTING IT?

A healthy lifestyle, of course. There's nothing you can do about the inherited risk factors or family history. But you can do something about your weight, the food you eat and a sedentary lifestyle. And if you smoke, you can quit.

Several studies around the world (in China, Finland, the United States and India, for example) have shown conclusively that people with prediabetes can delay or prevent the development of diabetes. All of these studies were based on people who made lifestyle changes. People increased their level of activity, ate a healthier diet and achieved modest weight loss (about 10–20 pounds). All these changes are achievable with a little effort, and the long-term benefit is enormous—not having to live with diabetes and reducing your risk of heart attack and stroke.

▪3▪

Understanding Heart Disease and the Metabolic Syndrome

UNDERSTANDING THE METABOLIC SYNDROME ✶

*I*f your doctor has told you that you have high blood pressure and "a touch of sugar" (prediabetes), you probably have the **metabolic syndrome**. This term describes the clustering of risk factors for heart disease, including

- diabetes or prediabetes
- central obesity
- high blood pressure
- high blood fats (triglycerides).

You may also see it referred to as Syndrome X or the Insulin Resistance Syndrome. Surveys show that 1 in 2 adults over 25 has the metabolic syndrome.

People with metabolic syndrome are three times as likely to have a heart attack or stroke as people without it, and they have five times more risk of developing type 2 diabetes (if it's not already present).

Insulin resistance is thought to be the reason these risk factors cluster, because tests on people with the metabolic syndrome show that insulin resistance is nearly always present. Each risk factor should be treated aggressively to reduce the risk of heart disease, and in this chapter we look at how you can do this.

RISK FACTOR 1
HAVING DIABETES OR PREDIABETES

High blood glucose levels increase the tendency for blood clots to form. The resulting increased risk of heart attack is a major reason why so much effort is put into helping people with diabetes achieve optimal control of their blood glucose levels, and why all people with diabetes should be checked for the other risk factors of heart disease. But you don't need to have diabetes to be at risk—having even moderately raised blood glucose levels hours after a meal has been associated with increased risk of heart disease in normal "healthy" people.

Here's how diabetes and prediabetes can cause inflammation and hardening of the arteries. A high level of glucose in the blood means:

- Excess glucose moves into cells lining the arteries, which causes inflammation, thickening and stiffening—the making of "hardened arteries"
- Highly reactive, charged particles called "free radicals" are formed; these destroy the machinery inside the cell, eventually causing cell death
- Glucose sticks to cholesterol in the blood, which promotes the formation of fatty plaque and stops the body from breaking down excess cholesterol, and
- Higher levels of insulin (which follow higher levels of glucose) raise blood pressure and blood fats, while lowering "good" (HDL) cholesterol levels.

RISK FACTOR 2
CENTRAL OBESITY

When you put on weight, the fat can be distributed evenly all over the body or stick around the middle: what is called middle-age spread, a pot belly or a muffin midriff. Fat around the middle part of your body (abdominal fat) increases your risk of heart disease, high blood pressure and diabetes.

A Healthy Waist

THE INTERNATIONAL DIABETES Federation has published criteria for defining the metabolic syndrome. A person with metabolic syndrome will have abdominal obesity plus at least two of the following other risk factors: high triglycerides, low HDL cholesterol, raised blood pressure and/or raised blood glucose. A basic guide to whether you have abdominal obesity is:

For people of European origin:

Men	37 inches (94 cm)
Women	31.5 inches (80 cm).

For people from South Asia:

Men	35.5 inches (90 cm)
Women	31.5 inches (80 cm).

For people from Japan:

Men	33.5 inches (85 cm)
Women	35.5 inches (90 cm).

These are the most recently published criteria from the International Diabetes Federation (2006).

For more information go to: www.idf.org/home.

In contrast, fat on the lower part of your body, such as your hips and thighs, doesn't carry the same health risk. In fact, your body shape can be described according to your distribution of body fat as either an "apple" or a "pear" shape:

There are significant health benefits in reducing your waist measurement, particularly if you have an "apple" shape.

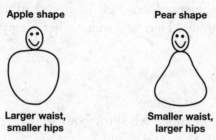

Apple shape   Pear shape

Larger waist,   Smaller waist,
smaller hips   larger hips

RISK FACTOR 3
HAVING HIGH BLOOD PRESSURE

High blood pressure (**hypertension**) is the most common heart disease risk factor. It is harmful because it demands that your heart work harder and it damages your arteries.

An artery is a muscular tube. Healthy arteries can change their size to control the flow of blood. High blood pressure causes changes in the walls of arteries which makes atherosclerosis more likely to develop. Blood clots can then form, and the weakened blood vessels can easily develop a thrombosis, or rupture and bleed.

About 1 in 3 American adults aged 20 years and older have hypertension, which is defined as having blood pressure above 140/90. This rises to more than 1 in 2 among adults over age 60. People with diabetes should aim to keep their blood pressure under 130/80. High blood pressure is especially dangerous because it often gives no warning signs or symptoms. Your blood pressure can be high and you feel on top of the world. That's why it is important to have it checked regularly by your doctor. If it is high, there are things you can do to lower it. Just as important, if your blood pressure is normal, there are things you can do to keep it from becoming high.

What can you do about high blood pressure?

A research study in the United States—the Dietary Approaches to Stop Hypertension (DASH) study—showed that you can reduce your blood pressure by eating foods rich in grains, fruits, vegetables and low-fat dairy products. Here are some other lifestyle characteristics that help:

▶ Be a nonsmoker
▶ Reduce your salt intake
▶ Achieve and maintain a healthy body weight
▶ Limit your alcohol intake, and
▶ Be active every day.

Tips for Reducing Your Salt Intake

■ Avoid salty foods such as processed meats, commercial sauces and soups (unless they are labeled low salt or reduced sodium), potato chips, salty fast foods and salty nuts.
■ When you buy foods in cans, bottles, jars, packages including stock cubes and wrapped bread, look for "no added salt," "low salt" or "reduced sodium."
■ Don't add salt when you cook. Use herbs, spices and salt-free seasoning blends instead.
■ Rinse canned foods when possible to remove some salt.

RISK FACTOR 4
HAVING HIGH BLOOD FATS (TRIGLYCERIDES)

Over half adult Americans have high blood fat levels. For people with diabetes, this increases the risk of having a heart attack or a stroke, or developing peripheral vascular disease (for example, in the lower limbs, particularly the feet).

What causes high blood fats?

Abnormal levels of blood fats are part and parcel of the metabolic abnormalities of diabetes and prediabetes. In particular, low levels of HDL cholesterol and high triglycerides are common. For some people, genetic factors are to blame, but for the majority, diet and lifestyle factors contribute.

Blood Fats

HDL CHOLESTEROL

HDL (high-density lipoprotein) cholesterol seems to protect against heart disease because it clears cholesterol from the arteries and helps in its removal from the body. So having low levels of HDL in the blood is a risk factor for heart disease.

LDL CHOLESTEROL

LDL (low-density lipoprotein) cholesterol does the most damage to blood vessels. It's a red flag for heart disease. LDL cholesterol comes from the liver to the rest of the body's organs, and can build up in the walls of blood vessels throughout the body.

TRIGLYCERIDES

The blood also contains triglycerides, another type of fat linked with increased risk of heart disease. Having too much triglyceride is often linked with having too little HDL cholesterol (high-density lipoprotein). Although this can be inherited, it's most often associated with being overweight or obese.

There is good evidence that people with diabetes have similar total and LDL cholesterol levels to the rest of the population. However, their average HDL cholesterol levels are approximately 7.8 mg/dL lower and their average triglyceride levels are around 30 percent higher than people without diabetes.

What can you do about high blood fats?

Moderate weight loss, regular exercise and good blood glucose control will all improve blood fat levels. Dietary factors that raise triglyceride levels include eating too many high-GI carbohydrates (see chapter 10), drinking too much alcohol and not eating enough omega-3 fats.

Should You Look Out for Foods That Claim to Be Low Cholesterol or Cholesterol Free?

OVERALL, IT IS more practical to focus on eating less saturated fat than on eating less cholesterol, because saturated fats have a more powerful effect on blood cholesterol levels, and many of the foods that are high in saturated fat are also high in cholesterol anyway.

If a food does say it is low cholesterol, check the amount of saturated fat in the nutrition panel. For oils, margarines and other similar foods that are nearly 100 percent fat, look for those with saturated fat content of less than 20 percent of the total fat. For other foods, if they have less than 1 gram per serving they are probably a good choice.

Most foods that are high in cholesterol are from animals, because cholesterol is manufactured in the liver. So low-cholesterol claims on rice and bread are pretty meaningless. However, some preprocessed plant-based foods have animal fats added to them when they are prepared (many cookies and cakes do), so some can contain significant amounts of cholesterol.

Omega-3 fats are found in oily fish, such as herring, mackerel, sardines, salmon and tuna. They are also found in certain nuts and seeds, and products made from them: flaxseed, canola, walnut and wheat germ for instance. You should try to eat two to three servings of fatty fish a week, a couple of handfuls of nuts (preferably walnuts) a week, and you should use margarines and oils. It is also helpful to eat a diet low in saturated fat by:

▶ Eating reduced-fat or low-fat milk, cheese, yogurt, ice cream and pudding

- Eating lean meat and chicken, and trimming off any visible fat before cooking
- Avoiding butter, lard, dripping, cream, sour cream, coconut milk, coconut cream and hard cooking margarines
- Limiting pastries, cakes, puddings, chocolate, cookies, and chips to special occasions
- Limiting the use of processed deli meats (such as bologna, luncheon meat, chicken loaf, salami), hot dogs and sausages
- Avoiding take-out foods such as French fries, fried chicken, batter-dipped fish, pizza and hot dogs, and
- Making and eating tomato and soy-based sauces and soups (rather than creamy ones).

What is insulin resistance?

Insulin resistance means that the body does not react in a normal way to insulin in the blood—it is insensitive, or "partially deaf," to insulin (the lock is faulty). Just as we may shout to make a deaf person hear, the body makes more insulin in an effort to make it work. So moving glucose into cells necessitates the release of large amounts of insulin. This is why high insulin levels are part and parcel of insulin resistance, which in turn leads to other abnormalities, such as high blood pressure, due to the effect of the high insulin levels on the kidneys.

While some insulin resistance is determined by your genes, what you do to your body is also very important. People who are overweight and do not exercise are usually insulin resistant.

How do you know if you have insulin resistance?

You probably have insulin resistance if you have two or more of the following:

- High waist circumference
- High blood pressure
- Low HDL (good) cholesterol levels
- Prediabetes
- High triglycerides, and
- High uric acid levels in blood.

Chances are your total cholesterol levels are within the normal range, which could give you and your doctor a false impression that your coronary health is okay.

You might also be normal weight but with a high waist circumference (more than 31.5 inches [80 cm] in women, more than 37 inches [94 cm] in men). This indicates excessive fat around the abdomen, which is a heart health risk.

But the red flag is if your blood glucose and insulin levels, after a glucose load, or after eating, remain high. Resistance to the action of insulin is thought to underlie and unite all the features of this cluster of metabolic abnormalities.

Why is insulin resistance so common?

The answer is that both genes and environment play a role. People of Asian and African American origin, and descendants of the original inhabitants of North and South America and Australia, appear to be more insulin resistant than those of Caucasian extraction, even when they are still young and lean. But regardless of ethnic background, insulin resistance develops as we age, probably because as we grow older we gain excessive fat, become less physically active and lose some of our muscle mass.

What we eat plays an important role, too. Specifically, eating too much fat, especially saturated fat, and too little carbohydrates can increase your insulin resistance. And if your carbohydrate intake is high, eating high-GI foods can make preexisting insulin resistance worse.

Why is it a big deal?

The higher your insulin levels, the more carbohydrates you burn at the expense of fat. This is because insulin has two powerful actions: one is to "open the gates" so that glucose can flood into the cells and be used as the source of energy; the other is to *stop* the release of fat from fat stores. The burning of glucose reduces the burning of fat, and vice versa.

These two things keep going on even if you have insulin resistance because your body overcomes the extra hurdle by just pumping out more insulin into the blood. Unfortunately, the level that finally drives glucose into the cells is 2–10 times more than is needed to switch off the use of fat as a source of fuel.

If insulin levels are high all day long, as they are in insulin resistant and overweight people, the cells are constantly forced to use glucose as their fuel source. They draw it from either the blood or stored glycogen. The blood glucose level (BGL) then swings from low to high and back again, playing havoc with appetite and triggering the release of stress hormones. And stores of carbohydrates in the liver and muscles also undergo major fluctuations over the course of the day.

When you don't get much chance to use fat as a source of fuel, it is not surprising that fat stores accumulate wherever they can:

- Inside the muscle cells (a sign of insulin resistance if you are not an elite athlete)
- In the blood (this means you have high triglycerides, and many people with diabetes or the metabolic syndrome have this)
- In the liver (nonalcoholic fatty liver), and
- Around the waist.

Insulin resistance gradually lays the foundations for heart attack and other diseases (stroke, polycystic ovarian syndrome, liver disease) and acne.

▪ 4 ▪

Coming to Terms
with Diabetes

PETER HOWARD

"NOTHING SUCCEEDS LIKE excess" was my mantra for many years, and boy did I live it with my job as a wine and food editor on national TV.

In 2004 I was diagnosed as having type 2 diabetes and my doctor told me in no uncertain terms that I had to mend my bacchanalian ways or suffer the consequences (and he graphically described what these were likely to be).

But even a couple of years into living with diabetes, I still find it hard to write the word "disease," because I want to ignore it or want it to go away. I know, however, that I do have a disease that won't go away but that I can manage it with diet, exercise and self-control. As it is for many other diabetics, this is a difficult, private battle. We have to forgive ourselves for arriving at this stage and just get on with life and our new-found lifestyle.

What has having diabetes meant? First of all it's been a real wake-up call and has strengthened my resolve to become healthy. I have had to find the determination to lose weight, exercise and completely cut back on drinking alcohol—essentially change my lifestyle completely. My intake of fruit and vegetables has certainly improved, as has my fiber intake, and I don't skip meals. I still have diabetes. I also have a lot more energy, my blood pressure has dropped, my blood glucose levels are sorting themselves out and my friends all comment on how well I look.

The really cold hard fact is that we people with type 2 diabetes have to take our lives into our own hands and accept the responsibility of living a healthier lifestyle.

COMING TO TERMS WITH DIABETES

Being told you have diabetes can come as a shock. It can be hard to accept that you have to take it seriously. And that it won't go away. Ever. As Peter Howard says, it's a "real wake-up call."

Changing the foods you eat, including more physical activity in your day, monitoring your blood glucose and/or taking diabetes medications or insulin can interfere with all the everyday activities you did before you were diagnosed with diabetes or prediabetes. Nothing will be the same again. And most people with diabetes experience some degree of loss—from the loss of the freedom to eat and drink whatever they like whenever they like, to the loss of a limb or vision. Many people go through a series of stages as they eventually learn to cope with their condition.

■

"This can't happen to me! No one in my family has ever had diabetes."

■

Denial

Many people respond to a diabetes diagnosis with a mixture of surprise, shock and disbelief. It's very easy to dismiss it when you have no major symptoms—as is often the case when you first find out. But it's not so easy to do if your eyesight has started to deteriorate, or you develop an ulcer on your foot because of poor circulation. What's most important at this stage is not to let your "denial" feelings get in the way of learning how to manage your diabetes.

■

"Why me? What have I done to deserve this?"

■

Anger

Anger can be healthy if you can express it without hurting yourself or others. Get it out in the open. It's better to find someone—a friend, family member or professional counselor—who can help you sort out your feelings than to bottle them up or dump them on those close to you.

Whatever you do, don't shut your family and friends out or turn them off; you need their love and support more than ever now.

Don't suppress your anger, as that can lead to other problems, such as channeling your resentment into resisting treatment. Not a good idea at all!

Find a way to work it out. Beat the stuffing out of your pillow, or use it to muffle a good yell, or simply go for a walk—the exercise will do you good too. Try to turn all that anger energy into motivation— refuse to let diabetes rule your life.

■

"If you'll just give me five years, God, I'll . . ."

■

Bargaining

Bargaining (for many of us) is essentially a last-ditch attempt to try to control life, to go back to things as they were. Dr. Elisabeth Kübler-Ross called it a period of "temporary truce." Some people address their pleas to a religious figure, some to their health professional, and others internalize their pleas. You'll find that as you sort out the day-to-day practical business of living with diabetes, you not only take responsibility for your health, you start getting back in control and things start to go your way again.

■

"How will I cope?"

■

Depression

Depression can be a significant problem for people with diabetes. Coming to terms with the changes that you have to make to accommodate diabetes has an impact. There may be times when you feel pretty distressed and unhappy with your situation. Making the transition from the "old, before diabetes self" to a "new, managing diabetes self" is difficult. Diabetes support groups, where you can talk to people who understand what you are going through, can really help you deal with low-level depression and anxiety. It's part of taking an active role in managing your diabetes, and this in itself can also be an antidote for depression.

DEPRESSION ISN'T JUST a fleeting feeling of sadness; it's a pervasive and relentless sense of despair. It is serious, and you need to ask for help. Common symptoms of depression include:

- A general lack of interest in life
- Marked changes in your sleeping patterns, including having trouble sleeping
- Ongoing fatigue and listlessness
- Changes in your appetite: either a loss of appetite or overeating
- Uncontrollable feelings of sadness, guilt, worthlessness or purposelessness
- An inability to concentrate on anything for longer than a few moments
- Suicidal thoughts, and
- Problems with sexual function (independent of any diabetes complications).

Talk to your doctor about getting professional help, or go to the following Web sites:

www.dbsalliance.org
www.depressionisreal.org
www.nami.org

However, some people are not able to overcome depression. If this is the case for you, seek help from a suitably qualified and experienced psychologist or psychiatrist.

"Yes, me!"

It isn't easy learning to accept as big a life change as diabetes, but when you start going through it, you start viewing life very differently. Once you've accepted your situation—that you have a chronic condition that isn't going to go away—it actually becomes much easier. But there are some issues that can arise. What follows are some guidelines for dealing with family, friends, colleagues, health professionals and the "diet police."

SOME OF THE THINGS YOU'LL NEED TO DEAL WITH

1. **Health professionals**

   The job of health professionals (general practitioner, diabetes educator, dietitian, endocrinologist) is to help you look after your diabetes yourself. If you think your healthcare providers are not treating you with the respect you deserve, talk to them openly about your feelings. If this does not lead to any improvement, politely ask to be referred to someone else.

2. **Telling others**

   Who needs to know that you have diabetes? There is no need to go around shouting to the world that you have diabetes; on the other hand, there is no need to be ashamed of it either. So how do you decide who to tell? While there are no hard and fast rules, these ideas might help you make up your mind.

   First, consider how often you see a person and what you do together when you meet. If you are to share a meal, why hide the fact that you have diabetes and need to check your blood glucose level (BGL) and take insulin or medication? You have nothing to be ashamed of—go ahead, tell them.

   On the other hand, if you just run into them from time to time and all you do is chat briefly, do they really need to know?

Schoolmates, colleagues, employers, or other people you see every day may need to know more. For example, if you take insulin or other diabetes medication that may make your blood glucose go low, you should tell your colleagues, because you may have to duck off and have a quick snack in the middle of something important—a game, a meeting, a class.

If you operate machinery or perform tasks that may put your or someone else's life at risk, you are morally obligated to let those who work with you know.

However, if you manage your diabetes or prediabetes just through healthy lifestyle, you probably do not need to tell your colleagues. If they ask you, though, it's wise to tell the truth.

3. The diet police

Let's face it—most people know, or have known, someone who has diabetes. If it was someone who was diagnosed just 10 years ago, chances are they were advised to avoid sugar in their diet as much as possible—this was the standard recommendation for all people with diabetes for most of the 20th century. That's why many people equate the management of diabetes with the avoidance of all sugar. But research has proven that people with diabetes can eat the same amount of sugar as the average person without compromising blood glucose levels. Of course "empty calories"—whatever the source: sugar, **starch**, fat, or alcohol—won't keep the engine running smoothly. "Moderation in all things" is a good motto.

■

"Should you be eating that? It's full of sugar."

■

How many times have you been asked this by an observer? While they have good intentions, it can be downright irritating. And wrong.

Beyond irritation, it can become dangerous if well-meaning individuals try to stop you from having dessert or a drink when you are having a hypo (blood glucose levels fall below normal)—there are more than a few stories of people having a potentially lifesaving "treat" snatched out of their hands!

But what can you do? If you are not having a hypo, you can politely explain that the recommendation to avoid sugar was based on experiments on dogs in the 1920s. We have known for the past 25 years that sugar does not upset blood glucose levels any more than a typical slice of bread.

Knowing why and how to look after yourself is very important, and once you are informed, you can enlighten other people about the modern management of diabetes.

Doesn't Sugar Cause Diabetes?

NO. THERE IS absolute consensus that sugar in food does not cause diabetes. Because the dietary treatment of diabetes in the past involved strict avoidance of sugar, many people wrongly believed that sugar was in some way implicated as a cause of the disease. While sugar is off the hook as a cause of diabetes, high-GI foods are not. Studies from Harvard University indicate that high-GI diets increase the risk of developing both diabetes and heart disease.

▪ 5 ▪

Understanding Diabetes Management

JOHN

I AM 64 and was diagnosed with diabetes at the end of May 2005. I was admitted to the hospital very ill—blood pressure 256/149; hemoglobin A1c 13.2; blood glucose 205; cholesterol 280; weight 250 pounds.

For several months I had been ill and showed all of the typical symptoms of diabetes—weight loss, craving for sweets, continual need to urinate, etc. But being a typical male, I refused to seek treatment until my condition was chronic. After 5 days in ICU and 3 in a recovery ward I was discharged with my blood glucose 8.2 and blood pressure controlled by medication. Fortunately, scans and tests revealed no abnormality to heart, lungs, liver or kidneys. Eyesight had deteriorated, but all pulses and nerves to extremities were normal. Eyesight has since restored itself and I use the same reading glasses I used before diagnosis.

I found out about the glycemic index and started the diet. I have now adopted this as a lifestyle. I have adhered to it for 6 months and intend to do so for the rest of my life. I have found the experience stimulating

and fulfilling and the dietary limitations minimal. In addition, I have a regimented regular exercise program of minimum of 30 minutes 5 days a
week on a treadmill at 4 mph. Over the past 6 months I have reduced
my insulin requirements, and for 4 weeks now I have stopped all insulin
injections. Random blood glucose readings vary between 81 and 115,
and this week I underwent my biannual medical, the results of which are
as follows: blood pressure 126/74, hemoglobin A1c (glycated) 99, cholesterol 127, LDL 48, HDL 61. All liver, kidney and urine tests normal.
ECG normal. Weight 220 pounds. I believe this is testament to the success of low-GI foods in the management of type 2 diabetes.

There are certain recommendations for good health for everyone
who has diabetes. Whether you have type 1 or type 2, keeping your
blood glucose levels as close as possible to the normal range (65–110
mg/dL) is the first step toward reducing the risk of complications. But
diabetes affects the whole body, so controlling your cholesterol and
blood pressure is the second step.

For some people with type 2 diabetes, all they have to do to achieve
this is manage their weight, maintain a healthy eating plan and be
active. Others need to take medicine as well and some may need
insulin (it depends on your number of surviving beta cells). People
with type 1 diabetes *must* have insulin injections.

Many women with gestational diabetes can be treated just by taking care with their diet, but some will require insulin injections. Other
diabetes medications are not used to treat gestational diabetes
because there is a chance that they may harm the baby.

Treating diabetes is a team effort. Ideally, on your team there will
be a doctor (and possibly an endocrinologist or specialist physician),
a diabetes educator, a dietitian, a podiatrist, an exercise specialist, an
eye doctor and a dentist. There may also be a counselor (psychologist
or psychiatrist) to help you cope with living with a chronic disease.

The most important member of your team is you, and knowledge is
your best defense. Only you can make sure you know as much as possible about your diabetes and only you can act on the advice that you
are given.

So, what do you need to aim for?

- Hemoglobin A1c (2–3 month average blood glucose)—under 7 percent
- Blood glucose levels 65–110 mg/dL (3.6–6.1 mmol/L)
- Blood pressure—under 130/80
- Cholesterol—under 156 mg/dL (4 mmol/L)
- Healthy weight
- Healthy eating plan
- Regular exercise
- Regular eye checks
- Regular foot examinations

If the combination of weight loss (if necessary), a healthy diet, physical activity and medication delivers near-normal blood glucose levels, your diabetes is well managed and your risk of complications is much lower. Unfortunately, it doesn't mean that your diabetes has gone away.

WORKING WITH A HEALTHCARE TEAM

Working with a healthcare team is the best way you can avoid the serious complications that diabetes can cause. That's the clear message from numerous studies of people with diabetes in recent years. And that's why you'll find the rest of this chapter is rather full of lists (sorry!).

What we have tried to do is give you as comprehensive a picture as possible of the sorts of tests and checkups you need, and how often you need them. If you find that you can't talk comfortably with anyone on your healthcare team, or that they don't give you the tests or information you need, go and find someone who will give you the care you deserve—and the answers to your questions. Don't hesitate to take this book (or a photocopy of the relevant pages) along with you to your appointments to refer to if it will help.

Seeing your family doctor

In most cases it's the family doctor who diagnoses diabetes and plays the central role in coordinating care. It is essential that you are happy with your doctor and feel comfortable talking to him or her, and that he or she understands what needs to be done.

What your doctor needs to do

First visit

- ▶ Give you general information about your diabetes so that you understand what it is and why effectively managing it is so important
- ▶ Measure your weight, height and waist
- ▶ Check your blood pressure
- ▶ Order blood tests to check your:
  - hemoglobin A1c (HbA1c) level, which is a measure of the average level of glucose in your blood over the last 2–3 months
  - cholesterol and triglyceride levels, and
  - creatinine level to see whether your kidneys are working properly
- ▶ Ask you to do a urine test to check for early signs of kidney problems
- ▶ Refer you to an ophthalmologist or optometrist to examine your eyes to check for early signs of diabetic eye disease (**retinopathy**)
- ▶ Refer you to a diabetes educator to give you more information about how you can manage your diabetes yourself
- ▶ Refer you to a dietitian to help you lose weight if you need to and determine the quantity and type of food you should eat at each meal
- ▶ Consider referring you to an endocrinologist, podiatrist, exercise specialist and/or other member of the diabetes management team, depending on your particular needs
- ▶ Talk to you about registering with American Diabetes Services or FreedoMed, so that you can buy cheaper test strips and needles if you need them

Even if your diabetes and any associated complications are being well managed, it is a good idea to have a checkup with your doctor every 3–6 months.

Checkups

- ▶ Check your blood pressure
- ▶ Check your weight

- Measure your waist circumference
- Order a blood test to check your hemoglobin A1c levels. HbA1c levels need to be checked every 3–6 months if you are using insulin, and every 6–12 months if you are not using insulin
- Check your cholesterol/triglyceride levels if they are above normal
- Help you set goals for managing your diabetes and discuss your progress towards achieving them, and
- Do a basic foot examination (every 6 months).

Each year
- Discuss how well you are managing your diabetes
- Check your cholesterol/triglyceride levels
- Ask you to do a urine test to check for early signs of kidney problems
- Discuss referral to an ophthalmologist or optometrist to have your eyes examined for early signs of retinopathy, and
- Refer you to an endocrinologist, diabetes educator, dietitian, podiatrist, exercise specialist and/or other health professionals as required.

Do You Need to See an Endocrinologist or a Specialist Diabetes Physician?

IF YOU HAVE type 1 diabetes you will generally need to see your endocrinologist annually for a checkup. Otherwise, your doctor may refer you to an endocrinologist or specialist physician if:

- Your hemoglobin A1c level is persistently over 8 percent
- You have been in the hospital for a diabetes-related problem
- You have other health problems associated with your diabetes, and/or
- You are pregnant or thinking of becoming pregnant.

Seeing a diabetes educator

The job of diabetes educators is to provide information, support and advice on diabetes management. They can instruct you on practical skills including how to monitor your blood glucose levels and manage your medication. This will be part of your diabetes management plan.

When should you see a diabetes educator?
▶ When you are first diagnosed with diabetes
▶ For an annual checkup, and
▶ If you change the way you manage your diabetes. For example, if you change from managing your diabetes simply by following a healthy lifestyle to taking diabetes medication, or from taking medicine to using insulin.
▶ It's also recommended you have a follow-up meeting if:
▶ Your HbA1c is persistently above 8 percent, and/or
▶ You are pregnant.

Finding a diabetes educator
▶ Your doctor or local hospital will be able to provide details on diabetes educators in your area. In the United States you can visit the American Association of Diabetes Educators Web site at www.aadenet.org.

What a diabetes management plan may cover
▶ How to monitor your blood glucose levels (and **ketones** if you have type 1 diabetes) and use the results to improve your diabetes management
▶ How to prevent, detect and treat high and low blood glucose readings and manage on sick days
▶ How to use your medications effectively on sick days
▶ How to manage your blood glucose, cholesterol and blood pressure levels
▶ What to do to reduce the risk of developing long-term complications of diabetes, including knowledge of risk-factor screening recommendations, ideal targets and personal targets

▶ Tips for communicating effectively with your diabetes healthcare team and negotiating your way through the healthcare system, and

▶ Advice on adapting your work, family and social life to live well with diabetes.

Seeing a dietitian

Dietitians can provide specific advice tailored to your current eating habits and food preferences, and will work with you to set realistic and achievable goals. They will help you understand the relationship between food and health and guide you toward making dietary choices that optimize your lifestyle.

When should you see a dietitian?

▶ When you are first diagnosed with diabetes, and possibly every 4 weeks for the first 3 months after you have been diagnosed, and then every 6–12 months after that

▶ Whenever you change the way you manage your diabetes

▶ If you are overweight

▶ If you are pregnant or thinking of becoming pregnant

▶ If your HbA1c is persistently above 8 percent

▶ If you have high blood pressure, cholesterol or triglycerides

▶ If you have diabetes and another condition such as heart disease, kidney impairment, **celiac disease**, or osteoporosis, and

▶ If you have problems managing your diabetes.

Finding a dietitian

Dietitians have professionally recognized qualifications in human nutrition. They practice as individual professionals and are available through most public hospitals and in private practice.

Call the American Dietetic Association's Consumer Nutrition Hotline (800-366-1655) or visit the ADA's home page: www.eatright.org. If you're in Canada, go to the Dietitians of Canada Web site at www.dietitians.org. Make sure that the person you choose has the letters RD after his or her name.

Seeing a podiatrist

Blood glucose levels that are high for long periods of time can damage nerves in the legs and feet, causing numbness or a burning sensation. If this happens, you can injure your feet without knowing it. If your diabetes is poorly managed, the blood vessels can become thick, rigid and narrow. Damage to the blood flow in your feet and legs can lead to problems such as infection, ulcers, and even gangrene. It's essential that people with diabetes practice good footcare. Hence, the recommendation to include a podiatrist in your healthcare team.

When should you see a podiatrist?

Annually for a routine diabetes foot check, and more often if you:

▶ Have a foot ulcer or have had one in the past
▶ Have had part or all of a foot amputated
▶ Have neuropathy (damage to the nerves in your feet)
▶ Have been told that you have problems with blood flow to your feet
▶ Have corns or calluses or other foot problems, including injuries that are slow to heal
▶ Have any problems or pain walking
▶ Have trouble finding shoes that fit you, and/or
▶ Can't look after your own footcare (can't reach your feet or have poor eyesight).

Seeing an exercise specialist

Did you know that you can improve your blood glucose levels, your blood fat levels and your body weight simply by being more active? A physiotherapist, exercise physiologist or ACSM (American College of Sports Medicine)-certified personal trainer can help you work out a program to improve your overall physical fitness, increase your total muscle mass and decrease your body fat.

When might you think about seeing an exercise specialist?

▶ When you are first diagnosed with diabetes
▶ If your HbA1c is persistently above 8 percent

- If you have high blood pressure, cholesterol or triglycerides
- If you have diabetes and another condition (such as problems with your heart or circulation)
- If you are overweight, and/or
- If you are having problems managing your diabetes.

Seeing an eye specialist

Everyone with diabetes is advised to have regular eye examinations with an eye specialist or optometrist, because early treatment can prevent the visual loss that can be part and parcel of diabetes.

When should you see an eye specialist or optometrist?
- When you are first diagnosed with diabetes, and
- At least every 1–2 years afterward.

Seeing a dentist

If you have diabetes, you are at greater risk of developing gum disease, including gingivitis and periodontitis (sore bleeding gums). Some studies also suggest that because gum disease is an infection, it can contribute to higher blood glucose levels. So it is important to keep your regular dental appointments. When you visit, remind your dentist that you have diabetes.

4 Steps to Preventing Gum Disease

- Brush your teeth twice a day and floss once a day
- Visit your dentist every 6 months for a checkup and cleaning to remove the buildup of tartar from areas your brush can't reach
- Manage your blood glucose levels, and
- Do not smoke—people who smoke are four times more likely to develop gum disease than people who don't.

Seeing a counselor

A psychologist or psychiatrist can help you make positive changes to your life that may make managing diabetes easier.

When might you think about seeing a counselor?
▶ If you suffer from stress because of your diabetes
▶ You are depressed or anxious, and/or
▶ You are having problems managing your diabetes.

Consumer health organizations such as the American Diabetes Association, (www.diabetes.org) or the Canadian Diabetes Association (www.diabetes.ca) can also play an important part in helping you manage diabetes, through membership, meetings, magazines and subsidized products.

Unfortunately, some people, despite their best efforts, find their diabetes difficult to manage and can't get the control they want. And again, despite hard work, some people still develop complications. This can be pretty discouraging. Just remember that if you do the best job you can day by day, you will reduce the risk of complications later on and slow the progress of complications that may be just beginning.

WHAT HAPPENS IF DIABETES IS NOT MANAGED WELL?

If blood glucose levels are not well managed, you can suffer damage to the blood vessels in the heart, legs, brain, eyes and kidneys. That's why heart attacks, leg amputations, strokes, blindness and kidney failure are more common in people with diabetes. Diabetes can also damage the nerves in your feet, causing pain and irritation in your feet and numbness and loss of sensation.

High blood pressure, high cholesterol, smoking and being overweight or obese can also lead to diabetes complications, especially damage to the blood vessels, which can in turn cause heart attacks, strokes and affect the circulation to the legs. That's why it's very important to deal with these problems and stay healthy.

PART 2:

What *You* Can Do

▪6▪

5 Steps to
Managing Diabetes

CLIFF

MY LOW-FAT, medium-protein, high-carb and low-GI diet has proved invaluable in helping me maintain tight glycemic control and long-term weight loss for some years. I now weigh 205 pounds—down from 260 pounds back in 1980, when I was 40.

I took early retirement for health reasons and because I knew that I needed to make some real lifestyle changes if I was going to have a life. Before that I had worked as an actuary, which is a very high-pressure, demanding job. At 46 I was diagnosed with diabetes, some three years later I had a mild heart attack, and in 1995 I needed to take insulin to manage my diabetes. My landmark year was 1997. I had successful six-artery bypass surgery and learned how to manage my diet using GI.

When I started using the low-GI approach, the first thing I had to learn was not to focus on the GI alone but to use it as a carbohydrate selection tool in meal preparation and when shopping (where label reading is of paramount importance). Memorizing which of my regular basic foods are low GI has been very useful for me, as I do not have to look up the GI and GL tables very often. Also, I find it essential to count my daily fat and carbohydrate intake using a simplified "portion" unit method, as I must not only monitor my GI but also my total energy intake.

To ensure good midmorning blood glucose readings, I find it necessary to confine breakfast to two pieces of low-GI fruit, rather than higher-energy-density cereal and milk with the same carbohydrate content—I eat bread and cereal later in the day when my insulin resistance is lower and I am consequently more at risk of having a "hypo."

I average five or six pieces of fruit per day (at the risk of having too little bread and cereal). And I have a large plate of microwaved vegetables (mainly home grown) and a side salad as part of my normal evening (fifth) meal, which is usually the only one including meat or seafood. My weekly dinner goal is 30 percent seafood, 30 percent vegetarian, 30 percent poultry, pork, veal and game meat, and 10 percent other red meat.

Portion control is an ongoing challenge, as is insidious nonhungry eating (I suffer from binge eating syndrome), especially in the evening.

From my experience, I must concede that my program would be rather difficult to maintain fully if I still worked full time in a demanding and stressful job. Being retired makes life much easier for a diabetic. But I am well and managing well. I have no serious diabetic complications— I have no eye or renal problems, and my heart health is stable. The main problem I have is moderate peripheral neuropathy.

Just for the record: my HbA1c is now 6.1, triglycerides 115.7, cholesterol—total 132.6, HDL 42.9, LDL 66.3, and VLDL 23.4.

MORE THAN ANY other chronic condition, diabetes requires a great deal of active input from people themselves. As much as 95 percent of diabetes care is self-care, and over the course of a lifetime, people will need a variety of skills and knowledge to enable them to manage their condition on a day-to-day basis and to modify their approach when circumstances change.

The Diabetes Information Jigsaw

The way you live will have a major impact on your diabetes, especially on your blood glucose levels. There are 5 key areas of your lifestyle/health to address in looking after diabetes. Not all the steps will apply to you. For example, if you don't need to lose weight or you don't smoke or drink alcohol, you may want to skip some of the chapters in this section.

STEP 1
EAT A HEALTHY, BALANCED DIET

Of course everybody should maintain a healthy, balanced diet. But it's not negotiable for people managing diabetes and associated diseases (such as atherosclerosis—hardening and narrowing of the arteries). In fact, many people can manage their type 2 diabetes or prediabetes simply by choosing the right kinds and amounts of foods (along with increasing physical activity)—they don't have to take any medication at all.

However, you can be forgiven for being confused about what eating a healthy balanced diet means. What is it? High carb or low? Lots of protein or moderate amounts? And where does the glycemic index (GI) fit into the picture?

For the answers to these and other questions, see chapters 7–16, which focus on **Step 1: Eat a healthy, balanced diet**.

STEP 2
BE ACTIVE EVERY DAY

We were made to move. But we don't do much of it these days in our push-button, "let your fingers do the walking" world. Too many of us lead busy but sedentary, desk-bound, commuting lives. We relax in front of the TV or computer and exercise infrequently or not at all.

Regular moderate physical activity is essential for managing diabetes or prediabetes and for reducing heart disease risk. Doing housework or gardening, or going for a brisk walk on a regular basis, all count toward increasing your activity level. Boosting them with regular, moderate-intensity exercise sessions can help you manage your blood glucose levels and reduce the risk of diabetes complications and heart disease.

How does it work? Exercise and activity increase glucose and insulin uptake and can:

- Help lower your blood pressure
- Reduce your heart attack risk
- Reduce your insulin requirements
- Help you stop smoking
- Help you manage your weight
- Increase your levels of good (HDL) cholesterol
- Help keep your bones and joints strong
- Improve your mood
- Ease depression
- Increase your stamina, and
- Increase your flexibility.

People who aren't active or who don't exercise have higher rates of death and heart disease compared with people who perform even mild to moderate amounts of physical activity (see chapters 17 and 18).

STEP 3
MANAGE YOUR WEIGHT

Besides making diabetes harder to control, being overweight puts you at a much greater risk of a range of health problems, including heart disease, high blood pressure, cancer, gout, gallstones, reproductive abnormalities and arthritis. Being overweight also interferes with sleep, because fat around the neck area and abdomen induces a dangerous form of snoring called sleep apnea, which means you could become tired and cranky as well! So losing a little weight, or at least stabilizing it if you are on the heavy side, has to be a priority.

The good news is you don't have to be "the biggest loser." Setting achievable weight-loss goals is the key. Research suggests that there are significant health benefits even when you lose just 5–10 percent of your body weight. For example, if you weigh 220 pounds, losing around 10–20 pounds over 12–24 weeks is realistic and safe—and enough to improve your health. If you achieve this and maintain the weight loss long term, your risk of developing other chronic diseases and the complications of diabetes will be substantially reduced.

> DID YOU KNOW that with our sedentary lifestyle, our energy needs are much lower than those of our parents and grandparents? We need about 30–50 percent less food energy than they did.

In chapter 19 we look more closely at body energy balance and what it takes to lose weight. We outline some workable approaches to weight management, setting realistic goals for body weight, and developing habits that may help you manage your weight.

STEP 4
DON'T SMOKE. IF YOU DO, QUIT

We all know that smoking is bad for our health—the warning label is on every pack. Smoking is most often associated with lung and other cancers, but it may also increase the risk of developing prediabetes or type 2 diabetes and many of the common complications of diabetes.

And did you know that smokers have more than twice the heart attack risk of nonsmokers and are much more likely to die if they suffer a heart attack? In fact, smoking is the most preventable risk factor for heart disease. Research has shown that smoking just one cigarette reduces the body's ability to use insulin by 15 percent! After a cigarette it takes 10–12 hours before the insulin resistance starts to improve.

In chapter 20 we look at smoking and diabetes.

STEP 5
LIMIT YOUR CONSUMPTION OF ALCOHOL

Like most things in life, moderation is the key. One or two drinks each day may actually help prevent or delay the development of diabetes, and some of its more common complications, by decreasing insulin resistance. It may also decrease the risk of developing heart disease, by providing small amounts of powerful antioxidants and thinning the blood. On the other hand, excessive amounts of alcohol may increase the risk of prediabetes and diabetes by contributing to weight gain— particularly if your drinking goes along with eating energy-dense foods.

If you have diabetes or prediabetes, it's important to limit your consumption of alcohol to no more than one standard drink a day if you are a woman and two standard drinks if you are a man.

In chapter 21 we look in more detail at alcohol and diabetes.

STEP 1

Eat a Healthy, Balanced Diet

$\mathcal{A}$ diagnosis of diabetes is a dietary wake-up call. Once you are diagnosed with diabetes, the question of what you eat is fundamental. It's time to learn from experience. Nutritional advice alone seldom motivates people to maintain a healthy eating plan.

So although we aim for this book to be informative and give you a better understanding of your diabetes, we also aim for it to be very practical to help you find the connection between what you eat and how you feel. We believe that once you've experienced the difference good nutrition can make in how you feel, you're in a great position to keep it up for the rest of your life.

In the following chapters we show you how you can eat a healthy, balanced diet that will keep you feeling fuller for longer, help keep your blood glucose levels on an even keel and reduce your risk of complications by helping you manage your blood pressure and blood fat levels.

·7·

Just Tell Me What to Eat

*T*here is no absolute "right" way to eat to manage diabetes. Only you can really tell what eating plan suits you best: you know what works for you and how you feel. People with diabetes are often "cheered up" when their dietitian says that "a diet that's good for people with diabetes is a diet that is good for everyone." What this really means is that you need to eat the same healthy foods that others eat (or they should start eating healthy foods like you). That way, when they have their cake, you can eat it too, if you want to.

It's tempting to simply try to write out lists of "what to eat" and "what not to eat." But it just can't be done. Take sugar, for instance. Any self-respecting person with diabetes would put it on the taboo list. Wouldn't they? Well, not necessarily. Eating well if you have diabetes isn't about good foods and bad foods, eating this and avoiding that. It's about enjoying *all* foods for nourishment and pleasure, just coupled with a knowledge of and respect for your body's needs (and if you're wondering how sugar fits in, check chapter 16).

There are three aspects of eating well for diabetes management:

▶ What you eat
▶ How much you eat, and
▶ When you eat.

Why what you eat is important

Your health and vitality depend on the quality of the food your body receives. Besides protein, fat and carbohydrates, you need vitamins to help your body convert food into fuel, minerals to carry oxygen in your blood, antioxidants to boost your defense system and phytochemicals to prevent disease (to name just a few).

Why how much you eat is important

Achieving or maintaining a healthy weight will help you manage your blood glucose. Too many **calories**, whether they are carbohydrates, protein or fat, will increase your body weight. Too much carbohydrate will raise your blood glucose levels. The trick is to find the amount and combination of healthy foods that's right for you.

Why when you eat is important

Eating regularly almost inevitably improves blood glucose levels, and there are probably several reasons for this. Most meal plans for diabetes include three meals each day. They may include snacks as well—there are no hard and fast rules about how many times a day you will need to eat.

Ten key dietary recommendations

Remember what we said at the beginning of this chapter: there isn't any one diet for everybody with diabetes. In fact, at the present, there is some controversy about what the best dietary approach should be for people with diabetes. The tussle is primarily between a traditional high-carbohydrate, low-fat diet and a lower-carbohydrate, higher-protein or higher-fat diet. And the GI story has put carbohydrate quality under the microscope.

What this means is that you actually have a great deal of flexibility in the overall makeup of your eating plan. It's a matter of discovering what suits you best while fitting within these 10 key dietary recommendations:

- ▶ Choose nutritious carbohydrate foods with a low GI as your staples
- ▶ Be aware of how much carbohydrate you eat
- ▶ Get plenty of fiber in your diet
- ▶ Limit foods that are high in saturated fat
- ▶ Eat lean protein foods to suit your appetite
- ▶ Eat fish once or twice a week: if you are a vegetarian, make sure you focus on including foods that contain quality proteins and are good sources of omega-3 fats
- ▶ Use **monounsaturated fats** (such as olive oil)
- ▶ Eat plenty of fruit and vegetables every day
- ▶ Limit your salt intake, and
- ▶ Limit your alcohol intake.

FROM FOOD TO FUEL:
A LITTLE BIT OF BASIC NUTRITION

The human body truly is a marvelous machine. It converts the energy found in food in a zillion different processes, from the micro level (molecular change) to the macro (your taking a step). Your body needs food for energy, just like cars need gasoline. However, unlike cars, which can run on just one type of fuel, your body needs three different fuel sources: protein, fat and carbohydrates (we can burn alcohol too, but it's an optional extra).

The energy available from these three fuels ranges from 4 calories per gram of protein or carbohydrate to 9 calories per gram of fat. It's kind of like standard fuel compared with super high octane. You get the most mileage from fat. (Unfortunately, though, most of us don't drive our bodies nearly as much as we drive our cars.)

There is a fuel hierarchy, too. That is, the body follows a particular order for burning the fuels you take in. If you drink, alcohol is at the top of the list, because your body has no place to store unused alcohol. Excess protein comes next, because we can store only a little.

Carbohydrates are third in line (we can store some), and fat comes off last (we have unlimited storage space for fat). In practice, the fuel mix is usually a combination of carbohydrates and fat in varying proportions. After meals, the fuel is predominantly carbohydrates, and between meals it is mainly fat.

Turning Food into Fuel

HERE'S WHAT HAPPENS to a piece of bread:

1. When you chew the bread in your mouth it combines with saliva. There's an enzyme in saliva that chops up some of the starch in the bread, breaking it down into smaller pieces.

2. When you swallow the bread, it lands in your stomach, where it gets pummeled and churned, pretty much the way clothes are in a washing machine. Once your stomach has squished it around, it spits out the bread into your small intestine. If the bread has viscous fibers in it (such as soybeans and oats), or is acidic (such as sourdough), your stomach empties more gradually.

3. Once the bread is in your small intestine, an avalanche of digestive juices attacks the starch and breaks it down into smaller and smaller chains of glucose, which then move toward the wall of the intestine. There is an oversupply of digestive juices—more than you really need—so this process can happen very quickly, depending on what kind of bread you've eaten.

4. At the intestinal wall, the short chains of glucose are broken down even further. The final results of digestion are monosaccharides (single sugars). They are absorbed from the small intestine through the intestinal wall into the bloodstream, where they are available to the cells as a source of energy.

5. Within minutes of eating, those glucose molecules appear in the bloodstream. The rate they appear at—in a big gush or as a little trickle—is determined by the rate of digestion, the rate of absorption through the intestinal wall and the rate at which food is emptied from the stomach.

WATER

Water is an often forgotten essential nutrient. It is critical for every bodily function. But for a lot of people, water is not part of their daily diet. We may not need the popularly recommended 8 glasses a day, but we all need some, and if we smoke, drink alcohol, consume caffeine or are physically active, we need more.

Drinking water is a habit, and it's one of the habits we want you to have. To get started, make it available. Whatever type of water you like—filtered, bottled or plain old tap water—make sure it's in front of you all the time. Then make a habit of drinking it.

The color of your urine tells you how well hydrated you are:

▶ Clear or very pale indicates good hydration, and
▶ Darker colored (except for first thing in the morning) suggests dehydration.

In the next chapter we take a closer look at each of the three main fuels—protein, fat and carbohydrates—to help you understand food better.

· 8 ·

Nutrition Basics
What You Need to Know About Protein, Fat and Carbs

PROTEIN

*P*rotein is part of every cell, and is therefore vital in the growth and repair of tissues throughout your body. It is made up of amino acids, which are the building blocks of the body. They form your hair, skin, muscles, hormones, blood cells, etc. Protein can also be used as a fuel. Indeed, any excess beyond your immediate needs (for amino acids) is quickly converted to energy.

Protein is found in lots of plant and animal foods. The foods with the most protein are meat (beef, pork, lamb, chicken), fish and shellfish. Dairy products such as cheese (especially cottage cheese), milk and yogurt are also rich sources. For vegetarians, legumes including soybeans and their products (tofu), nuts and grains are significant sources. Protein foods, especially meat, are also rich sources of micronutrients such as iron, zinc and vitamin B_{12}, and fish is a source of omega-3 fats.

Protein and blood glucose

Protein does not directly affect blood glucose levels, but just like carbohydrates, it does stimulate secretion of significant amounts of insulin. Up to half the protein we eat will eventually be converted to glucose via a process called "gluconeogenesis" (which literally means the creation of new glucose). After you eat a protein-rich meal, your glucose concentrations do not rise and fall in any marked way because your body balances the rate of glucose production with the rate of glucose burning.

How much do you need?

When we grow, so do our protein needs. That's why children, adolescents and pregnant women need more protein than healthy, full-grown adults. It's the same scenario if you are recovering from an injury (healing burns or wounds), from a major illness, or repairing or building muscles (as athletes or weekend warriors do)—your protein needs are greater.

When your blood glucose levels are high, as they are in type 1 and type 2 diabetes, there is an increase in your protein turnover, and this in turn increases your body's protein needs slightly. However, because most people already consume much more protein than they physically need, eating even more protein is not usually recommended.

Most people with diabetes can stick with their regular protein intake: it usually provides about 15–20 percent of their total energy intake. This means eating enough protein to provide about 1 gram of protein per 2 pounds of your healthy body weight. It isn't hard to do. As long as you have enough food to eat, you will be getting enough protein, because it is so widely available in our food supply. Unfortunately, this is not the case for many people living on the African continent.

Should you eat a high-protein diet?

In the last few years, researchers have discovered many potential benefits of a high-protein diet, especially for weight management. In particular, protein has been found to be more satiating than carbohydrates and fats—it makes you feel fuller for longer. Not only are you more satisfied after eating; it also reduces your hunger in between meals.

Protein has another benefit for weight management. It increases your metabolic rate for 1–3 hours after meals. Although the effect is only small, it may make a difference to your weight over the long term.

Some studies show that **insulin sensitivity** and blood glucose levels improve in people with type 2 diabetes following a high-protein diet. However, a recent study from the University of Sydney showed that a high-carbohydrate diet was superior when weight loss and cardiovascular risk were considered together.

There is also a question about high protein intake and the kidneys. While high protein intake does not appear to contribute directly to the development of diabetic kidney disease (**nephropathy**), it does increase the workload of the kidneys, because the waste products of protein breakdown need to be excreted quickly via urine. This is why high-protein diets aren't recommended for people with diabetes, particularly those who have any signs of nephropathy.

Perhaps the greatest concern about protein is the company it keeps. Slabs of fatty steak, a plate of eggs and bacon and chunks of cheese and salami are high in protein, but they also contain lots of saturated fat. This is one of the main reasons why a high-protein diet is not recommended for people with diabetes.

FAT

You're about to butter your toast at breakfast and then you hesitate. Would margarine be better? Or natural butter? Maybe you shouldn't use anything at all? But dry toast isn't very appealing.

In 1927, Elliot P. Joslin, a professor at the Harvard Medical School wrote: "with an excess of fat, diabetes begins, and from an excess of fat, diabetics die." Although Joslin wrote that nearly 80 years ago, he was right. Excess body fat definitely contributes to the development of type 2 diabetes. The increasing prevalence of both obesity and diabetes supports that. And there is good evidence linking a high saturated fat intake to the complications of diabetes. But is a low-fat diet the answer? Scientists disagree.

What's the problem with fat?

One problem with fat is the amount we eat (sometimes without knowing it). Fat provides a lot of calories (more than any other nutrient per gram) and is the least satiating nutrient. This is great for someone who's starving, but it's a real disadvantage for those of us who constantly verge on eating too much. Fat provides 9 calories per gram—more than twice the energy of protein or carbohydrates. And the main form in which our bodies store those extra calories is—you guessed it—fat. Indeed, scientists can tell what sort of fat you've been eating by analyzing a slice of your body fat.

Another problem is heart disease. As we explained earlier, people with diabetes have a greatly increased risk of **cardiovascular disease**—heart disease and stroke are 2–3 times more likely in people with diabetes than in those without, and almost 70 percent of people with type 2 diabetes die of cardiovascular disease. High levels of LDL (bad) and total cholesterol are a known risk factor for cardiovascular disease, and reducing total fat—and in particular saturated fat—lowers both total and LDL cholesterol, and therefore decreases this risk.

Whatever the fat content of your diet (low or moderate), the type of fat you eat matters—monounsaturated fats (found in nuts, seeds, olive oil, avocado, etc.) should dominate. Eating more fat from these sources gives you a nutritional profile more like a Mediterranean diet, which will also help you lower your triglyceride levels and increase your HDL (good) cholesterol. However, you need to remember that the Mediterranean diet carries a risk of weight gain (if it's not calorie controlled), and in the long run may not benefit your **glycemic** control.

What happens when we eat fat?

The digestion of fat is a slow process compared with the digestion of protein and carbs—it doesn't really begin until the fat reaches your small intestine. Here bile works rather like detergent in the dishwasher, breaking up fats into small droplets that are cleaved apart by an enzyme from the pancreas. About 3 hours after eating, the digested fat is fully absorbed. Once absorbed, the fat circulates in your bloodstream as triglycerides.

What are triglycerides?

Triglycerides are the white fat you see on meat. They come from fats we eat in foods, but they are also made in the body from excess glucose, and they circulate in our bloodstream after meals. Calories that are in excess of our body's needs can be converted into triglycerides and transported to fat cells to be stored. Excess triglycerides in the blood are a common characteristic of diabetes and have a bad effect on metabolism. They also, of course, contribute to the increased risk of heart disease, stroke and liver disease.

Triglyceride levels rise gradually after a meal, and in a person who doesn't have diabetes, they return to premeal levels after 4–6 hours. But in people with type 2 diabetes, the clearance of triglycerides from the circulation is delayed, and having high levels in your bloodstream for a long time is harmful. Here's what high triglycerides do:

- They impair insulin's action, thus suppressing glucose uptake and use by muscles, which means that glucose hangs around in the bloodstream
- They stimulate the liver to make more glucose, raising blood glucose levels even further
- They cause the liver to form fatty particles that are toxic to blood vessels
- They accumulate in the liver and cause "fatty liver," and
- They impair insulin secretion (possibly by accumulating in the pancreas and impairing beta cell function).

All in all, this means a high-fat meal can be pretty bad news for your diabetes.

WHAT FAT IS THAT?

The most concentrated sources of fat in our diet are butter, margarines and oils. Although all fats provide about the same number of calories per gram (and so are theoretically as fattening as each other), there are differences in the nature of the fatty acids they contain, and those differences have major implications for your health.

Fats are broadly classified into three groups—polyunsaturated, monounsaturated and saturated. The classification is based on the chemical structure of the fat and the type of fatty acid that is dominant.

What's a Fatty Acid?

A FATTY ACID is a chain of carbon and hydrogen atoms bonded together. Most fats contain three fatty acids joined by a glycerol back-bone to form one fat molecule or triglyceride.

Polyunsaturated fats

These are found in seed oils. They are liquid in nature. The most common examples are safflower, sunflower, soybean and cottonseed oils, which are rich in omega-6 fats. These fats all have cholesterol-lowering properties, but like saturated fats, we can eat too much of them.

Omega-3 fats are another form of polyunsaturated fats. Very long chain forms are found in significant quantities in fish, and a shorter form is found in some plant oils, including canola, linseed (flaxseed) and walnut oils. They can reduce your risk of cardiovascular disease too, mostly by reducing your triglyceride levels. Many of us don't get the recommended quantities of the omega-3 fats we need.

Monounsaturated fats

These are found in virtually all edible fats, but canola and olive oils, margarines made from these oils, nuts and avocados are particularly rich sources. These fats can protect you against heart disease and increase HDL (good) cholesterol levels. Although olive oil doesn't have a lot of omega-3 fatty acids (which are good), it has the advantage of not providing a lot of omega-6 fats. It also has the longest history of safe and healthy use and is rich in antioxidants if it is "cold pressed" (look for "first cold pressing" on the label).

Saturated fats

These are solid at room temperature—the more saturated fatty acids there are in the fat, the harder it is at room temperature. Saturated fats are generally bad for our health. They decrease the effectiveness of insulin, increase LDL cholesterol levels and increase heart disease risk. Eating foods rich in certain saturated fats promotes the formation of too much LDL cholesterol in our blood. High blood cholesterol is strongly associated with heart disease risk.

Dripping (fat from beef and lamb), lard (fat from pork), butter and cream are largely saturated fat. Two plant oils, coconut and palm kernel oil, also contain fats that can promote higher blood cholesterol.

Trans fats

These are formed in food manufacturing when vegetable oils are processed and made more solid. Think of them as saturated fats, because they damage the body in a similar way. Commercial baked goods (such as crackers, cookies and cakes) and fried foods (such as doughnuts and French fries) are likely to contain trans fats.

How much fat do you need?

Not everyone has to cut down on their fat intake. If you are at a healthy weight now (and have no problems maintaining it), you may not need to reduce the amount of fat you eat at all. So how much fat is enough? And how much is too much?

Minimum: The World Health Organization recommends that men get at least 15 percent of their energy (calories) from fat and women of reproductive age get at least 20 percent.

Maximum: The upper level for adults is 35 percent of their energy. This translates to about 50–60 grams of fat daily for a sedentary adult, not more than 10 grams of which should be saturated.

■

Did you know that breastfed infants get 50–60 percent of their energy intake as fat?

■

We all need some fat because:

▸ It is part of all our cell membranes
▸ It is a carrier of fat-soluble vitamins A, D, E and K and many antioxidants
▸ It is an integral part of many hormones
▸ It is an energy source, and
▸ It provides insulation, for warmth and protection of vital organs like the kidneys.

The absolutely essential fatty acids that we must get in our diet—because our body can't make them—are alpha-linolenic acid (ALA) and linoleic acid (LA). ALA is an omega-3 fat found in flaxseed, canola, walnuts and some dark green leafy vegetables. LA is an omega-6 fat found in corn, safflower and sunflower oils.

Giving the bad fats the brush-off

Saturated and trans fats are some fats that we all need to avoid. An intake of less than 10 percent of your total calories per day from saturated fats and less than 2 percent from trans fats is what's recommended. For an average diet of 2000 calories, this means a maximum of 15–20 grams of saturated fat per day.

Limit these foods
▸ Fatty meats and meat products—sausages, salami, bologna, pepperoni (average 10 grams saturated fat per serving)
▸ Full cream (full fat or whole) dairy products—milk, cream, sour cream, cream cheese, cheese, ice cream (average 8 grams saturated fat per serving)
▸ Coconut milk and cream and palm oils (about 20 grams saturated fat per serving)

▶ Solid frying oils, cooking margarines (average 7 grams saturated fat per 2 teaspoon serving)
▶ Potato chips, tortilla chips, packaged snacks (6 grams saturated fat per average serving)
▶ Cakes, cookies, slices, pastries, pies, pizza (10 grams saturated fat per average serving), and
▶ Deep-fried foods—fried chicken, French fries, spring rolls, tempura, batter-dipped foods (around 10 grams saturated fat per serving, depending on the oil used).

Choosing the good fats

A healthy balance of fats means including *some* polyunsaturated oils that are rich in omega-6 fats (such as corn, soybean and safflower oils) and more sources of omega-3 (such as fish, canola, flaxseeds, walnuts, pecans and soybeans). A monounsaturated fat such as olive oil is a good general oil to use.

Include these sources of mono- and polyunsaturated fats

▶ Olive and canola oils
▶ Mustard seed oil
▶ Margarines and spreads made with canola, sunflower or other seed oils
▶ Avocados
▶ Fish, shellfish, shrimp, scallops
▶ Walnuts, almonds, cashews, pecans
▶ Natural muesli (not toasted), and
▶ Linseeds (flaxseeds).

The Benefits of Omega-3

DID YOU KNOW that people with large amounts of omega-3 fats in their diet are less likely to have type 2 diabetes or prediabetes? What's more, these fats are a must for a healthy heart—and they don't upset your blood glucose levels. There are lots of ways omega-3 fats can help you:

- They make your platelets less sticky and lower fibrinogen levels (fibrinogen is a blood-clotting factor). This means they decrease the chance of forming blood clots throughout your body, thus reducing the likelihood of a heart attack, stroke or embolism (clot).
- They make your red blood cells more flexible so your blood flows more easily, lowering your blood pressure and improving delivery of nutrients and oxygen to your cells.
- They lower blood fats (especially triglycerides) and increase HDL (good) cholesterol levels.
- They stabilize your heartbeat, preventing abnormalities (arrhythmia) that can lead to cardiac arrest.
- They may reduce microalbuminuria (an abnormally high amount of protein in the urine) and thus help patients on dialysis (a process used to filter the kidneys).
- They may elevate your mood, lift depression and improve your ability to deal with stress.
- They reduce inflammation and can relieve symptoms of arthritis.
- They may reduce the output of the stress hormone adrenaline.

How to Get Your Omega-3 Fats

- Eat oily fish—salmon, ocean trout, sardines, mullet, herring, mackerel, tuna or canned fish (especially red salmon, sardines and mackerel) at least twice a week.
- Choose omega-3-enriched foods in place of the regular variety.
- Eat an omega-3-rich egg three or four times a week.
- Use canola oil in cooking and dressings.
- Eat plenty of dark green vegetables.
- Include walnuts, pecans, linseeds (flaxseeds), wheat germ and soy products in your diet.

The American Heart Association recommends 2–3 servings of fish per week.

If you don't eat fish, consider a fish oil supplement, but consult your dietitian or doctor first.

CARBOHYDRATES

Carbohydrates are a part of food. Starch is a carbohydrate; so are sugars and most types of fiber. Starches and sugars are nature's reserves, created by energy from the sun, carbon dioxide and water. Carbohydrates come mainly from plant foods, such as cereal grains, fruits, vegetables, and legumes (peas and beans). Milk and yogurt also contain carbohydrates, in the form of milk sugar (lactose). The following foods are good sources of carbohydrates:

- **Cereals and grains** such as wheat, rice, corn, oats, barley, bread and breakfast cereals. These are rich in starch and vary from 20 to 85 percent carbohydrates by weight.
- **Legumes** such as navy beans, lentils, chickpeas and split peas are also rich in starch and contain 55–65 percent carbohydrates.
- **Some root vegetables**, such as potatoes, sweet potatoes, yams and cassava contain 10 to 25 percent starch. Most other vegetables (broccoli, zucchini, tomatoes, etc.) contain no starch and only minor amounts of natural sugars.
- **Fruits** range from 5 to 15 percent carbohydrates (berries to bananas, respectively) in the form of sugars. Bananas are the only ones containing some starch in the ripe state.
- **Milk** is around 5 percent carbohydrates, in the form of the sugar lactose.
- **Honey** is 75 percent sugars (**fructose**, glucose, sucrose).
- **Processed foods** may contain large amounts of added sugars to satisfy consumer desire for sweetness. Examples are fruit yogurt (18 percent sugars), cookies (35 percent sugars) and chocolate (56 percent sugars).

Why do you need it?

Carbohydrates are the body's main energy source and an essential source of fuel for the brain—which is the most energy-demanding organ in your body. Unlike muscle cells, which can burn either fat or carbohydrates, the brain cannot burn fat. Strictly speaking, humans can "get by" on as little as 50 grams of carbohydrates a day. But your muscles and brain will complain: you'll tire easily and feel headachy. In time, your body might adjust, but nutritionally speaking, it's not ideal.

Sugars, Starches and Dietary Fibers

Sugars: The simplest form of carbohydrates is a single sugar molecule called a monosaccharide (mono meaning one, saccharide meaning sweet). Glucose is a monosaccharide that occurs in food (as glucose itself, and as the building block of starch); it is the most common source of fuel for the cells of the human body.

When two monosaccharides join, the result is a disaccharide (di meaning two). Sucrose, or common table sugar, is a disaccharide, as is lactose, the sugar in milk. As the number of monosaccharides in the chain increases, the carbohydrate becomes less sweet. Maltodextrins are oligosaccharides (oligo meaning a few) that are five or six glucose units long; they are often used as a food ingredient. They taste only slightly sweet.

Starches: At least half the glucose in your body comes from starches in your food. Starches are long chains of sugar molecules joined together like pearls in a necklace. They are called polysaccharides (poly meaning many). Starches are not sweet-tasting at all. When you eat starches your body breaks them down into glucose units, rather like chopping up the string of pearls at random. Amylose and amylopectin are common forms of starch.

Dietary fibers: These are usually large carbohydrate molecules containing many different sorts of monosaccharides. They are different from starches and sugars in that they do not get broken down by human digestive enzymes. Fibers reach the large intestine without change. Once there, bacteria begin to ferment and break them down.

Different fibers have different physical and chemical properties. Soluble fibers can be dissolved in water. Some soluble fibers are very viscous (syrupy) when they are in solution, so they slow down the speed of digestion. Other fibers, such as cellulose, are insoluble (do not dissolve in water) and do not directly affect the speed of digestion.

If you fast for 24 hours or decide to limit your carbohydrate intake, your brain relies first on the stores of carbohydrates in the liver, but within hours these are used up and the liver begins creating glucose from noncarbohydrate sources (including amino acids from muscle tissue). It has only a limited ability to do this, however.

We now know that any shortfall in glucose availability affects brain function, and not in a good way. People with diabetes have firsthand experience of this if they've ever suffered **hypoglycemia** or low blood glucose. Confusion, trembling, dizziness, nausea, incoherent rambling speech, and lack of coordination are what happen when the brain and central nervous system are not getting enough glucose.

How much do you need?

The current recommendation from health authorities around the world is to aim to meet 45–65 percent of your energy requirements with carbohydrate foods. However, you need to take into account your personal food preferences and your overall eating patterns when working out how much carbohydrate is right for you. Also, a person's total energy requirements differ according to age, gender, body size and activity level.

How much carbohydrate should you eat?

Having diabetes doesn't mean that you need less carbohydrate than anyone else. It just means that how much you need takes more careful thought, because:

- If you have type 1 diabetes, increasing your carbohydrate intake increases your insulin requirements, and
- If you have type 2 diabetes or gestational diabetes, too much carbohydrate may be bad for your glycemic control because of your relative insufficiency of insulin.

See part 3 for details on the daily carb needs for different types of diabetes.

As a starting point, you have to consume enough carbohydrates to easily meet the needs of your brain, central nervous system and red blood cells. At the same time, you want to minimize loss of body muscle (protein can be broken down to make glucose) and usually, you want to prevent ketosis.

Ketones, Ketosis and Ketoacidosis

AT ALL TIMES, our bodies need to maintain a level of glucose in the blood that will serve the brain and central nervous system. When necessary, the brain will use ketones, a by-product of the breakdown of fat, as fuel. Ketones occur in higher concentrations when the body can't use glucose as a fuel because there is not enough insulin.

Ketones are strong acids. They are normally released into the urine, but if levels are very high or if the person is dehydrated, they may begin to build up in the blood.

High levels of ketones in the blood can cause fruit-smelling breath, loss of appetite, nausea or vomiting, fast, deep breathing (to blow off the acid in the form of carbon dioxide) and excessive urination (to eliminate the extra acid). In severe cases, it may lead to coma and death.

In a pregnant woman, even a moderate amount of ketones in the blood may harm the baby and impair brain development. The excessive formation of ketones in the blood is called ketosis—the metabolic state when the body is burning mostly fat for fuel. Large amounts of ketones in the urine may signal diabetic ketoacidosis, a dangerous condition caused by very high blood glucose levels.

We know that eating less than 50–60 grams of carbohydrates per day (or 7–10 percent of your total calorie intake) can lead to ketosis. You need around 100 grams per day (or 15–20 percent of your total calories) of carbs a day to be sure to prevent this.

The current United States dietary reference intake for carbohydrate is 45–65 percent of energy, with a minimum of 130 grams per day for healthy adults. Most Americans get only 50 percent of their energy from carbohydrates—the lower end of the requirement.

Carbs and glucose tolerance

You might wonder why a relatively high-carb diet was ever recommended for people with diabetes when this is the very nutrient they have difficulty metabolizing. There are two important reasons.

One is that your glucose tolerance, or carbohydrate tolerance, improves the higher your carbohydrate intake. The reason for this is increased insulin sensitivity—the more carbohydrates you eat, the better your body gets at handling them. This effect is particularly apparent at high carbohydrate intakes (greater than 200 grams a day). This led to the general health recommendation to eat at least 250 grams of carbohydrates a day for maximum glucose tolerance and insulin sensitivity.

Second, if you don't have a high carbohydrate intake, you run the risk of eating a high-fat diet instead (because when the level of carbohydrate falls, the level of fat rises). This can increase your insulin resistance and make your blood glucose levels worse. What's more, diabetes means a *greatly* increased risk of cardiovascular disease. We know that a low fat intake, particularly a low saturated fat intake, reduces this risk.

What we now know is that not all carbs were created equal. In the next chapter we cover various approaches to the diet for diabetes, including carb exchanges and carb counting, and explain what's wrong with a low-carb diet. And in chapter 10 we look at carbohydrate quality and the glycemic index (GI).

·9·

Carb Quantity:
Getting a Grip on the Eating Plan for Diabetes

For over two thousand years, people with diabetes have been given advice on what to eat. Many diets were based more on what seemed like logical (although unproven) theories, rather than actual research. The emphasis was on carbohydrates—either cutting them out altogether or seriously restricting them. The diet was also high in fat, so it's no surprise that cardiovascular disease was the most frequent cause of early death.

It was not until the 1970s that carbohydrates were first considered a valuable part of the diet for diabetes. To their surprise, researchers found that not only did the nutritional status of patients improve with a higher carbohydrate intake, their blood glucose levels did as well.

Carbohydrates are an important part of your diet: they help keep your body sensitive to insulin and gives you stamina. Carbohydrate is also the only part of food that directly affects your blood glucose levels. As we have explained, when you eat carbohydrate foods, they are broken down into glucose and this lifts your blood glucose levels. Your body responds by releasing insulin into the blood. The insulin clears the glucose from the blood, moving it into your muscles, where it is used for energy, so the blood glucose level (BGL) returns to normal.

In the face of a lack of insulin (type 1) or of effective insulin (type 2), too much carbohydrate will result in high blood glucose levels. This is why dietary tools for people with diabetes focus on carbohydrates. Dietary approaches to a healthy way of eating for diabetes today will usually incorporate guidance regarding how much, what type and when to eat carbohydrates.

The two main approaches to quantifying carbohydrates in the diet are:

- A carbohydrate exchange system, or
- Carbohydrate counting.

CARBOHYDRATE EXCHANGES

With the exchange approach, carbohydrate foods are identified in specific quantities known as exchanges or portions. You then eat a certain number of carbohydrate exchanges for each meal over the day. The aim is to promote consistency in the amount of carbohydrates you eat from day to day. The system was developed in the 1950s, long before research on the GI appeared (in 1981). The emphasis is on carbohydrate quantity rather than quality.

A carbohydrate exchange is an amount of food typically containing 10 or 15 grams of carbohydrates (depending on where you live) such as:

- 1 slice of bread
- 1 cup (8 ounces) milk, and
- 1 small piece of fruit

Carbohydrate exchange lists are available that detail serving sizes for different types of breads, cookies, breakfast cereals, fruit, starchy vegetables and dairy products that provide 15 grams of carbohydrates. A dietitian will then recommend a certain number of carbohydrate exchanges for each meal over the course of the day.

Although this system has been widely used around the world, many people with diabetes have difficulty using it. It can be a tricky concept to get your mind around at first, and estimating carbohydrate exchange amounts in a plate of food isn't easy, particularly if the food is unfamiliar or doesn't fit readily into one of the carbohydrate exchange groups. Take a lavash wrap filled with breaded pieces of chicken, chickpeas and salad, for example. Where do you start!

Another problem with the exchange system is that it doesn't take into account the physical nature of the carbohydrates in a food and what actually happens in your body when you eat it. It assumes that the glycemic potency of each carbohydrate exchange is the same.

CARBOHYDRATE COUNTING

Carbohydrate counting means what it says—simply counting the actual number of grams of carbohydrates in the foods you eat by using food composition tables, the nutrition labels on food packages or an experienced estimate.

With this method (and with the exchange system) you really need to get familiar with household measures like cups and tablespoons and have a set of kitchen scales at home. You also need to learn how to interpret food labels, and how to access other sources of information (like Web sites and books) on the carbohydrate content of foods.

Memorizing the percentage of carbohydrates in common foods such as rice, bread, dry cereal, fruit, potato and milk can also help you judge your carbohydrate intake. For example, bread averages 50 percent carbohydrates, so if you know the weight of the bread you're eating, you'll know you have half that amount of carbohydrates, in grams.

With a system of carbohydrate counting, your carbohydrate choices aren't limited by the extent of whichever exchange list you use, so it does allow more dietary freedom. In this regard it's a good idea to be mindful of basic nutrition principles. Depending on your knowledge of the carbohydrate content of foods, carbohydrate counting tends to be a more accurate way of monitoring your actual carbohydrate intake than carbohydrate exchanges and is therefore widely used by those using an insulin pump. Like carbohydrate exchanges, it does not take into account differences in the type of carbohydrates.

■

**The secret to the diet for diabetes is not just the
quantity but also the *type* of carbohydrates you eat.**

■

WHAT ABOUT LOW-CARBOHYDRATE DIETS?

Low-carbohydrate diets are either high protein or high fat or both.
They cannot be anything else, because you have to get your energy
from something (and alcohol in large amounts, the only other energy
source for humans, won't keep you alive for long).

There are at least two variations of carbohydrate intake on a low-
carbohydrate diet. There are those that are:

- ▶ *Very low* in carbohydrates, containing less than 100 grams of
  carbohydrates per day, or
- ▶ *Extremely low* in carbohydrates, containing as little as 20–30
  grams of carbohydrates per day (ketogenic diets).

The "extremely low" variation is often found in the "kick start"
phase of popular diet books. It is not recommended for anyone with
diabetes.

A recent review of low-carbohydrate diets in type 2 diabetes conclud-
ed that they are safe and effective in terms of weight loss in the short
term but there are potential risks with them in the long term (more than
6 months). Little research has been done on people with diabetes.

**Some problems you can have if you don't have enough carbohy-
drates in your diet**

- ▶ Muscle fatigue, causing moderate exercise to be an enor-
  mous effort
- ▶ Insufficient fiber intake, causing constipation
- ▶ Headaches and tiredness due to low blood glucose levels, and
- ▶ Bad breath due to the breakdown products of fat (ketones).

A major concern, however, with low-carb diets is the possibility of eating too much saturated fat. Even a single meal high in saturated fat can have a bad effect on your blood vessels. And the long-term effect would be an increase in your LDL (bad) cholesterol.

Also, your intake of fruit, vegetables and cereal grains would be low on a low-carb diet so you probably need to take supplements, particularly to meet folate and fiber requirements.

Low-carbohydrate diets may also be high in protein. High protein loads long term (over 6 months) may speed up a decline in your renal (kidney) function and increase your calcium loss in urine, and this could predispose you to osteoporosis, kidney stones and other kidney problems. Scientists do not agree on the dangers of low-carbohydrate diets, and long-term studies are needed.

The evolution of the dietary recommendations for people with diabetes

Before the advent of insulin in the 1920s, most people with type 1 diabetes did not live for more than one year after their diagnosis. While people with type 2 diabetes generally lived longer, their lifespan was still much shorter than average.

OVER 3,500 YEARS AGO

Believe it or not, the first mention in recorded history of symptoms of what we now know as diabetes was by the Egyptians. In an ancient text known as the Ebers Papyrus, dated around 1550 BCE, higher-carbohydrate foods such as wheat grain, fruit and sweet beer were recommended to stop a condition characterized by "the passing of too much urine."

AROUND 230 BCE

The next mention of the symptoms of diabetes was around 230 BCE by the Greeks, who thought diabetes was caused by a weakness of the kidneys and loss of excess moisture from the body. They prescribed a remedy of mostly low-carbohydrate foods such as pot-herbs, endive, lettuce, rock fishes, juices of knotgrass, elecampane in dark-colored wine, and myrtle.

AROUND 150 CE

In Greece, around 150 CE, a follower of Hippocrates, who was perhaps the ancient world's most famous doctor, prescribed higher-carbohydrate foods such as milk, gruel, cereals, fruits and sweet wines to help manage diabetes.

AROUND 500

Around 500 in India, "sweet urine" was thought to be caused by eating too much rice, flour and sugar, and it was recommended that people with the condition restrict their eating of these high-carbohydrate foods.

AROUND THE 1600s

Much later, in England around the 1600s, milk, lime water, blood pudding, rancid meats and low-carbohydrate vegetables were prescribed as a treatment for diabetes, along with opium (to suppress the appetite).

LATE 1700s AND EARLY 1800s

The first scientific approach to the treatment of diabetes was developed in England and Germany in the late 1700s and early 1800s. Doctors observed that by reducing the consumption of carbohydrates to a bare minimum, most of the sugar in the urine was eliminated. They found that the intake of carbohydrates from food, and their digestion, was directly related to increases in the amount of sugar in the urine. As a result, patients were treated using a diet that was high in fat and protein and low in carbohydrates.

LATE 1850s

Some French physicians were advising their diabetes patients to eat extra-large quantities of sugar as a treatment for diabetes, perhaps with the aim of replacing what was being lost in the urine.

AROUND 1870

A French physician recognized that foods containing protein and carbohydrate increased urination. He recommended an "austere" diet with very little carbohydrate or protein, but allowed the liberal use of fats. Apparently the diet was so unappealing that patients were sometimes locked up for up to 5 months to force them to follow it!

BETWEEN 1900 AND 1915

A range of higher-carbohydrate "fad" diabetes diets began to appear. They included the "oat cure," in which the majority of the diet was made up of oatmeal, and the "milk diet," the "rice cure," and "potato therapy," all of which worked along similar lines. Many of these diets were "supplemented" by the liberal use of opium, again to suppress the appetite.

1912

In the United States, Dr. Fred Allen developed a 1,000-calorie per day "starvation" diet. People became emaciated and weak, and were later described as looking like "concentration camp survivors." The diet started with a 7-day fast, after which other foods were gradually reintroduced. Patients were advised to boil their low-carbohydrate vegetables three times in water to remove starch. A very-low-carbohydrate diet indeed!

1920s

Research on pancreatectomized dogs by Dr. Fred Allen led him to the conclusion that glucose was more rapidly absorbed than starch. This principle was expanded to include all simple sugars. Based on this research, low-sugar diets were recommended for people with diabetes throughout the world for most of the remainder of the 20th century.

Doctors began recommending high-fat diets for their diabetic patients. Unfortunately, most of the fats that were commonly used were animal fats—high in saturated fat and cholesterol. They didn't know about the potential dangers of a high-animal-fat diet, but they did know that fat didn't break down to become blood glucose. We now know that high-fat diets, particularly high-saturated-fat diets, speed up the development of heart disease, which is the most frequent cause of death among people with diabetes in modern times.

1921

Insulin was discovered by the Canadians Drs. Frederick Banting and Charles Best in 1921, and became commercially available toward the end of 1922. It revolutionized the management of diabetes throughout the world.

1923

As early as 1923, Dr. H. Rawle Geyelin, in the United States, demonstrated that a higher-carbohydrate diet did not upset blood glucose levels as long as enough insulin was supplied. Despite this, most doctors were recommending low carbohydrate intakes—15–40 percent of total calories—until the late 1940s.

1950

The American Diabetes Association and American Dietetic Association developed and published the first set of "carbohydrate exchange lists." The lists focused on six food groups that had similar macronutrient (carbohydrates, fat and protein) levels, operating on the assumption that any foods within a group were interchangeable because they would have the same impact on blood glucose levels. The exchanges were also designed to reduce people's carbohydrate intake to a minimum. Despite the fact that we now know that all foods within a food group do not have similar effects on blood glucose levels, people with diabetes worldwide are still encouraged to use exchange lists.

1970s

The world's major diabetes associations began to review their dietary recommendations due to the increasing number of deaths of people with diabetes from heart and blood vessel diseases. Until this time, people with diabetes simply hadn't lived long enough to develop diabetic complications, but insulin therapy meant that people who would have in the past died within a few years of diagnosis were living relatively normal lives and lifespans. Recommendations for dietary fat dropped to less than 35 percent of calories and carbohydrate recommendations went up to 55–60 percent of calories. Researchers found that the nutritional status of patients improved with a higher carbohydrate intake, and their insulin sensitivity improved as well.

1981

Dr. David Jenkins, Dr. Thomas M. S. Wolever and their colleagues at the University of Toronto developed the concept of the glycemic index (GI) of foods. In the light of this new research, major diabetes associations around the world cautiously began to revise their restrictions on simple sugars, but as you will see, it has taken two decades for most of them to recommend the use of the GI as a tool for general diabetes management.

1994

The American Diabetes Association in 1994 completed a major revision of its dietary guidelines for people with diabetes, which acknowledged that there was no "one" right diet. It recommended that 10–20 percent of calories come from protein and 60–70 percent of calories come from a combination of monounsaturated fat and/or carbohydrates, depending on personal and cultural preferences. This was due to increasing evidence that high-carbohydrate diets may increase triglycerides and decrease HDL (good) cholesterol levels, increasing the risk of heart and blood vessel disease. It's important to note that, most of the research at this stage did not take the GI of the high-carbohydrate diets into account. However, specific recommendations to limit the amount of simple sugars were dropped from the American Diabetes Association guidelines.

1997

In its highly influential report on carbohydrates in human nutrition in 1997, the World Health Organization/Food and Agriculture Organization recommended that the terms "simple sugars" and "complex carbohydrates" should no longer be used to describe carbohydrate foods. They recommended the use of the GI as the best guide to the effect of carbohydrate foods on blood glucose levels.

The concept of **glycemic load (GL)** was developed by researchers at Harvard University, and diets with a high GI were for the first time linked to the development of type 2 diabetes and heart and blood vessel disease in women and men.

2004

All the scientific research from around the world that looked at the optimal diet for the management of diabetes was combined and analyzed as a whole. The results supported the recommendation of a higher-carbohydrate, lower-GI diet. The medical nutrition therapy recommendations from the major international diabetes associations now closely reflect the results of this research.

2006
The American Diabetes Association fully revised its guidelines for the nutritional management of diabetes and included the use of the GI as one of the recommendations.

▪10▪

Carb Quality:
What You Need to Know About the Glycemic Index (GI)

LEIGH

I WAS A high-profile TV and radio journalist and newscaster for over 30 years. One day in the summer of 1998 my life turned upside down. A simple virus took me into the wilderness of chronic fatigue syndrome for more than 2 years — until I found low GI.

I was sent off for some blood tests, which showed I'd contracted a viral form of hepatitis. I was told to take two weeks off work and I'd be fine.

However, I kept returning to the doctor for weeks—months— struggling to describe a body and brain that were both running on empty. It seemed like something toxic was flowing through my veins. I was overwhelmed by crushing fatigue and weakness.

I remained in this "wilderness" for another year until a doctor friend discovered some research which said that for a proportion of CFS sufferers, it's worth looking at their metabolism. I went for a glucose tolerance test, where both glucose and insulin were tested, and for once, "abnormal" readings came back—in the "prediabetic" range.

A dietitian put me on a low-GI diet, with graded activity, then graded exercise, with a prediction that in 2 weeks I'd notice an improvement in my health! Two weeks later I returned to see her and announced— "You've given me a life again!"

Today, 5 years later, I'm still on the low-GI diet and swimming 3 miles a week again, and I continue to revel in good health. I'm not back to 100 percent—I'm probably 90–95 percent.

In the last chapter we looked at the evolution of the dietary guidelines for diabetes, the importance of observing the quantity of carbohydrates you eat and techniques that may help you do this. It's also important to be choosy about the type of carbohydrates you eat, because their **glycemic potency** varies—different carb foods will have dramatically different effects on your blood glucose levels. The tool to use to help you choose the right type of carbs is the glycemic index, the GI.

The GI of a food reflects how fast its carbohydrates hit the bloodstream. It is based on scientific testing of real foods in real people, in the state in which they are normally consumed:

▶ Carbohydrates that break down quickly during digestion, like those in white bread, have high-GI values—the blood glucose response is fast and high, and

▶ Carbohydrates that break down slowly during digestion, like those in pasta, whole grains and legumes, release glucose more gradually into the bloodstream and have a low GI.

The GI is a dietary tool that gives you a scientifically based measure of carb quality. It compares carbohydrates in different foods gram for gram. Don't confuse it with the *quantity* of carbohydrates in a food. You need to know about that too if you have diabetes. Research on the GI shows that *both the quantity and quality* of the carbohydrates you eat determines your blood glucose and insulin levels for many hours after you have eaten.

THE GI REVOLUTION

GI research has turned some widely held beliefs upside down. Historically, carbohydrates were described by their chemical structure: they were simple or complex. Sugars were simple and starches were complex for no better reason than sugars were small molecules and starches were big. By virtue of their size, complex carbohydrates were assumed to be the slowly digested goodies, causing only a small rise in blood glucose levels. Simple sugars, on the other hand, were assumed to be the villains of the piece—digested and absorbed quickly, producing a rapid rise in blood glucose.

But these were just assumptions. And research has proved them wrong. We now know that the concept of simple versus complex carbohydrates is not a useful or true guide to how carbohydrates behave inside our bodies. **And that's why the GI caused a revolution.** And while the GI still has its critics, it is widely accepted as a useful dietary tool for **helping** people with diabetes.

> THE GI is a measure of how fast carbohydrates hit the bloodstream. It compares carbohydrates weight for weight, gram for gram.

Today we know the GI of hundreds of different food items that have been tested in healthy people and people with diabetes (see the GI tables at the back of the book for some examples). The findings rocked the boat in many ways.

The first surprise was that the starch in foods such as bread, potatoes and many types of rice was digested and absorbed very quickly—not slowly, as had always been assumed.

Second, scientists found that the natural and refined sugars in foods such as fruit, dairy products and ice cream did not produce more rapid or prolonged rises in blood glucose, as had always been thought. The truth was that most of the sugars in foods, regardless of the source, actually produced moderate blood glucose responses, lower than most of the starches. Why? Because sugars are a mixture of molecules, and some of them have a very slight effect on blood glucose levels.

So forget the old distinctions between starchy foods and sugary foods, or simple versus complex carbohydrates. They are no help at all when it comes to managing your blood glucose levels. By learning about the GI you can base your food choices on sound scientific evidence that will help you choose the right type of carbohydrates for your long-term health and well-being.

> IN 2003, SCIENTISTS pooled results of 20 years' research on GI and its effect on people with diabetes and demonstrated that the use of the GI can lead to on average a 0.5 point decrease in HbA1c. This is equal to the effect that many diabetic medications and insulins have on blood glucose levels in people with diabetes. A drop in HbA1c of 0.5 points reduces the risk of diabetic complications by 10–20 percent—a highly significant reduction.

HOW CAN STARCHY FOODS BE DIGESTED QUICKLY?

As we said earlier, foods containing carbohydrates that break down quickly during digestion have the highest GI values. Most modern starchy foods, especially processed ones such as breads and breakfast cereals, are high-GI foods because the starch is fully gelatinized. This means it is highly soluble in digestive juices and easy for them to attack. Because the digestion of starch produces its own weight as glucose, starchy foods can have a major impact on blood glucose levels. Just like a flash flood when there's too much rain over a short space of time, rapid starch digestion results in blood glucose levels that rise quickly and create what you could call a "metabolic flood."

On the other hand, foods that contain carbohydrates that break down slowly, releasing glucose gradually into the bloodstream, have a low-GI value. The starch in these foods is only partially gelatinized, and so it is more resistant to attack by digestive juices. The slow and steady digestion of low-GI foods produces a smoother blood glucose curve, greater feelings of fullness and reduced metabolic disturbance. To show you the difference we have drawn a diagram—a picture can be worth a thousand words. The figure below shows the different effects of slow and fast carbohydrates on your blood glucose levels.

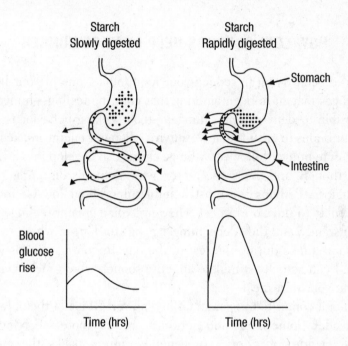

The most important factor that determines the GI of a food is the final physical state of the *starch* (not the sugars). If the starch granules have swollen and burst (think puffed and flaked cereal products), they will be digested in a flash, even if the fiber content is high. On the other hand, if the starch is still present in "nature's packaging" (think whole *intact* grains and legumes), the process of digestion will take longer.

Over the last 50–100 years, advances in food processing such as high-speed milling, high-pressure extrusion cooking and puffing technology—have had a profound effect on the carbohydrates we eat: they are much more rapidly digested and absorbed than the carbs our grandparents ate. It's one of the reasons why type 2 diabetes is far more common now than it was in the past.

But you don't have to eat only low-GI carbs to get the health benefit. We know that when a low- and a high-GI food are combined in one meal (such as lentils and rice), the overall blood glucose response is between the two. You can keep both your glucose and your insulin levels lower over the course of a whole day if you choose at least one low-GI food at each meal.

HOW LOW-GI FOODS HELP MANAGE HUNGER

If you've been trying to reduce your food intake, one of your biggest challenges may have been ignoring that gnawing feeling—hunger. It's impossible to deny extreme hunger—food-seeking behavior is wired into our brains to ensure that we survive when our energy intake is low.

Extreme hunger followed by binge eating can develop into a vicious cycle, though, and that's one reason why dietitians discourage rapid weight loss. Perhaps the most helpful thing about low-GI foods is their ability to stave off hunger. They give you a greater feeling of fullness instantly, and they delay hunger pangs for longer, which reduces your food intake during the rest of the day. In contrast, foods with a high GI can actually stimulate appetite sooner, which means you eat more at your next meal.

When it comes to hunger and filling power, GI is not the only thing to consider. Some foods and nutrients are just more satisfying than others, calorie for calorie. In general, protein packs the greatest punch, followed by carbohydrates and then fat. But within the carbohydrate group, the low-GI versions of foods have more filling power than their high-GI counterparts. So a low-GI breakfast based on traditional rolled oats has more filling power than a high-GI breakfast based on bran or wheat flakes, and a low-GI rice meal has more punch than a high-GI rice meal.

Why is this so? One explanation is that low-GI foods spend longer in the gut and reach much lower parts of the small intestine, triggering receptors that produce natural appetite suppressants. It doesn't take a genius to see that a food that empties rapidly from the stomach and gets digested and absorbed in minutes won't satisfy you for long.

A second reason is that high-GI foods may actually, in an indirect way, stimulate hunger. They produce a rapid rise and then a fall in blood glucose levels. Stress hormones such as adrenaline and cortisol are released when the levels are low, and both those hormones stimulate appetite, because they aim to reverse falls in blood glucose levels.

Third, some low-GI foods may increase feelings of fullness after eating simply because many are naturally high in fiber and water, which increases their bulk without increasing their energy content.

WHAT CAN THE GI DO FOR PEOPLE WITH DIABETES AND PREDIABETES?

We know from research that a diet based on low-GI carbohydrate choices will:

▶ Reduce blood glucose "spikes"
▶ Improve markers of average blood glucose levels (that is, HbA1c)
▶ Improve insulin sensitivity
▶ Improve blood cholesterol levels, particularly LDL cholesterol
▶ Increase feelings of fullness after eating
▶ Reduce hunger between meals
▶ Increase the rate of weight loss (compared with a conventional diet)
▶ Reduce waist circumference (abdominal fat), and
▶ Help prevent weight regain over the longer term.

PUTTING THE GI INTO PRACTICE

The easiest way to put the GI into practice is to use the "this-for-that" approach, swapping high-GI foods for low-GI foods within the food groups you are already eating. So if your normal breakfast cereal has a high GI, swap to a low-GI one. If your usual bread is high GI, change to a low-GI one. Remember, two key dietary recommendations for the eating plan for diabetes are to

▶ Choose carbohydrate foods with a low GI, and
▶ Be conscious of the quantity of carbohydrates you eat.

The tables at the back of this book will help you identify the GI of the major carbohydrate foods and include the carbohydrate content in grams. In the Daily Food Guides you'll find carbohydrate-rich foods in serving sizes that contain approximately 15 grams of carbohydrates (i.e., carbohydrate exchanges).

For the GI of your favorite carbs, check the tables in this book or go to the GI database at www.glycemicindex.com.

SOME THINGS TO KEEP IN MIND ABOUT THE GI

1. **The GI relates only to carbohydrate-rich foods**

   The GI applies only to high-carbohydrate foods. It is impossible to measure a GI value for foods that contain almost no carbohydrates. These foods include meats, fish, chicken, eggs, cheese, nuts, oils, cream, butter and most vegetables. There are other nutritional aspects that you could consider in choosing these foods, such as the amount and type of fats they contain.

2. **It is not intended to be used in isolation**

   The GI of a food does not make it good or bad for us. High-GI foods such as potatoes and whole wheat bread still make valuable nutritional contributions to our diet. And low-GI foods such as pastry that are high in saturated fat are no better for us because of their low GI. The nutritional benefits of different foods are many and varied, and we suggest you base your diet on a wide variety of foods that are low in salt and saturated fat, high in fiber *and* have a low GI.

3. **You don't need to avoid all high-GI foods**

   There is no need to eat only low-GI foods. While you will benefit from eating low-GI carbs at each meal, this doesn't have to mean excluding all others. A meal that includes a high-GI food such as a potato and a low-GI food such as corn will result in a medium GI overall.

4. **You don't need to add up the GI each day**

   The GI value of a food can be altered by the way it is processed or cooked, so we don't believe it is possible to calculate a precise GI value for recipes or to predict the GI of a menu for the whole day. That's why we prefer simply to categorize foods as low, medium or high GI in most circumstances. We have also seen the benefits people gain by simply substituting low-GI foods for high-GI foods in their everyday meals and snacks without more complicated dietary changes.

What's Glycemic Load?

YOUR BLOOD GLUCOSE LEVEL (BGL) rises and falls when you eat a meal containing carbs. How high it rises and how long it stays high depends on the quality of the carbs (the GI) as well as the quantity. Glycemic load, or GL, combines both the quality and quantity of carbohydrates in one "number." It's the best way to compare blood glucose values of different types and amounts of food. The formula for calculating the GL of a particular meal is:

GL = (GI × the amount of carbohydrate) divided by 100.

Let's take a single apple as an example. It has a GI of 38 and it contains 13 grams of carbohydrates.

$$GL = 38 \times 13 \div 100 = 5$$

What about a small baked potato? Its GI is 85 and it contains 14 grams of carbohydrates.

$$GL = 85 \times 14 \div 100 = 12$$

So we can predict that our potato will have twice the glycemic effect of an apple. Think of GL as the amount of carbohydrates in a food "adjusted" for its glycemic potency.

Although the GL concept has been useful in scientific research, it's the GI that's been most helpful to people with diabetes. That's because a diet with a low GL, unfortunately, can be a "mixed bag," full of healthy low-GI carbs in some cases, but low in carbs and full of the wrong sorts of fats (such as meat and butter) in others.

If you choose healthy low-GI foods—at least one at each meal and monitor the amount of carbohydrates—chances are you'll be on the right track to blood glucose control.

Use the GI to identify your best carbohydrate choices, then watch your portion size to control the overall GL of your diet.

•11•

How to Change the Way You Eat

BOB HAS JUST been told by his doctor that he has diabetes. He leaves the doctor's surgery and heads to his local bar. He feels bad. There he begins to down the first of six pints of beer. As he sits and drinks, his mind is raging—anger, denial, depression and guilt go round and round in his head. His doctor told him he would need to lose weight, cut back on fried food, but Bob barely heard this. He is not thinking about his dietary habits at all.

This stage of change is **precontemplation**.

Some time later Bob is walking into a diabetes education center on his doctor's referral. He listens to a lecture about food and diabetes and hears that he's supposed to eat regularly, cut back on fat and eat more fruit and vegetables. He's heard many of these ideas before. He thinks about eating breakfast, buying fruit to take to work. After the visit he changes nothing, although he starts to notice things—like his pot belly and the amount of food he eats. He sees some colleagues eating fruit during a break and imagines himself doing the same. He thinks about the money he would save if he ate less fast food. Bob is thinking about food choices more and entertaining the idea of change.

This is typical of the *contemplation* stage of change.

Bob's next appointment is with a dietitian. He was of two minds about attending, but he's made the effort. Half of him feels positive with the anticipation of getting healthier; the other half feels resentful about even needing to think about this. The dietitian asks him about what he eats and what he thinks he can change. She suggests they start with breakfast and some healthier options for buying lunch. She suggests a reduction in alcohol. Bob agrees to try breakfast. They talk about what he will need to do to make this happen—the shopping, the time plan, what to have.

This is the stage of *preparation*.

Talking and thinking about what to do is one thing. The next step for Bob is putting the plans into action. This requires buying breakfast foods, setting the alarm clock, getting up when the alarm goes off, and actually eating breakfast as planned. It's unlikely that this will work out all the time. Obstacles like not having time to shop and sleeping in will turn up. At times Bob won't feel like the cereal he usually has and his skill at coming up with a healthy alternative will be tested. The way Bob reacts to these obstacles and to his lapses predict whether he's likely to reach the **maintenance** stage where breakfast is a daily habit.

"Get regular exercise." "Eat a healthy balanced diet." "Quit smoking." "Easier said than done," you say.

Yes, it's much easier said than done. For most people, no matter whether they have type 1, type 2, gestational or prediabetes, managing what they eat and getting enough physical activity are the most challenging aspects of diabetes care, because these really are lifestyle changes.

Limiting your food intake in the midst of plenty and getting more exercise in today's world are huge tasks on their own, let alone combined. That's why we've included a chapter that's devoted entirely to how to go about behavior changes when it comes to your eating habits. (And in chapter 17, we cover ideas for activating your day [Step 2].)

Your current food habits are the product of many factors: your cultural and family background, childhood experiences, personal tastes, family preferences, budget, the season, food availability, appetite, mood. And that's just to name a few. That's why changing what you eat is more than simply putting something else on your plate. Changing what you eat can challenge your beliefs, relationships and resourcefulness.

Although you have to make the decision to change, you'll most likely benefit from some outside help and support. That's why we suggest that everyone with diabetes see a qualified dietitian. As you saw in chapter 5, when we ran through what's involved in a diabetes management plan, it recommended you see a dietitian when you are first diagnosed, and have routine follow-up. Because you are looking at managing a lifelong condition, it makes sense to find someone you are comfortable seeing regularly. A good place to start is to ask your doctor for a recommendation.

When you have diabetes, you have it for the rest of your life, but the health complications, such as blindness, kidney failure or heart disease, take years to develop, so it can be hard to focus on the changes that you need to make here and now.

TRIED AND TRUE TIPS
FOR CHANGING EATING AND ACTIVITY HABITS

▶ **Aim to make changes gradually.**
▶ **Acknowledge your stage of change.**
   People don't make changes instantaneously; they work up to it. For some, the first step is increasing awareness of their eating habits by keeping a food diary. This can really help you identify obstacles such as lack of time, traveling, socializing or working late. Once you have identified the obstacles, you can do something about them.
▶ **Try the easiest changes first.**
   Start with something easy that is realistic and that's achiev-

able. There's not much point aiming to eat fresh fish three times a week if it's not readily available where you live. Nothing inspires like success, so start with changing a habit that will give you confidence to go on. A track record of small successes will give you the momentum you need for the challenges ahead.

▶ **Break big changes into a number of smaller ones.**

Don't try to change everything at once. Trying to quit smoking and drinking, start eating better, and exercising all at the same time could leave you feeling discouraged and ready to give up. Break the change down from a large behavior (quitting smoking) into smaller ones (not buying cigarettes, smoking fewer and fewer each day, eliminating the after-dinner cigarette, etc.).

▶ **Accept lapses in your habits:** it's part of being human.

Don't expect 100 percent success. Giving up comfort foods can cause depression and resentment, so factor in a little treat every now and then. And don't be too hard on yourself when you can't resist that piece of cheesecake. Lapses are a natural part of developing new habits. Falling over is easy, but getting up, dusting yourself off and keeping on takes real effort. Watch toddlers learning to walk and take a leaf out of their book.

OVERCOMING BARRIERS
TO CHANGING EATING BEHAVIOR

We hear many reasons for people not wanting to change their lifestyle. Sometimes the time is just not right for change—often there are real (or perceived) barriers in the way. Most barriers to change are rooted in some type of fear: fear of the unknown, fear of pain, fear of anger, fear of failure, fear of embarrassment. Recognizing your own barriers is a step towards overcoming them. You aren't alone. Here are some of the common barriers we hear about when talking to our clients.

"I'll never be able to do this."

Not believing you can do something is often based on fear of failure. People often put off making changes in their life—changing jobs, or beginning a new sport, for instance—because of this fear. Rome wasn't built in a day. Begin with the little things and build on them. It isn't smart to set yourself up for failure, so be realistic in what you're aiming for. You may be 60 pounds overweight, but it's unrealistic to think you have to lose all this just because your best friend did. If your goal is simply to eat better than you do now, or lose a little bit of weight, you will probably succeed, but if your goal is to "cure" diabetes or eat "perfectly," the fear of failure is likely to hold you back.

"I want to do it but I don't have time to change."

The excuse of lack of time is often really a fear of changing your priorities. For decades, you've put work and family ahead of yourself. Perhaps you have valued your ability to manage everything, and making time will mean you have to ask for help or delegate. Perhaps you're afraid of asking for help, or perhaps you feel guilty taking time for yourself.

Try not to make too many changes at once. Little changes usually take less time, but they can add up. Here are some other ideas about how to save time:

- Learn ways to manage your time better—a book, a course.
- Cut back on time-wasters like watching TV (the average person watches 31 hours per week!).
- Assess the demands on your time—work, family, friends, hobbies—and be realistic about where dietary and exercise changes can fit in. Don't overcommit.
- Make good investments in time and you will reap the rewards later on. For example, skim through some cookbooks and make a list of quick, healthy meals that you can cook. Stick this up on your fridge for when you're stuck for what to cook.
- Share the grocery shopping and cooking where possible. Others may like to help out.

"Healthy foods are too expensive."

The idea that healthier foods cost more may be underlined by a fear that you will be unable to afford to eat the way you think you ought to. Also, perhaps you are avoiding prioritizing your spending differently. It is possible to eat well on a tight budget; you just need to know how. Dietitians have lots of ideas on how to eat well on a budget if they are aware you have this need. Here are a few options to consider:

▶ Eat unprocessed cereals such as rolled oats rather than commercial varieties like instant oatmeal packets
▶ Buy long-life skim milk, rather than fresh
▶ Take your pantry to work. Lean ham, tomatoes, a salad bag and bread can create a sandwich. Taking leftovers from home will also save you money, and
▶ Look out for weekly food specials in supermarket circulars and make a shopping list that you stick to.

"I don't like healthy foods."

This reason, or variations of it—"I don't eat vegetables," "I won't drink watery milk," etc.—reflect fear of the foreign or unknown. But your tastes can change. Thirty years ago, only health freaks ate yogurt, but now it's as common as milk in supermarket carts. Overcoming your fear of new things requires commitment to change. This doesn't mean giving up your favorite foods; it might just mean changing how often you eat them. Making a new behavior a habit usually takes at least 3 months. Decide to withhold your judgments about what you like and dislike in foods until you have given the new foods a chance.

How you feel about foods has a strong influence on whether you eat them or not. And don't advertisers know it! Chocolate bars have millions of dollars behind them to push them into your field of acceptance, but little old lettuce has nothing. By learning the benefits of healthy foods you can change your perception of them and feel as eager to try a new combination stir-fry as a creamy dessert.

"I would feel silly eating health food."

Many people are held back from changing their eating habits because of how they think it will appear to others. You might think "People will make fun of me," or "I don't want to draw attention to myself," but these thoughts are really just an indication of low self-esteem.

It could help to mix with others who are also working on their diet—a night class on healthy cooking, a diet club Web site, or a diabetes education group. Not only will you realize you're not alone, you could share some good ideas. You may be surprised to see how many other people have diabetes when you open up about it yourself.

In the commercial food sector, "health food" is the new fashion, so don't be afraid to make special requests when you're eating out. And don't trust what other people tell you is "good" for you. Make sure you're informed on what are good choices and don't be afraid to ask the nitty-gritty questions, such as what type of oil is used.

Fear of asserting yourself may also make it difficult for you to make healthy food choices when your family or friends aren't. "I eat white bread because that's what everyone else likes" is a common one. Take a look at what you value and what the real problem is. When it comes to breaking the mold, someone has to go first. Involving your family in your dietary changes can result in an improvement in their diet too.

HELPING YOURSELF TOWARDS HEALTHIER EATING HABITS

Become aware of nonhungry eating

Food is part of socializing, celebrating and comforting, and eating gives us something to do when we are bored. We eat food for a whole range of reasons that have nothing to do with hunger. We eat:

- So as not to offend a host
- Because we feel anxious or depressed
- To finish off what the kids have left
- Just because it looks good, or because it's there, and
- Because we feel we have to leave nothing on our plate.

Nonhungry eating isn't wrong, but it can contribute to overeating, and you need to be aware of it if you are going to do anything about it. Try to identify what triggers you to eat when you're not particularly hungry, and work on eliminating or reducing those triggers. If an argument with your partner sends you to the cookie jar, deliberately do something else—taking a walk, for instance—to work out the emotion instead of suppressing it with food.

Think about what to eat, rather than what not to eat

What happens if someone asks you to imagine a pink elephant? You imagine it, right? The future is what we imagine. So rather than thinking of what you don't want to eat, think of what you do. If you crave chocolate, have some, but buy only one tiny bar of your favorite and relish it.

Planning the meals you are going to eat reduces the likelihood that you'll go off track. Plan the week's entrées and shop once for the ingredients you'll need. Make a shopping list of healthy foods, including some favorites that you always buy. Two of our favorites are nut bars and fruit-and-muesli bread. The bread is a satisfying snack anytime at home and the bars are great for food on the go.

Eat regularly

Have you ever noticed that the hungrier you are, the more tempting high-calorie foods like chocolate, cookies and French fries are? And the harder it is to stop at one? You'll find it easier to eat normally if you learn to graze on low-GI carbs.

Make overeating as hard as you can

When you go to have a slice of bread, take out one slice, then seal up the bag and put the loaf away. Put the spreads and toppings away before you sit down to eat. Out of sight generally means out of mind. Keep those occasional foods out of sight—better still, don't buy them routinely.

If it's healthy, keep it handy

In your face and ready to eat! Keep washed, shiny apples or crunchy snow peas in an attractive bowl in the fridge; dried fruit in a jar on your desk; packaged instant salads for convenience; presliced tomato and cucumber in the fridge, ready to use on sandwiches.

These are just a few of the ways you can increase your chances of eating the types of foods you planned to eat.

Minimize distractions while you're eating

If you're sitting in front of the TV with a bag of chips or a bar of chocolate, it is very easy to absent-mindedly eat it all. Focus on and savor what you are eating.

Get support from others

Whether it's from your family, friends, work colleagues or health professionals, get as much help as you can. Find a buddy who also wants to get into shape. When your motivation dips, theirs will pull you along. If someone seems to be sabotaging your efforts, let them know how they could help. For example, they could agree to change to low-GI bread. There are things you may need to negotiate. Be prepared to lead by example, and to ignore the hecklers . . . and you may convince others you are onto something good.

Coping with stress (without using food)

Stress can take many forms. It can appear emotionally as anxiety, worry or depression. Or you can experience it physically, as pain or illness. Situations such as a confrontation with another person or a near-miss accident can trigger the so-called fight-or-flight response, which is associated with the release of stress hormones.

For people with diabetes, stress often results in elevated blood glucose levels, because these stress hormones trigger the release of stored glucose. This energy-mobilizing effect helps people who don't have diabetes deal better with their environment, but it is no help for people with diabetes. They find it harder to regain normal glucose equilibrium. This can lead to chronic high blood glucose.

If you have diabetes, you need to find ways to manage your stress without resorting to the cookie jar, alcohol or cigarettes. Here's a list of some of the things you can do to help yourself manage stress better:

- **Self-knowledge**. Get to know your body's normal reactions so that you can recognize when you are tense. Shallow breathing and a fast pulse are often an indication of your body's reaction to stress.
- **Relax**. Deep breathing is a natural relaxant. Try to take several deep breaths each hour.
- **Talk**. Talking to other people can be a valuable way to deal with your problems and reduce the stress associated with them.
- **Walk**. Physical activity will help you reduce tension and can be a great way to clear your mind.
- **Smile and laugh**. It's therapeutic, so take any opportunity you can to do it.
- **Make lists**. This will help you sort out your priorities and give you a feeling of control over what you want to do. Make a list of ten things that make you happy—a cup of coffee? A good book? A hot bath? Make sure you indulge occasionally.
- **Have fun**. Learn to play a little. Keep up your hobbies and try to get out of the house regularly, even if it's only for short outings.
- **Explore**. New activities may help you relax. Try massage, listening to music, meditating or yoga.
- **Believe**. Your religious or spiritual beliefs could be very supportive and help you to see a way forward.
- **Be aware of your needs**. Give priority to meeting them when you can. Take time to rest when you are tired, to eat when you're hungry. Be kind to yourself.

If none of these solutions seems to help, it's a good idea to see a trained counselor. Behavioral stress management programs do work.

HERE'S A TECHNIQUE TO TRY FOR PROBLEM SOLVING

When things become so overwhelming that you can't see a way out, try sitting down quietly somewhere, taking a few deep breaths and looking at things objectively:

▶ Look at all the different causes of your tension and identify one that you want to do something about.

▶ List all the possible options and solutions that you can think of, even the ones that seem silly, and remember that doing nothing can also be an option.

▶ Select one solution that's realistic and that you feel has a fair chance of succeeding.

▶ Give it an honest try, and

▶ After a reasonable period of time, sit back again and evaluate what happened.

• 12 •

Putting Together
Healthy Meals

*I*n this chapter we show you two approaches you can use (by themselves or together) to put you on track to a healthy diet to manage your diabetes. The techniques give you an idea of:

▶ What your dinner plate should look like (see "Planning meals using a plate model"), and
▶ What your food choices—or exchanges—are (see "Your daily food guide").

Then we show you how to put it all together in "1, 2, 3 . . . steps to a balanced meal," with ideas for breakfast, lunch and dinner and quick and easy desserts—something sweet to give your brain the all-important satiety (fullness) signal it needs.

PLANNING MEALS USING A PLATE MODEL

A basic entrée, whether it's traditional foods or foods with a Mediterranean or Asian twist, consists of some sort of meat with vegetables and potato, or rice or pasta, for the majority of people in the United States and Canada. There's nothing wrong with this as a starting point; a little fine-tuning of the proportions to match the plate model will ensure a healthy, balanced meal.

What is the plate model? We didn't create it, but we use it and recommend it because it is simple and it works. It's an easy-to-learn aid to visualizing what to put on your plate. It is adaptable to different cuisines and handy to take to restaurants. You can use it for any sized servings as long as you keep the food to the proportions shown.

You can use the plate model alongside other dietary tools you find helpful, such as the daily food guide or carbohydrate counting (see chapter 9). And as long as you choose foods that fit into the key recommendations—upping the good fats, cutting back on saturated fat and being choosy about your carbs—you're on track to a healthy diet for managing your diabetes and losing weight (if you need to).

In our experience, there are some situations where people find the plate model particularly useful. They are:

- When you have just found out you have diabetes and you feel overwhelmed by all the dietary changes you need to make
- When you want a simple diet plan to follow
- When you are having a hard time understanding other diet methods, such as using a food guide for diabetes (similar to the food guide pyramid), counting carbohydrates in your diet, or using lists that group foods according to nutrient content (diabetic exchange lists)
- If you have difficulty reading
- If you learn best by visualizing, and
- When you are eating away from home.

If you are already using other methods, the plate model might be another dietary tool to help you plan interesting, well-balanced meals, especially when you are trying out new recipes or a different cuisine.

   With Asian meals, where food is typically served in individual bowls, the same principle applies—imagine three bowls: a small bowl each for the rice or noodles and for the protein part of the meal and a large bowl for the vegetables.

   With the plate model there are just three simple steps to a healthy meal.

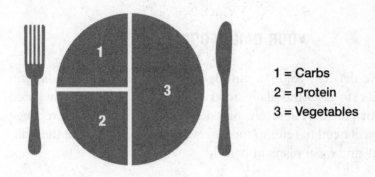

1 = Carbs
2 = Protein
3 = Vegetables

On the plate

   1. **Carbohydrate-rich foods**
      How much? One quarter of the plate
      What? Bread and cereals (choose low-GI types) and other starchy foods such as potatoes, sweet potatoes, yams, legumes, sweet corn, pasta, noodles and rice
   2. **Protein-rich foods**
      How much? One quarter of the plate
      What? Meat, chicken, fish, eggs, tofu and alternatives such as legumes, milk or yogurt
   3. **Vegetables**
      How much? Half the plate
      What? Brighten your plate with a variety of colorful vegetables. Try leafy green and salad vegetables, green beans and peas, broccoli and cauliflower, zucchini and baby squash, onions and leeks, fennel and asparagus, for starters. Think of vegetables as free foods that are full of fiber and essential nutrients, and that fill you up without adding extra calories.

Note: When it comes to vegetables, potato, sweet corn, sweet potato, yams and legumes count as carbohydrate foods.

Outside the plate

Fruit and/or milk products as a beverage or dessert on occasion.

YOUR DAILY FOOD GUIDE

For a more detailed guide to putting together meals over the day you may prefer to use the daily food guides that we have included throughout part 3. These are based around the following exchange lists. You will need to refer to these serving size guides to use the sample menus and meal plans in part 3.

HOW MUCH IS A SERVING?

Within each of the different food groups you will find serving sizes of foods that are nutritionally similar. For example, 1 slice of bread is nutritionally equivalent to ⅓ cup of cooked rice (roughly). Within one group, foods can be swapped or exchanged for another. For example, two servings of *breads, cereals and other starchy foods* could be taken as ⅔ cup of muesli or 1 cup of corn kernels.

Breads, cereals and other starchy foods
1 slice of bread
⅓ cup natural muesli
¼ cup raw rolled oats
½ cup All-Bran
⅓ cup cooked rice
⅓ cup pearl barley
½ large ear of corn
½ cup corn kernels
½ cup cooked pasta or noodles
½ cup cooked chickpeas, kidney beans, white beans, etc.

¾ cup cooked lentils

1 cup cooked split peas

¾ cup diced sweet potato

2 small new potatoes or 1 medium sized

½ cup mashed potato

Fruit

1 medium-sized piece of fruit (e.g., apple, orange, banana)

2 small pieces of fruit (e.g., apricots, plums, kiwifruit)

½ cup diced pieces or canned fruit

1 ounce dried fruit (e.g., 1½ tablespoon raisins, 6 dates,
   6 apricot halves)

4 prunes

½ cup fruit juice

Milk & milk products

1 cup low- or reduced-fat milk

1 cup calcium-fortified soy drink

1 cup low-fat yogurt

1 cup buttermilk

Meat & alternatives

3½ ounces raw lean meat or chicken

5 ounces raw fish

3½ ounces drained, canned fish

3½ ounces tofu or cooked soybeans

2 omega-3-enriched eggs

2 ounces reduced-fat hard cheese

4 slices (packaged) (3 ounces) reduced-fat processed cheese

Fat-rich foods

2 teaspoons mono- or polyunsaturated margarine

2 teaspoons mono- or polyunsaturated oil

3 teaspoons peanut butter

½ ounce nuts

1–2 tablespoons oil based salad dressing

¼ avocado

Vegetables

½ cup cooked vegetables

1 cup raw leafy salad vegetables

1 cup vegetable soup or pure vegetable juice

1, 2, 3 . . . STEPS TO A BALANCED MEAL

Breakfast basics

Breakfast really is the most important meal of the day. It speeds up your metabolism after an overnight fast and recharges your brain. We know that the people who eat the biggest breakfasts eat fewer calories over the whole day.

A long interval between dinner the night before and breakfast the next day may trigger hormones that drive food-seeking behavior. Furthermore, the longer you maintain your fast, the more insulin resistant you become. This means that whatever you eat next will require an elevated insulin response, making life harder for your beta cells and probably resulting in an elevated blood glucose.

No doubt you know that it's a good idea to eat breakfast if you want to keep healthy, but did you realize that your food choices may also be a critical factor? Firing up your engine with high-GI cornflakes or soft white toast gives you a short-lived fuel supply, and you'll be looking for a pick-me-up within a few hours. If you want something to nourish your body and sustain you through the morning, follow our basic breakfast tips. Choose foods from each group: carbohydrates (opt for low-GI choices where possible), protein, and fruit and vegetables.

Start with a low-GI carbohydrate such as muesli, whole-grain toast or a commercial low-GI breakfast cereal.

Add some protein, such as low-fat milk or yogurt, soy milk, eggs, reduced-fat cheese, tofu or sardines.

Plus fruit and/or vegetables: the choice is yours—a freshly squeezed juice, a handful of diced fruit, a sprinkling of dried fruit or sautéed vegetables, for example.

> **SOMETHING TO THINK ABOUT . . .**
> AT THE SAME time that obesity in American adults doubled, the proportion of adults skipping breakfast almost doubled.

Muesli and fruit breakfast

Carbohydrate: natural muesli
Protein: skim milk*, low-fat natural yogurt
(* if you normally use whole full-fat milk, start with a reduced-fat milk and work your way gradually to skim milk)
Fruit: strawberries
To make: add a little skim milk to a bowl of natural muesli to moisten it, then add a generous dollop of a good low-fat natural yogurt and top with a handful of chopped strawberries (or any other fruit).

Hot oatmeal breakfast

Carbohydrate: traditional rolled oats
Protein: skim milk
Fruit: raisins, pure floral honey
To make: cook traditional rolled oats according to the instructions on the package in skim milk instead of water for a creamier oatmeal and serve topped with a scattering of raisins and a drizzle of honey.

Big cooked breakfast

Carbohydrate: healthy German-style bread, such as Mestemacher or Feldkamp
Protein: eggs
Vegetables: mushrooms, parsley, tomato
To make: take a generous handful of button mushrooms, slice and cook in a little olive oil. When softened, add some fresh chopped parsley and season with salt and pepper if desired. Serve on toasted flaxseed bread with poached or dry-fried eggs. A grilled tomato alongside makes a nice addition.

Light and low, the smart carb lunch

While most people agree that eating a healthy lunch is important, 63 percent of Americans skip it at least once a week, according to a recent study by the National Restaurant Association. "Too busy" is the mantra of lunch-skippers. Not enough time, too many errands to run, and not being hungry are other main complaints.

Taking time to refuel properly is critical to maintaining health, managing weight, boosting energy levels and simply feeling better overall. It will also help maintain your productivity and concentration through the afternoon and reduce your chance of snacking on something indulgent later in the day.

Lunch does not need to be a big meal. In fact, if you find yourself feeling sleepy in the afternoon, cut back on the carbs and boost the protein and light vegetables. (Of course a cup of tea or coffee might help.)

Try these light meal suggestions for lunch—or for dinner if you prefer to eat your main meal at lunchtime.

Start with a low-GI carb such as whole-grain or sourdough bread, pasta, noodles, sushi rice, sweet corn, lentils or mixed beans.

Add some protein, such as fresh or canned fish, lean meat, sliced chicken, reduced-fat cheese or egg.

Plus vegetables and/or fruit salad to help fill you up. A large salad made with a variety of vegetables would be ideal. Round off the meal with fruit.

A sandwich from a deli, sandwich shop or salad bar

Carbohydrate: ask for mixed-grain, flaxseed or seeded bread with a smear of mustard, mayonnaise or avocado in place of margarine

Protein: canned salmon, tuna, hard-boiled egg or skinless chicken

Vegetables: as many salad items as possible, such as tomato, sprouts, grated carrot, onion, beet, mixed salad greens, lettuce, cucumber, coleslaw, etc.

Tortilla and beans

Carbohydrate: Mexican beans (canned red kidney beans in a tomato and mild chili sauce), corn tortilla
Protein: reduced-fat cheese, red kidney beans
Vegetables: avocado, shredded lettuce, sliced tomato
To make: warm ½ cup beans and serve in a corn tortilla with 2–3 avocado slices, lots of shredded lettuce, tomato slices and grated reduced-fat cheese.

Simple long soup

Carbohydrate: vermicelli noodles, creamed sweet corn
Protein: chicken stock, chicken, egg
Vegetables: carrot, scallions (shallots/green onions)
To make: bring 2 cups of chicken stock to a boil, add a handful of dry vermicelli noodles and 1 carrot, finely diced. Cook the noodles and carrot for 3–4 minutes then stir in ½ cup of creamed corn, strips of cooked chicken (a great way to use leftovers) and chopped scallions. Heat through. Beat 1 egg and slowly pour it into the boiling soup in a thin stream, stirring quickly.

Make Lunchtime an Opportunity to Increase Your Vegetable Intake

- Add plenty of salad vegetables to your sandwich—try tomato, lettuce, cucumber, sprouts, beet, grated carrot and peppers.
- For toasted sandwiches, go for tomato, pepper, sweet potato, zucchini and eggplant with cheese.
- In colder weather try vegetable soup—butternut squash, sweet potato, lentil, split pea, minestrone, or tomato.
- Salads are a great way to fill up at lunchtime—don't stay with lettuce, tomato and cucumber; try adding snow peas, peppers, corn, green beans, asparagus, roasted sweet potato, a few cubes of avocado and olives. But make sure you have your protein and carbs too.
- Coleslaw and tabbouleh are great salad inclusions.

Dinner

It's great to turn off the TV, sit down at the dining table and take time over one big meal every day. But what to make for dinner? It's the perennial question. Most people know that eating well is important, but it can be hard to get motivated to cook at the end of a long day. You don't have to spend hours preparing, though. If your cupboards and refrigerator are stocked with the right foods (see "Pantry revamp" in chapter 15), you should be able to put a healthy balanced meal together in 30–45 minutes.

Start with a low-GI carb such as sweet potato, pasta, noodles, sweet corn, legumes (beans, chickpeas, lentils).

Add some protein, such as lean meat or chicken, fish or seafood, eggs, tofu or legumes.

Plus plenty of vegetables and salad to help fill you up— remember the plate model. A large salad made with a variety of vegetables would be ideal.

Round off the meal with fruit.

Peppered steak with sweet potato purée
Carbohydrate: sweet potato
Protein: lean fillet, rump or topside steak
Vegetables: mushrooms, green beans, salad vegetables, including tomato
To make: sprinkle the steak with pepper seasoning and barbecue or pan-fry. Serve with steamed sweet potato mashed with low-fat milk, sliced mushrooms cooked in a little olive oil, steamed green beans and a crisp salad tossed in a vinaigrette dressing.

Spicy fish with rice and vegetables
Carbohydrate: basmati rice
Protein: fish
Vegetables: frozen vegetable combination (peas, carrots, beans, sweet corn, etc.)

To make: brush firm white fish fillets with your favorite curry paste blended with some lemon juice. Pan-fry and serve with basmati rice and steamed vegetables.

Spaghetti with tomato salsa and feta
Carbohydrate: spaghetti (or your favorite pasta shapes)
Protein: feta cheese
Vegetables: tomato, onion, basil, olives, salad vegetables
To make: finely chop 4 tomatoes, ½ a red onion, a bunch of basil leaves and ½ cup of pitted kalamata olives. Combine in a bowl to make the salsa. Toss cooked spaghetti with a little olive oil and top with salsa and ⅔ cup of crumbled feta. Serve with a crispy green salad.

Make Dinner an Opportunity to Increase Your Vegetable Intake

CONSIDER VEGETABLES OR SALAD a crucial part of entrées. Remember, three basic parts: carbohydrate + protein + vegetables.

- Try them steamed or microwaved, seasoned with fresh or dried herbs, olive oil dressing, lemon juice, balsamic vinegar, garlic or a few shaves of parmesan cheese.
- Keep frozen or ready-diced vegetables to add to pastas and stir-fries.
- If you don't like vegetables on their own, add them to mixed dishes like stir-fries, curries, casseroles, and grated into ground meat.
- Try vegetable-based takeouts such as vegetarian pizza, vegetarian lasagna or a falafel kebab.
- Serve meals with a side salad—either individual bowls or a large salad in the center of the table.

Dessert

There's no reason why you can't enjoy a dessert if you have diabetes. Something sweet is sometimes all you need to send your brain the all-important satiety signal. Low-GI options like fruit and low-fat dairy foods (such as yogurt or pudding) help you get all the nutrients you need each day. If you're concerned that it will add too much carbohydrate to your meal, wait for a couple of hours after dinner and have your dessert as your evening or bedtime snack.

Quick and easy fruit and dairy combos

▶ Low-fat ice cream and strawberries
▶ Sliced banana and low-calorie pudding
▶ Canned plums with a dollop of natural yogurt and sprinkle of crunchy muesli, and
▶ Fresh or canned fruit with low-fat fruit yogurt.

•13•

Snacks—
Why? What? What Not?

*T*here are some who overdo it, some who don't want to do it at all and some who aren't aware that they are doing it. What? Snacking—taking a bite to eat between meals, refreshments, nibbles.

Diet sheets for people with diabetes often include a recommendation to eat little and often, including between-meal snacks. This can cause a lot of concern.

If you take some types of insulin or other diabetes medications, you may need to eat some form of carbohydrates between meals to stop your blood glucose from dropping too low (though newer forms of medication make it less likely that you will need to do this). Besides preventing hypos, this chapter looks at some of the reasoning behind eating more than three times a day.

WHY SNACK?

Even if you're not taking any diabetes medication, lots of people with diabetes or prediabetes want to know whether it's better to eat many small meals rather than less-frequent large meals.

There's no doubt that snacks can make a significant contribution to a healthy diet, and for little children in particular, they're recommended—it's harder for them to get sufficient calories. Even for adults, regular snacks can prevent extreme hunger and hopefully reduce the amount of food eaten at meals, which can be helpful for blood glucose levels.

Studies examining the metabolic effects of small, frequent meals ("grazing") versus two or three large meals have found that blood glucose and blood fat levels may improve when meal frequency increases. There's also some evidence that you will reap metabolic benefits by eating at set times rather than at different times on different days.

This doesn't mean eating more food.

It means spreading the same amount of food over more frequent and smaller meals. It seems that if you spread the nutrient load more evenly over the day, you reduce the load on the beta cells and maximize insulin sensitivity. Researchers have seen this effect in people without diabetes, too. Although it has not yet been proven in controlled trials, it may also be that small, frequent meals lower the risk of developing diabetes by reducing the periodic "surges" in insulin that follow large meals.

CLIFF

WHAT WORKS BEST for me is to have 6 small meals daily, each with two or three carbohydrate portions, depending on my blood glucose level (BGL) 2 hours after the previous meal and my current level of physical activity. (I know that this is very compulsive, but it works for me as a disciplined daily routine that does not unduly inhibit my quality of life.) Equally important is for me to average at least 1 hour's walking, or equivalent exercise, daily.

There's also evidence that eating foods with carbohydrates in them at regular intervals can improve your mood and your mental performance. A steady supply of glucose from snacks has been shown to improve short-term memory and has been linked to better attention and number recall.

What happens if you're not a snacker and you don't feel hungry between meals? Although you may be able to last for several hours without eating because you are busy or preoccupied, going a long time between meals generally means you will be hungrier when you do eat and therefore driven to more energy-dense (more calories per bite) foods.

The jury is still out on whether or not snacking is good for your weight. There are pros and cons. There is circumstantial evidence that eating three meals a day may help you manage your weight. The French, for example, generally eat only three meals a day, with little or no snacking between, unlike Americans, who tend to eat small quantities of food fairly often. However, there's another big difference in eating habits between the French and the Americans that may be even more important: in France, meals are more often prepared and eaten in the home, not on the run.

It is possible that healthy snacking on low-fat, high-carbohydrate, high-fiber foods will stave off your "hunger pangs" and help you stick to moderate servings at meal times. Grazing can be a healthy way to live and still maintain or lose weight—but it depends on what you eat and how much you eat. Very physically active people should probably graze on high-carbohydrate snacks to make sure a continual supply of carbohydrates is available to their hard-working muscles.

However, snacking is definitely bad news for your teeth. Each time you eat, the bacteria in plaque attack your tooth enamel. For your dental health, you need to leave a minimum of 2 hours between drinks or snacks.

Slowly sipping sweetened or acidic drinks (and this includes diet soft drinks) also has harmful effects on your teeth, because it causes "dental erosion" (loss of tooth enamel caused by acid attack). It's better for your teeth to drink relatively quickly, and give your teeth a period of at least 2 hours for "rest and recovery."

In the end, it is your overall food intake that counts with weight matters, not whether you only eat breakfast, lunch and dinner or graze throughout the day.

Snacking: the bottom line

People who snack and eat regularly:

▶ Have a reduced risk of low blood glucose levels (hypo-glycemia)
▶ Show improved insulin sensitivity with lower postprandial (after-eating) insulin levels
▶ May have lower blood cholesterol levels
▶ Perform better in memory and problem-solving tasks, and
▶ May be less likely to overeat at meals.

WHAT TO SNACK ON

What to choose for snacks can be a real challenge given the huge (and tempting) range of individually packaged snack bars, cookies, fries, puddings and dairy desserts, muffins and drinks on the market, most of which have eye-catching packaging that tells you they have some vital nutritional benefit.

In reality, the best snack foods don't usually come in packaging at all—but it may boost their sales if it did. The best snacks are portable, inexpensive, nutritionally faultless foods. What are they? Fresh fruit, of course. An apple, a banana, a bunch of grapes, a pear or a nectarine or a mandarin or orange. However, if you're looking for some variety beyond fruit, look no further than our lists below.

Breads, muffins and cereals

▶ a slice of raisin toast lightly spread with poly- or monounsat-urated margarine
▶ a slice of whole-grain toast lightly spread with marmalade or jam
▶ a fruit-and-nut bakery muffin
▶ 2 large whole-grain crackers topped with smoked salmon,

mustard or mayonnaise and a sprinkle of chopped parsley
- a slice of grainy bread spread with peanut butter (no butter)
- 4 whole-grain crackers topped with flavored cottage cheese and sliced tomato
- ½ of a "salad" sandwich (made with 1 slice of grainy or sourdough or soy and flaxseed bread)
- a sliced pear with a wedge of reduced-fat cheese
- ½ of a whole-grain English muffin
- 4 cups of air-popped popcorn—ideal to take along on a hike or long walk
- 1½ tablespoon of hummus with mini tomatoes and fresh vegetable sticks (crudités)
- a bowl of whole-grain cereal such as traditional rolled oats, shredded wheat or muesli.

Topping off your low-fat dairy intake (or calcium-enriched soy alternatives)

- a glass of low-fat milk
- a skim milk latte
- ½ cup of low-fat, fruit yogurt
- a small iced coffee with a scoop of low-fat ice cream
- 2 scoops of low-fat ice cream in a glass of diet soda
- 1–1½ scoops of low-fat ice cream in a small cone
- 2 teaspoons of Quik in a cup of low-fat milk

Fruity fillers

- 2 tangerines
- a small banana
- a 2-ounce package of dried fruit and nuts
- 6 dried apricot halves
- a handful of grapes
- frozen orange quarters
- ½ cup of canned fruit
- a small box of raisins
- a small cup of fruit salad
- a commercial 100 percent fruit bar

- 10 dried apple rings
- a large wedge of fresh melon

Think ahead

It is a good idea to plan between-meal snacks ahead of time. If you leave your snacks to chance, you probably won't make the best choice when you walk in the door at the end of the day, ravenous. Dinner won't be ready for at least another hour, so what do you do? Well, it depends:

- If you've kept some nutritious snacks in your workplace, car or bag, you could have taken the edge off your appetite with something healthy on the way home.
- You might have prepared a plate of chopped fruit, carrot and celery sticks with hummus in the morning and popped it into the fridge.
- You might have bought some low-fat yogurt, crackers and low-fat cheese or roasted nuts and seeds.

Sweet treats with a low glycemic impact

Allow yourself small indulgences. It's okay to give yourself a sweet treat a couple of times a week, but you don't need a kingsize Snickers bar every day to satisfy a craving for chocolate. Go for a smaller-sized chocolate—and resist those cravings as often as you can. One of the things that makes snacks a treat is keeping them as rewards for healthy eating. Here are some suggestions:

- a 1.7-ounce package of sugar-free candy
- a single ice cream cone
- a 1.7-ounce bag of M&Ms
- 5 squares of chocolate, or
- a Twix.

WHAT NOT TO SNACK ON

Have you ever opened up a bag of chips or nuts, thinking you'll eat just a few, and before you know it you're licking the salt off your fingers and wondering where they've all gone? The problem with snacking is control. That's one reason why it can be one of the worst dietary habits.

It's the way we snack that can be the problem—what we choose, when we have it and why we're eating it. Beware of triggers that lead you to snack on something you hadn't planned on. The TV commercial late at night (or at the movies) for some delectably creamy ice cream; the bag of chips that jumps into your hands from a vending machine as you are walking by; the chocolate bars that gleam and smile at you when you stop to buy gas.

Risky snacking scenarios

- Replacing meals with snacks because you don't have the time or the food preparation skills, or you're feeling lazy and unmotivated
- At sporting events
- At the movies
- Watching TV
- When you're upset—emotional, nonhungry eating
- Eating when you're away from home, such as when you're out shopping

Q&A

Is it true that people with diabetes should eat between-meal snacks and supper before going to bed?

Children and adults with type 1 diabetes and those with type 2 who are using insulin often need to have between-meal snacks to prevent experiencing hypoglycemia.

People with prediabetes or type 2 diabetes probably don't need to snack to help with blood glucose control, though there may be individual exceptions.

In today's calorie-dense environment, there is mounting evidence that poorly chosen between-meal snacks lead to weight gain, which may in turn make your diabetes worse.

You should aim to have three moderate-sized meals based around low-GI carbohydrates to keep your blood glucose levels stable throughout the day. If you find you are going low between main meals, ask your diabetes team to review your blood glucose–lowering medications.

The "Bad" Snack Habit

FOR MANY OF us, poor snacking is just habit. Common elements to bad snacking are:

- Inactivity
- Self-indulgence
- Easy finger food
- Food that doesn't require preparation
- A long-term habit

For some people, giving up these "bad" habits is about all that's needed to turn their diet around. Consider these actual scenarios that we've heard:

Don, 35, eats a bag of potato chips while watching TV most nights.

Reg, 49, buys a chocolate bar or carton of ice cream at a convenience store on the way home from work.

Paul, 55, loves chocolate ice cream and indulges himself most nights with a bowl of it in front of the TV.

Wendy, 42, makes her children sandwiches for a snack when they come home from school and usually ends up eating 2–3 herself.

Lesley, 37, buys a hot chocolate at the station on her way to work each morning.

Sally, 51, regularly eats a handful of cookies during the day while she is at home doing housework.

If you choose snacks carefully and replace poor snack choices (high in fat and sugar) with healthy snacks (fruit and vegetables), and maintaining a healthy eating plan will be much easier.

·14·

Renovate Your Recipes

*M*anaging diabetes doesn't mean you have to throw out your favorite cookbooks and head to the local bookstore for new ones. Many recipes can easily be adapted to suit healthy eating guidelines. In this chapter we set out four key strategies to use when modifying recipes and four sample recipe makeovers to inspire you to put on an apron, pick up a wooden spoon and take charge in the kitchen!

A note of caution: modifying recipes can involve a certain amount of trial and error. And it certainly helps if you have some cooking experience and an idea of what's likely to work and what definitely won't (read: be prepared for some flops). But you'll reap the reward when your health—and your family—thank you for a superhealthy, superdelicious "re-creation." And you can have a lot of fun in the kitchen experimenting.

With diabetes, the general aims in modifying a recipe are to:

▶ Reduce the amount or improve the quality of the fat—or both.

- Lower the GI.
- Boost the fiber content.
- Reduce the salt content.

So how do you go about it? There are four basic strategies you can use. You may need to use one or all four, depending on the recipe:

1. *Substitute* healthier versions of ingredients: replace full-fat milk with low-fat milk, for instance.
2. *Add* low-calorie ingredients to make a higher-calorie dish go further: use vegetables as part of the filling in a quiche or frittata, for example.
3. *Eliminate* the ingredient you're trying to avoid: leave the cream out, for example.
4. *Reduce* the amount of the ingredient you're trying to cut back on: use one strip of bacon instead of two, for example.

FAT—HOW TO REDUCE THE AMOUNT AND IMPROVE THE QUALITY

Delectable ingredients such as butter, cream, bacon, cheese and chocolate need to stay on the supermarket shelf and out of your shopping cart if you're going to create anything approaching a heart-friendly recipe.

Substitute
- Olive oil for butter when sautéing
- Lemon juice and black pepper as a dressing for steamed vegetables rather than melted butter
- Canola oil for butter or margarine when baking
- Avocado, hummus or reduced-fat mayonnaise on a savory sandwich instead of butter
- Low-fat evaporated milk, buttermilk, low-fat natural yogurt or skim milk thickened with cornstarch in place of cream for savory sauces
- Reduced-fat cheese (even partially) for regular full-fat cheeses (NB: most mozzarella is lower in fat than many other cheeses)

▶ 2–3 sheets of filo pastry brushed with milk or a little olive oil for regular puff or short crust pastry.

Add

▶ Slivered nuts, sunflower seeds or pumpkin seeds instead of bacon bits to salads
▶ Avocado instead of cheese or margarine to a sandwich
▶ Low-fat natural yogurt instead of sour cream to a salad dressing
▶ A handful of nuts to stir-fries or in baked goods such as muffins and cakes.

Eliminate

▶ Fat from meat before cooking by trimming it away, and removing the skin from chicken pieces
▶ Fat from soups and stews by cooking ahead, chilling, then skimming the fat from the top
▶ Fat from cooking by using parchment paper or pan liners when frying, and using low-fat cooking methods such as steaming, grilling or microwaving.

Reduce

▶ The amount of oil when stir-frying by adding a splash of water or stock (don't add them at the same time!)
▶ The amount of cheese by using half the amount of a sharper flavored type like parmesan, or by replacing slices of block cheese with a sprinkle of grated cheese
▶ The amount of oil used when roasting vegetables by partially cooking them in the microwave first, then spraying or brushing them with oil and baking until crisp
▶ Saturated fat by using reduced-fat sour cream, low-fat yogurt, buttermilk or reduced-fat ricotta cheese as an alternative to full-fat sour cream
▶ Baked cheesy toppings by using half the cheese, mixed with traditional rolled or stone-ground oats, bread crumbs or wheat germ
▶ Margarine or butter in cakes by experimenting with fruit puree or egg whites as a partial substitute.

Keep fat in perspective

Sometimes you can't replace a high-fat ingredient or switch to a low-fat cooking method without compromising the end product. Not all the food you eat has to be low fat. The key is balance. As well as modifying some of your existing recipes, you can also find new recipes that are similar to your recipes but have less fat and more nutritious ingredients.

■

And remember, there's another way to control your fat intake. Reduce the amount of food you normally consume and fill up with vegetables instead.

■

GI—HOW TO REDUCE THE GLYCEMIC IMPACT AND LOWER THE GLYCEMIC LOAD

Substitute

- Unprocessed oat bran (as a partial substitute) for flour in baked muffins and cakes
- Low-GI alternatives such as sweet corn, lentils or cannellini bean mash, or washed whole small new potatoes cooked in their skin, for high-GI foods such as mashed potato
- A pure floral honey, maple syrup or agave nectar for sugar as a sweetener
- Sourdough or low-GI bread for regular white bread
- Soy flour or chickpea flour as a lower-GI alternative to whole wheat flour if making flatbreads
- Basmati rice for regular rice.

Eliminate

- Fluffy high-GI white breads: go for dense whole-grain or low-GI white types instead
- Large servings of high-GI foods and ingredients, including potatoes and floury products
- Light crispy crackers and chips: eat fruit or a low-fat dairy product instead.

Add

- Something acidic to the meal or dish, such as vinaigrette over salad, lemon juice over vegetables, yogurt or buttermilk in baked goods
- Dried fruit or fresh diced apple or pear to a muffin mix
- Natural low-fat yogurt to a curry and rice meal
- A low-GI food to a high-GI food to give you something in between
- Legumes to meals: bean mix to a salad, lentil mash, chick-peas to a casserole, for instance
- **Alternative sweeteners** instead of sugar—see chapter 16 and the "What Sweetener Is That" section at the back of the book for a comprehensive list of what's available and suited for use in your cooking.

Reduce

- The amounts of sugar added to recipes: look at the overall quantity of sugar in relation to how many servings (½ cup of sugar in a recipe that serves 10 people will have very little effect on your blood glucose levels, for example)
- Your serving size of rice- or pasta-based meals (add extra vegetables to fill the gap)
- Snacks of cookies, crackers, bagels, muffins, cakes, high-GI white bread and rolls: replace them with fruit, low-fat yogurt, nuts and vegetable sticks.

FIBER—HOW TO BOOST

Substitute

- A mixture of whole wheat and white flour or add a little bran: you may need to add a little extra liquid to keep the recipe moist
- Whole-grain bread, whole-grain bread crumbs, grainy muffins, whole wheat flatbread, whole wheat rolls, low-GI white bread wherever you've previously used plain white
- Dried fruit for sweet treats.

Eliminate
- ▶ Low-fiber, high-GI cereals from your breakfast shelf.

Add
- ▶ Extra vegetables to casseroles, soups and sauces
- ▶ Leave the skin on fruits and vegetables (such as apples or potatoes) when using them in recipes.
- ▶ Fresh or dried fruit in bread and cookie recipes
- ▶ Legumes (beans, chickpeas and lentils, home-cooked or canned) to meals
- ▶ A small amount of processed wheat bran cereal to rissoles, meat loaf or even a breakfast smoothie
- ▶ Sautéed mushrooms, other vegetables or some lentils in a spaghetti sauce.

Reduce
- ▶ The number of times you buy high-GI white bread, white bread rolls, muffins and frozen waffles, which are usually low-fiber forms of these foods.

SALT—HOW TO REDUCE THE AMOUNT YOU EAT

Substitute
- ▶ A salt substitute (such as potassium chloride) in cooking or an alternative with iodized salt
- ▶ "Reduced sodium" or "no added salt" varieties for regular canned foods
- ▶ Spices such as freshly ground black pepper, chili, paprika, mustard and cardamom for salt.

Eliminate
- ▶ Salt from the dining table
- ▶ Sea salt, rock salt, vegetable salt, celery salt, garlic salt, chicken salt: they are not suitable substitutes for salt

Add
- ▶ Other flavorings, such as fresh herbs (try parsley, basil,

oregano, chives, rosemary, cilantro, mint, sage, thyme, tarragon and marjoram)

▶ Lemon juice, onions, ginger, shallots, vinegar, wine as flavorings.

Reduce

▶ Your intake of foods high in added sodium
▶ Canned and instant soups
▶ Canned vegetables
▶ Bottled sauces, including tomato, BBQ, Worcestershire, soy and fish sauce
▶ Stock cubes and powders
▶ Salty snack foods such as chips, pretzels, roasted nuts or savory crackers
▶ Olives and pickles
▶ Deli meats, bacon and other cured meats
▶ Cheeses
▶ Restaurant and take-out foods.

RECIPE MAKEOVERS

Many of us whip up our favorite recipes time and again without thinking about how we could change them. But there are often ways to prepare food that can make it taste better than ever. So it's out with the old and in with the new . . .

Recipe makeover 1: Big breakfast for one	
OLD	NEW
2 x eggs	2 x eggs rich in omega-3 fats
3 x breakfast bacon strips	2 x rindless, short-cut bacon strips, trimmed
1 x sausage	1 cup (3½ oz) field mushrooms and ripe tomatoes
2 x white toast	2 x whole-grain toast
Butter	A little oil

To make:

▶ Brush a sautée pan lightly with oil.

▶ Add the bacon and the halved tomatoes (cut side up) to the heated pan and cook until the bacon is lightly golden. Remove the bacon to a plate and keep warm.

▶ Add the mushrooms to the pan and turn the tomatoes. Drizzle a little oil over the mushrooms and pan-fry. Once done to your liking, plate with the bacon and keep warm.

▶ Break the eggs into the pan, adding half an eggshell of water as well. Cover and steam the eggs for 1–2 minutes, or until done to your liking.

▶ While the eggs are cooking, toast the bread. Put the toast onto plates and top with the eggs, adding the bacon, tomato and mushrooms alongside.

Recipe makeover 2: Finger food for a party

OLD	NEW
Shoulder of ham chunks, beef jerky, salami and mortadella	Cigar rolls of pastrami, leg ham, deli roast beef or pork
Cheddar cheese cubes with seasoned crackers	Baked ricotta, homemade lavash crisps and antipasto vegetables. Spread lavash bread with a blend of olive oil and crushed garlic. Sprinkle with sesame seeds and grill until crisp.
Cream cheese dip with salty, fatty crackers	Guacamole, hummus or tomato salsa with vegetable sticks (bell pepper, carrot, baby corn, celery, cucumber, radish)
Potato chips	Nuts (not salty roasted)
Pizza and pigs in blankets	Satay chicken sticks (marinated breast chicken threaded onto skewers, grilled and served with dipping sauce)

Recipe makeover 3: An alternative to quiche

QUICHE LORRAINE	HAM AND VEGETABLE BAKE
4½ oz butter + 4½ oz cream cheese	4 omega-3-rich eggs
3 eggs + ¾ cup cream	14-oz can corn kernels
4 strips of bacon	1¾ oz leg ham, diced
6½ oz cheese	½ cup reduced-fat grated cheese
1 small onion, chopped	2 zucchinis, grated
	2 carrots, grated
	1 onion, grated
	½ cup whole wheat self-rising flour

This traditional recipe for quiche packs in 53 grams of fat (33 grams saturated) per serving.

In comparison, the ham and vegetable bake (which is much easier to make) contains only 7 grams (3 grams saturated) per serving. Both provide 18 grams of carbs per serving.

To make:
- Whisk the eggs.
- Add the corn, ham, cheese, zucchini, carrot and onion then sift in flour and combine. Spoon into a greased pie or lasagna dish and press down to flatten top. Bake in a preheated oven (300°F) for 40 minutes, or until browned and set.

Recipe makeover 4: Cheesecake

TRADITIONAL CHEESECAKE	FRESH FRUIT CHEESECAKE
9 oz shortbread cookies	9 oz oatmeal cookies
3½ oz butter, melted	3½ oz poly- or monounsaturated margarine, melted
	2 tsp gelatin
	2½ tbsp boiling water
cream	8 oz low-fat fruit yogurt
9 oz cream cheese	9 oz low-fat pineapple cottage cheese
½ cup sugar	¼ cup honey
½ tsp vanilla	½ tsp vanilla
strawberries to decorate	1 cup chopped fresh fruit, such as apple, cantaloupe, grapes, pear, strawberries

There's the same carb content per serving in each of these (34 grams per serving if cut into 8 slices), but there's three times the fat in the traditional version.

To make:
- For the base, mix together the cookie crumbs and margarine in a bowl until well combined. Press into a 9-inch pie dish. Bake at 350°F for 10 minutes, then cool.
- Sprinkle gelatin over boiling water in a cup and stir until dissolved. Cool slightly.
- Process the cooled gelatin with the yogurt, cottage cheese, honey and vanilla in a blender or food processor.
- Arrange chopped fruit over the cooled base of the crust; pour over the yogurt mixture and chill for 1 hour, or until set.

Think small

We are all eating too much. Nobody needs a "family size" bar of chocolate. Serving sizes are increasing at the expense of our waistlines. Bulk-sized packs may be less expensive ounce for ounce, but the cost to your health can be considerable. Individual portions are more convenient, more practical, and a healthier option when you need to watch how much you're eating.

- Keep the refrigerator stocked with portable bottles of water, small cartons of low-fat milk (long-life type), small containers of low-fat yogurt, and a bowl of small washed apples and pears.
- Keep mini boxes of raisins, nuts and other dried fruits in the pantry.

If you prefer to buy in bulk, repackage the items in individual portion sizes at home—break down a 2-pound bag of nuts or raisins into ready-to-go snack bags.

Create attention-grabbing snacks

First, get rid of the mini packs of potato chips or chocolate treats. Then:

▶ Place a bowl of easy-to-eat fresh fruit on the kitchen counter.
▶ Snip washed grapes into snack-size portions.
▶ Keep chopped melon chunks, ready-to-eat vegetables, and a small bowl of low-fat dip on the most visible shelf in the refrigerator.

Use health-promoting appliances

Pay attention to how you're cooking as well as what you're cooking:

▶ Toss the deep fryer and buy a good nonstick frying pan.
▶ Use a vegetable steamer to steam a big batch of vegetables so that you can add them to lunches or dinners.
▶ For low-fat cooking, consider a wok or a slow cooker, both of which let you cook without a lot of added fat.

·15·

Smart Shopping

*M*ost people with diabetes would probably appreciate a simple "stamp of approval" on healthy products, but what would you do if your favorite brand of salad dressing didn't carry it? Or if you want to buy the locally made pasta sauce, and it doesn't have it either? You've got no choice—you have to read the label.

Food labels are strictly regulated to help you make informed decisions about the foods you choose. But you have to know how to read them.

BEFORE YOU GO SHOPPING

It may sound like stating the obvious, but what you buy is what you eat. That's why it's essential to plan meals for a few days or even a week ahead and make a list of the ingredients you will need before you go shopping—rather than hoping for inspiration when you hit the aisles. Planning helps you resist impulse purchases based on price, advertising, shelf position, etc. Not that these factors won't affect your food choices, but planning gives nutrition a higher priority in your food choices and so makes healthier eating easier to achieve. It also helps you stick to your budget.

■

Remember, if you don't buy it, you can't eat it.

■

Reading between the lines

The three main sources of nutrition information on a package are:

▶ Nutrition claims
▶ Ingredient lists
▶ The nutrition information panel

Can I Believe What It Says?

THE CENTER FOR Food Safety and Applied Nutrition is a government organization responsible for developing standards for food labeling. Their key role is to protect our health through maintaining a safe food supply. For more information, visit www.cfsan.fda.gov/label.html.

NUTRITION CLAIMS

At first glance, it may seem that everything on the shelves is either "fat free" or "diet" or "lite" (usually spelled incorrectly). These are nutrition claims. Nutrition claims are marketing tools that manufacturers are permitted to use on their packaging and in their advertising to draw attention to a special nutritional feature of their product.

They can't just say what they like—they are supposed to abide by a code of practice for food labels and advertisements that spells out very specific conditions under which claims can be made. In the near future all manufacturers will need to abide by the food law, which will give consumers even greater protection.

At the moment, these claims usually highlight only the positive nutritional properties of a food, and they are frequently misinterpreted. What they say and what it means . . .

"Light" or "lite" can be used to describe various properties of the product (even its color), but is often taken by consumers to mean low in fat or calories. Manufacturers should describe what the "light" refers to, but this is sometimes overlooked or in very small print.
What to do? Check the nutrition panel to find out what's been lightened—fat, or energy (calories) or something else.

"Cholesterol free" does not mean no fat or healthy. Many foods can be cholesterol free and still relatively high in saturated fat— and therefore blood cholesterol–raising. It is often a ridiculous claim because it's used on foods (such as plant foods and products made from them) that are naturally cholesterol free—even coconut and chocolate fat are cholesterol free. It's not a guide to a healthy choice.
What to do? Check the nutrition panel for total fat and saturated fat per serving.

"No sugar added" or "unsweetened" on fruit juices, for example, means no sugar has been added, but the product may contain just as much natural sugar as a soft drink and may still affect your blood glucose level (BGL).
What to do? Check the nutrition panel for total carbs and energy (calories).

"97% fat free" really means 3 percent fat. Although only low-fat foods (3 percent fat or less) can make this claim, it still doesn't tell you how much fat is in one serving—or what type it is.
What to do? Check the nutrition panel for total saturated fat per serving.

"No trans fat" does not mean zero trans fat—FDA regulations allow up to 0.5 grams of it to count as no trans fat—and the servings can add up.

What to do? Check the nutrition panel for "hydrogenated or partially hydrogenated oil."

THE INGREDIENT LIST

All packaged foods must carry a list of ingredients in descending order according to their proportion by weight. This means that the ingredient at the top of the list is the one in the product in the greatest amount.

The percentage of *characterizing ingredients* must also appear. These are ingredients that appear in the name or are emphasized on the label of the food. For example, in "raisin cookies," the percentage of raisins must be listed.

Use the ingredient list to determine the basics of what you're buying and compare brands for value for money.

- Canned tuna, for example, can vary from around 48 percent tuna to 98 percent tuna, depending on the liquid, flavorings and dressings included in the can.
- When you're buying chicken breast you're buying 100 percent chicken, but if you buy chicken cutlet you're buying about 50 percent chicken and 50 percent bread crumbs, and possibly paying the same price per pound.
- If you're concerned about the sugar listed in the nutrition information panel, you can identify its source as milk, fruit or refined sugars from the ingredient list.

Ingredients that represent carbohydrates—dextrose, glucose, fructose, sucrose, lactose, maltose, sugar, brown sugar, molasses, honey, starch, corn starch, maltodextrin, high fructose corn syrup, corn syrup solids, invert syrup, liquid glucose, flour, thickener—are also listed. They all raise blood glucose levels, by varying amounts.

Gluten, shellfish, eggs, fish, milk, nuts, sesame, soybeans, added sulphite in high concentrations, royal jelly, bee pollen or propolis must be also declared, because many people are allergic to one or more of these things.

Serving Size and Servings per Container—What It Means

THE SERVINGS PER container or package tells you how many servings (as defined by the manufacturer) are in the whole package. So if the package contains 4 fillets of fish and serves 2, then the manufacturer has decided that each serving is 2 fillets.

At the top of the nutrition information panel you'll see a serving size description. This serving size is the amount of food you would need to eat to get the amount of listed nutrients. It may be described by weight or by a common measure such as a cup.

The serving size of the food in the nutrition information panel is not necessarily a recommended serving size. It is chosen by the manufacturer and is usually based on common sense, but it may be very different from the amount you eat. You may need to scale up—or down—the nutrition information per serving according to your serving size. If there are two servings in the package, and you eat the entire package in one go, for instance, your serving will be double the amounts of nutrients per serving listed on the package.

THE NUTRITION INFORMATION PANEL

The nutrition information panel on food packaging lists the amount of energy (calories), protein, fat, saturated fat, total carbohydrates and sugars and sodium in a food. Typically this information is shown in two columns, per serving and percentage of the daily value.

The daily value allows you to make a direct comparison between foods—you can compare one cheese with another, for example. In a particular food category, such as granola bars, you will find that there are significant differences in nutrients such as fat, fiber and salt content from one brand to another. Knowing these differences lets you make the best choice for your own health needs. Some products list the types of fat (polyunsaturates, monounsaturates, saturates, trans and cholesterol) and the types of carbohydrates (sugars, dietary fiber). The content of particular vitamins and minerals in the food may also be listed.

If you like to keep some numbers in your head when you're shopping, the following details are for you. They are a general guide only, so don't use them on their own to exclude or include foods in your diet.

Energy

This may sound as if it's a measure of how much get-up-and-go you'll have after eating the food, but it is not. Energy measured in calories is an indicator of how much fuel the food gives your body. Most of us need less fuel than we are getting (because we eat too much). We need to eat more foods with a lower energy density (fewer calories per bite) and combine them with smaller amounts of higher-energy foods. To assess the energy density, look at the serving size in grams and calories per serving. A low energy density is when the number of calories is less than the number of grams.

Protein

The protein content of the food is listed in grams. Much of the human body—including muscles, skin, and the **immune system**—is made up of protein, so it's something we need in our diet for healthy growth and repair, but it's also a nutrient we tend to get enough of without having to seek it out.

Fat, total

This number indicates how much fat, in grams, is in a single serving of food. Fat is the most energy dense nutrient in food, so if the total fat content is high, the energy density will be too. How high is high? Well that depends on a lot of factors, but for most people 20 grams per serving would be high. A food has to contain less than 3 grams of fat per serving to be allowed to be labeled as low fat.

Saturated fat

The amount of saturated fat appears below total fat. Saturated fats and trans fats are often called "bad fats" because they raise cholesterol and increase your risk of developing heart disease. Look for a low saturated fat content, ideally less than 20 percent of the total fat. This means that if the total fat content is 10 grams, you want saturated fat to be less than 2 grams. A food can be labeled as low in saturated fat if it contains less than 1 gram of saturated fat per serving.

Carbohydrates, total

This is the starch, plus any naturally occurring and added sugars in the food. There's no need to look at the sugar figure separately because it's the total carbohydrates that affects your blood glucose level (BGL). You can use this figure if you are monitoring your carbohydrate intake and to calculate the GL of your serving of the food.

The GL = grams of total carbohydrates $\times$ GI + 100.

Sugars

Sugars, which includes all naturally occurring and added sugars (table sugar, honey), are listed under total carbohydrates on food labels. If you asked people with diabetes about this figure, two out of three would probably say it was important that it is low. In fact, that's not the case: it's the **total** carbohydrates figure that counts when it comes to blood glucose. Sugars are found in healthy foods like mangoes and grapes and are an important source of glucose for our bodies. It isn't necessary to distinguish between sugars and starches when you have diabetes (see chapter 16). But for the sake of consistency, you do need to monitor the total carbs.

Dietary fiber

Most foods have very low fiber content—if there's any at all. Breakfast cereals and breads are valuable sources of fiber in our diet, so generally the higher the better. Fiber promotes bowel health and is a necessary part of a balanced diet.

According to Food and Drug Administration (FDA) regulations, a "good" source of fiber contains at least 2½ grams per serving and a "high" or "excellent" source has more than 5 grams per serving.

Sodium

Sodium is a component of salt. We need small amounts of sodium to keep our body fluid in balance. It also helps with the transmission of electrical signals through nerves. But too much sodium can worsen water retention and high blood pressure in people who are sensitive to it. Almost all foods naturally contain small amounts of sodium.

Our bodies need some salt, but most of us consume way more than we need. Many processed foods—canned foods in particular—are high in sodium. Check the sodium content per serving on the label next time: a low-salt food contains less than 140 milligrams of sodium per serving. Many packaged foods and convenience meals are well above this. As a guide, aim for less than 450 milligrams per serving.

NB: Our guidance on figures on the nutrition panel are an arbitrary recommendation to help you shop for healthier packaged foods. They should not be substituted for individualized dietary advice.

HOW DO YOU KNOW IF A FOOD IS LOW, MEDIUM OR HIGH GI?

To find the GI of your favorite brands you can:

- Look for the GI-tested symbol on the product
- Check the nutritional label—some manufacturers now include GI
- Visit www.glycemicindex.com and search the free database
- Check out the tables in this book, or your *Shopper's Guide to GI Values* (an updated edition is published at the beginning of every year), and/or
- Contact the manufacturer and ask (hound) them to have the food tested by an accredited lab.

The GI symbol program

When you see this international symbol you will know that the food has been assessed by the experts.

GI symbol

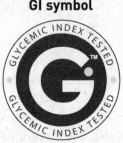

This symbol means that the food is healthy and has been glycemic index (GI) tested by the approved method. It's your guarantee that the GI value stated near the nutrition information table is reliable. Foods that carry the GI symbol have also been assessed against a range of nutrient criteria (calories, fats, fiber and sodium) so you can be sure that the food is a healthy nutritional choice for its food group and suitable for people with diabetes and prediabetes.

For more information go to www.gisymbol.com

THE FOOD CERTIFICATION PROGRAM
AND HEALTH CHECK

American Heart Association's heart-check mark (and the Health Check in Canada) is another tool that can be helpful in selecting healthier foods. Products that carry the heart-check mark or Health Check are independently tested to meet the program's strict standards for nutrients such as saturated and trans fat, sodium (salt), cholesterol and dietary fiber.

Carbohydrates are not specifically considered for the program so people with diabetes need to keep this in mind.

The heart-check mark or Health Check is found on a wide range of foods, including milk, cheese, fish, meat, poultry, grains, legumes, nuts and seeds. And the mark is also found on dairy foods and egg substitutes to help people choose the ones that are lower in saturated fat and sodium.

For more information, and to see the check marks, visit www.heartcheckmark.com or www.healthcheck.org.

PANTRY REVAMP

Healthy eating isn't an accident. It's only going to happen with planning and preparation. Rethinking how you shop, store and prepare food can improve the whole household's eating habits. Here are some tips to make preparing healthy meals easier.

Your checkout choices: the healthy home shopping list

Here is a practical shopping list to stock your fridge, pantry and freezer.

First, plan a day where you remove all the "junk" foods normally kept in your pantry—the cakes, cookies, snacks, chocolates, etc. Go shopping in the afternoon (don't go hungry) for healthy substitutes, as suggested below.

What to keep in your pantry

Asian sauces—chili, hoisin, oyster, soy and fish sauces are a good basic range. Look for reduced-sodium versions.

Barley—one of the oldest cultivated cereals, barley is highly nutritious and high in soluble fiber. Look for pearl barley to use in soups, stews and pilafs.

Black pepper—buy ground pepper or grind your own peppercorns.

Bread—low-GI options include grainy, soy and flaxseed, stone-ground whole wheat, pumpernickel, sourdough, English-style muffins, low-GI white, flat bread and pita bread.

Breakfast cereals—these include traditional rolled oats, natural muesli and low-GI packaged breakfast cereals.

Bulgur wheat—use it to make tabbouleh, or add to vegetable burgers, stuffings, soups and stews.

Canned evaporated skim milk—this is an excellent substitute for cream in pasta sauces.

Canned fish—keep a good stock of canned tuna packed in spring water, and canned sardines and salmon.

Canned fruit—have a variety on hand, including peaches, pears, apples and nectarines. Choose the brands labeled with "no added sugar" fruit juice syrup.

Canned vegetables—sweet corn kernels and tomatoes can help boost the vegetable content of a meal.

Couscous—ready in minutes; serve with casseroles and braised dishes.

Curry pastes—a tablespoon or so makes a delicious curry base.

Dried fruit—such as apricots, raisins, prunes and apples.

Dried herbs—oregano, basil, ground coriander, thyme and rosemary can be useful.

Honey—try to avoid the commercial honeys or honey blends, and use "pure floral" honeys, which have a much lower GI.

Jam—a dollop of good-quality jam (with no added sugar) on toast has fewer calories than butter or margarine.

Legumes—stock a variety of legumes (dried or canned), including lentils, chickpeas, split peas and beans; there are many bean varieties, including cannellini, butter, white, kidney and soybeans.

Mustard—seeded or whole-grain mustard is useful as a sandwich spread, and in salad dressings and sauces.

Noodles—many Asian noodles, such as hokkien, udon and rice vermicelli, are low to medium GI because of their dense texture, whether they are made from wheat or rice flour.

Nuts—try them sprinkled over your breakfast cereal, salad or dessert; try unsalted nuts as a snack as well.

Oils—try olive oil for general use; extra virgin olive oil for salad dressings and marinades; sesame oil for Asian-style stir-fries; and canola or olive oil cooking sprays.

Pasta—a great source of carbohydrates and B vitamins. Fresh or dried, the preparation is easy: cook in boiling water until just tender (al dente), then drain and top with your favorite sauce (not made with cream) or mix in plenty of vegetables and a sprinkle of parmesan cheese.

Quinoa—this whole grain cooks in 10–15 minutes and has a slightly chewy texture. It can be used as a substitute for rice, couscous or bulgur wheat; it is very important to rinse the grains thoroughly before cooking.

Rice—basmati or Japanese sushi rice (koshihikari) varieties are good choices because they have a lower GI than, for example, jasmine rice.

Rolled oats—besides oatmeal, oats can be added to cakes, cookies, breads and desserts.

Spices—most spices, including ground cumin, turmeric, cinnamon, paprika and nutmeg, should be bought in small quantities because they lose pungency with age and incorrect storage.

Stock—make your own stock or buy long-life ready-made products; to keep the sodium content down with ready-made stocks, look for reduced-sodium ones.

Tomato paste—use in soups, sauces and casseroles.

Vinegar—white or red wine vinegar and balsamic vinegar are excellent as vinaigrette dressings in salads.

What to keep in your refrigerator

Bacon—bacon is a valuable ingredient in many dishes because of its flavor. You can make a little bacon go a long way by trimming off all fat and chopping it finely. Lean ham is often a more economical and leaner way to go. In casseroles and soups, a ham or bacon bone gives great flavor without much fat.

Bottled vegetables—sun-dried tomatoes, olives, grilled eggplant and roasted red peppers are flavorsome additions to pastas and sandwiches.

Capers, olives and anchovies—these can be bought in jars and kept in the refrigerator once opened. They are a tasty (but salty) addition to pasta dishes, salads and pizzas. Use sparingly.

Cheese—any reduced-fat cheese is great. A block of parmesan is indispensable and will keep for up to a month. Reduced-fat cottage and ricotta cheeses have a short life so are best bought as needed; they can be a good alternative to butter or margarine in a sandwich.

Condiments—jars of minced garlic, chili or ginger will spice up your cooking in an instant.

Eggs—to increase your intake of omega-3 fats, we suggest using omega-3-enriched eggs. Although the yoke is high in cholesterol, the fat in eggs is predominantly monounsaturated, and therefore considered a "good fat."

Fish—try a variety of fresh fish.

Fresh fruit—almost all fruit makes an excellent snack. Try apples, oranges, pears, grapes, grapefruit, peaches, apricots, strawberries and mangoes.

Fresh herbs—these are available in most supermarkets and there really is no substitute for their flavor. For variety, try parsley, basil, mint, chives and cilantro.

Meat—try lean beef, lamb fillets, pork fillets, chicken (breast or drumsticks) and ground beef.

Milk—skim or low-fat milk is best, or low-fat calcium-enriched soy milk.

Vegetables—keep a variety of seasonal vegetables on hand, such as spinach, broccoli, broccoli rabe, cauliflower, Asian greens, asparagus, zucchini and mushrooms. Peppers, scallions and sprouts (mung bean and snowpea sprouts) are great to bulk up a salad. Sweet corn, sweet potato and yam are essential to your low-GI food store.

Yogurt—low-fat natural yogurt gives you the most calcium for the fewest calories. Have vanilla or fruit versions as a dessert, or use natural yogurt as a condiment in spicy dishes. If using yogurt in a hot meal, make sure you add it at the last minute, and do not let it boil.

What to keep in your freezer

Frozen berries—berries can make any dessert special, and frozen berries mean you don't have to wait until berry season. Blueberries, raspberries and strawberries are a fantastic source of antioxidants and Vitamin C.

Frozen vegetables—keep a bag of peas, beans, corn, spinach or mixed vegetables in the freezer; these are always handy to add to a quick meal.

Frozen yogurt—this is a fantastic substitute for ice cream and some products even have a similar creamy texture, but with much less fat.

Ice cream—reduced- or low-fat ice cream is ideal for a quick dessert, served with fresh fruit.

▪16▪

Sugar and Sweeteners:
The Real Deal

*D*o you feel guilty every time you enjoy something sweet? Do you think diabetes equals no sugar? Join the club. Many people think that if something tastes good, it must be bad for them. And many people with diabetes, and even their doctors, mistakenly believe that sugar consumption is the most important explanation for high blood glucose readings.

While we now know that's not the case, old habits die hard. Traditionally, people with diabetes have been told to replace all sugar with an artificial sweetener and to drink diet soda. It's enough to make some people with diabetes turn their backs on all dietary advice.

But wanting something sweet is instinctive, and hard to ignore. It is part of our "hardwiring." In our hunter-gatherer past, fruits, berries and honey were our only source of carbohydrates.

■

**"There is a charm about the forbidden that makes
it unspeakably desirable."**

Mark Twain

■

You'll be relieved to know that most diabetes organizations all
around the world no longer advise strict avoidance of refined sugar or
sugary foods. This is one of the happy spin-offs from research on the
GI—recognition that both sugary foods and starchy foods raise your
blood glucose.

Furthermore, dozens of studies indicate that moderate amounts of
added sugar in diabetic diets (for example, 30–50 grams per day) does
not result in either poor control or weight gain. Yes, a soft drink can
be a concentrated source of calories, but so can a fruit juice or an
alcoholic drink.

But a word of caution: there is increasing evidence that energy in
liquid forms (both soft drinks and fruit juices) may sneak past the
brain's appetite center. For example, if you give people 100 extra calories as solid jelly beans, they unconsciously compensate by consuming fewer calories over the rest of the day. But if you feed them 100
calories in a soda, fruit juice, beer or other liquid, they don't reduce
their intake much at all. Those extra calories can head straight for the
waistline. In a recent study at Harvard University, the children who
became overweight over time were the ones who were greater consumers of soft drinks and fruit juices.

■

**A healthy diet is *not* a diet that requires a ton of
sacrifice and self-discipline.**

■

You can enjoy refined or "added" sugar in moderation—that's about
6–10 teaspoons (30–50 grams) a day—an amount that most people
consume without trying hard. Try to include sweetened foods that
provide more than just calories—dairy foods, breakfast cereals, oatmeal with brown sugar, jam on whole-grain toast, etc. Even the World
Health Organization says "a moderate intake of sugar-rich foods can

provide for a palatable and nutritious diet." So forget the guilt trip and allow yourself the pleasure of sweetness.

WHAT ABOUT ALTERNATIVE SWEETENERS?

Alternatives to sugar are widely used by people with diabetes to sweeten drinks (tea and coffee) and foods (breakfast cereals); to sweeten recipes (for cakes and desserts); and in low-calorie commercial products (soft drinks, fruit punch, jams, jellies and yogurts).

They do give you sweetness with fewer calories, and usually with less effect on blood glucose levels, but there are differences between them.

Not all alternative sweeteners are the same—some have just as many calories as sugar, others have no calories at all; some are thousands (yes, thousands) of times sweeter than sugar; others are not very sweet at all. One thing they all have in common, however, is that they are more expensive than sugar.

There are lots of brands of sweeteners on the supermarket shelves, but essentially there are two main types:

▶ Nutritive sweeteners, and
▶ Nonnutritive sweeteners.

What's the difference?

Nutritive sweeteners

Nutritive sweeteners are simply those that provide some calories. Sugar, for example, is a nutritive sweetener, but so are things like sorbitol and maltodextrin. They have differing effects on blood glucose levels. In What Sweetener Is That? at the back of the book we list the key properties of commonly used nutritive sweeteners so that you can check out the differences at a glance.

Old-fashioned table sugar stands up well under scrutiny—it is the second sweetest after fructose, has only a moderate GI, is the best value for money and is the easiest to use in cooking. And because it generally has a lower GI than the refined flour used in baking, it can actually lower the GI of many recipes!

The sugar alcohols, such as sorbitol, mannitol and maltitol, are generally not as sweet as table sugar, provide fewer calories and have less of an impact on blood glucose levels. To overcome their lack of sweetness, food manufacturers usually combine them with nonnutritive sweeteners to help keep the calorie count down and minimize the effect on blood glucose levels. This will be shown in the ingredients list on the food label.

The nutritive sweeteners such as sorbitol, mannitol, xylitol and maltitol, and maltitol syrup, may have a laxative effect or cause gas or diarrhea if you consume them in large amounts. Foods that contain more than 20 grams of these alternative sweeteners, or more than 50 grams of sorbitol, isomalt, or polydextrose, carry warning statements about the possible laxative effect on their labels. These products can be a particular problem for children and adolescents, because of their smaller body size.

Used in sensible quantities, fructose certainly rivals table sugar as a good all-around sweetener. It stands out from the crowd, being sweeter than sugar, providing the same number of calories, but having only one-third the GI. So you can use less fructose to achieve the same level of sweetness, and as a result, consume fewer calories and experience a much smaller rise in your blood glucose levels. Its main drawback is cost.

If you have read alarmist reports about fructose and blood fats and/or insulin resistance, remember that this research was on rats and mice fed excessive quantities—more than someone with even the sweetest tooth could tolerate. There is no evidence that fructose has adverse effects in people with diabetes consuming normal quantities.

Nonnutritive sweeteners

Nonnutritive sweeteners (such as Equal, Splenda or saccharin) are all much sweeter than table sugar and essentially have no effect on your blood glucose levels because most are used in such small quantities and are either not absorbed into or metabolized by the body. Because they are only used in minute amounts, the number of calories they provide is insignificant.

What's best to use for cooking?

The nonnutritive sweeteners that are made of protein molecules often break down when heated at high temperatures for long periods, thus losing their sweetness. For this reason, they are not always ideal for baking. The best nonnutritive sweeteners to cook with are Splenda, and saccharin, and to a lesser extent Equal Spoonful.

Are they safe?

As a group, nonnutritive sweeteners have been studied more thoroughly than any other type of food additive. Questions about the safety of saccharin were raised when it was first discovered over 125 years ago, and its effect on human health has been monitored ever since. The same is true of more recent sweeteners such as aspartame and sucralose. There is no convincing evidence so far that any of the nonnutritive sweeteners on the market have any negative effects on our health.

While the nonnutritive sweeteners available in North America are considered safe for everyone, some health professionals opt for caution and recommend that pregnant women avoid saccharin and cyclamate. This is because both of them cross the placenta into the growing fetus and can also be found in breast milk.

What about Stevia?

THE LEAVES OF this semitropical herb of the aster family are around 30 times sweeter than table sugar but with no calories. As an herb, they can be used fresh or dried. In the dried form, less than 2½ tablespoons of crushed leaves can replace 1 cup of table sugar, although it's hard to be specific, because its actual sweetness can vary. Stevioside, its extract, is 250–300 times sweeter than sucrose and is currently not approved for use as a food but is a dietary supplement in the United States and Canada (see also What about Herbal Therapies? in chapter 40). Stevia (*Stevia rebaudiana*), native to the mountains of Brazil and Paraguay, first came to the attention of the Western world in the 1800s, but remained relatively obscure until it was used as an alternative sweetener in England during World War II.

Also, studies in rats have shown an increased risk of bladder cancer due to saccharin use and kidney disease due to cyclamate use. To put this in perspective, remember that saccharin and cyclamate were both used widely after World War II because there was a worldwide sugar shortage, and we did not see an increase in bladder or kidney cancer over that period. So it seems unlikely that either sweetener is a problem for pregnant women or those who are breastfeeding. However, some women still choose to avoid these two nonnutritive sweeteners.

Phenylketonuria and Aspartame

FOODS AND BEVERAGES in the United States and Canada that contain aspartame must carry a warning for people with phenylketonuria. Phenylketonuria is a rare genetic disease, which is characterized by an inability of the body to utilize the essential amino acid, phenylalanine. About 1 in 10,000 newborn babies is affected with the condition. Managing this disease includes sticking to a low-protein diet, with particular emphasis on avoiding foods high in phenylalanine. As aspartame contains a significant amount of phenylalanine, it is not recommended for people with phenylketonuria.

Blends: the best of both worlds?

Splenda Sugar Blend for Baking is a blend of ordinary table sugar and sucralose, a nonnutritive sweetener. By adding sucralose to sugar, you get the best of both worlds: an intense sweetener with fewer calories, but the cooking properties of sugar. Its only downside is its cost—nearly three times that of table sugar.

WHAT SHOULD YOU DO?

Replacing table sugar with alternative sweeteners may have some health benefits but these come at a cost. To achieve the best of both worlds we suggest that you use your favorite alternative sweetener in those dishes that normally require a significant amount of added sugar (half a cup or more). For the rest of the time, just have a teaspoon or two of sugar and enjoy it.

STEP 2

Be Active
Every Day

$\mathcal{P}$hysical activity is one of the cornerstones of managing diabetes and prediabetes.

■

"The single thing that comes close to a magic bullet, in terms of its strong and universal benefits, is exercise."

Associate Professor Frank Hu, Harvard School of Public Health

■

·17·

Activate Your Day

"IN THE BOTTLE before you is a pill, a marvel of modern medicine that will regulate gene transcription throughout your body, help prevent heart disease, stroke, diabetes, obesity, and 12 kinds of cancer—plus gallstones and diverticulitis (inflammation of the intestines). Expect the pill to improve your strength and balance as well as your blood **lipid profile**. Your bones will become stronger. You'll grow new capillaries in your heart, your skeletal muscles and your brain, improving blood flow and the delivery of oxygen and nutrients. Your attention span will increase. If you have arthritis, your symptoms will improve. The pill will help you regulate your appetite and you'll probably find you prefer healthier foods. You'll feel better, younger even, and you will test younger according to a variety of physiologic measures. Your blood volume will increase and you will burn fats better. Even your immune system will be stimulated. There is just one catch.

"There's no such pill. The prescription is exercise."

Jonathan Shaw, *Harvard Magazine* (March–April 2004)

It doesn't really matter who you are, or what type of diabetes you have: if you want to be around and in good shape to enjoy your life, your family and your friends, you have to get some exercise.

"I'm active," you say. "I'm on the go all day, walking here and there, in and out of the car, up and down stairs, doing the housework, always busy."

That's great for starters. But what we're talking about here is deliberate muscle movement sessions that add up to at least 150 minutes of physical activity a week, plus making being active and exercising regularly a way of life.

In this chapter we set out the benefits of exercise to get you motivated; and to get you on the move we discuss the kinds of activities you might do and the precautions you need to take when you are doing them, including managing your food and medication during exercise.

If you're already exercising regularly, that's great, but could you do more, or try something different? Whatever the case, you'll find lots of practical ideas here.

■

There are really only two requirements when it comes to exercise. One is that you do it. The other is that you continue to do it.

■

WHY PUSH YOURSELF TO EXERCISE?

Exercising muscles need fuel and the fuel they need most is glucose. So as soon as you start moving your muscles they'll start burning up glucose. First they'll use their own stores of glucose (that's glycogen); then they'll call on the liver for some of its stores, all the time drawing the glucose out of the blood and lowering your blood glucose levels.

Here are some of the other benefits (in no particular order) you can get from regular exercise:

▶ More energy
▶ Better sleep

▶ A better mood: exercise produces feel-good chemicals in the brain called endorphins, which will help you cope better with stress
▶ Better digestion
▶ Improved immunity
▶ Stronger bones
▶ Increased insulin sensitivity: exercise increases the number, sensitivity and binding capacity of insulin receptors
▶ Lower blood pressure
▶ Less of the bad cholesterol (LDL) and more of the good (HDL)
▶ Better circulation so less risk of diabetic complications (including impotence)
▶ Better weight management and less fat. After about 30 minutes of continuous exercise the body turns to using fatty acids as a fuel. This clears fats out of your blood and gets some movement happening in the flabby bits
▶ Fewer hospital admissions or visits to the doctor, and
▶ Fewer pills to take—medications related to diabetes, blood pressure and cholesterol could be reduced

Plus, you'll be able to do things you haven't done for years, such as climb a flight of stairs without puffing.

And don't underestimate the positive impact on those around you—you'll be a role model for your family, friends and colleagues!

Exercise Can Help You Live Longer

A STUDY OF nearly 4,000 people with type 2 diabetes found that after an average of 18 years, nearly 40 percent had died—two-thirds of them from cardiovascular heart and blood vessel disease. When participants were grouped according to the levels of physical activity they did, those who engaged in moderate to high activity in their leisure time, at work, or while commuting (riding a bike to work, for instance) had half the risk of dying at an early age.

ACTIVATING YOUR DAY

Start with extra incidental activity

Having to do 30 minutes of exercise every day of the week can seem impossible. What? How? Before thinking about more serious exercise, work on increasing your incidental activity.

Incidental activity means the short bouts of physical activity of 5–10 minutes you accumulate as part of your normal daily routines—making the bed, doing chores, walking to the bus stop, popping out for a coffee, parking the car and walking to the shops or office. If you make a conscious effort to increase this kind of physical activity in your day, it eventually becomes second nature. Just by adding a little more each day, you will have accumulated the benefits of more exercise by the end of the week.

■

Think of incidental activity as an opportunity not an inconvenience.

■

BETTY

WHEN I WAS recently diagnosed with type 2 diabetes, at the age of 75, I was horrified when my doctor suggested I go for a walk each day. "Walk? The farthest I ever walk is to the driveway!" I said. But I wanted to manage my diabetes and to do that I really had to lose some weight, so I began walking every morning, with my husband. After six weeks I could walk 40–50 minutes a day easily. And I had lost more than 10 pounds. I feel so much better for it and I can do things I haven't done in years.

Here's how, with just a little extra effort, you can build more incidental activity into your life and reap the benefits. You have probably seen lists like this before—we aren't inventing the wheel here. Use our suggestions as a start, then add your own ideas:

- Use the stairs instead of taking the elevator (Jennie's 83-year-old father lives in a 6th-floor apartment and never takes the elevator)
- Don't stand still on the escalator—walk up and down (holding the rail)
- Take the long way around whenever you can—running down to the corner store, getting a drink from the office water cooler, going to the bathroom
- Make the time to walk the children or grandchildren to school
- Meet your friends for a walk rather than coffee and cake
- Walk the dog instead of hitting tennis balls for him to chase and retrieve
- Get rid of the leaf blower (your neighbors will thank you) and rake the leaves or sweep the yard, and
- Park the car 100 yards away and walk to the corner store, ATM, post office or dry cleaners: it all adds up.

Getting more serious about exercise

Here are two tips to help you activate your day:

1. Set a schedule, keep a daily log and stick to it! Make the commitment to exercise just the way you make any other important appointment. Remember, habits are developed through practice, and
2. Find a pleasant setting for exercise, because this will help keep you motivated. Try a park near work where you can walk, or find a clean, comfortable attractive fitness center, an attractive walking buddy, a radio or MP3 player with earphones, etc.

■

Before you begin, have a medical checkup.

■

If you're planning on doing anything more vigorous than brisk walking you should have a medical checkup first. Now's the time to talk to your doctor about the type of exercise you have in mind and whether or *not* it is safe for you. Because everyone with prediabetes or diabetes has an increased risk of heart disease, your doctor may want you to do an exercise stress test.

If you have:

Proliferative retinopathy (a noninflammatory disease of the retina), strenuous exercise or excessive straining is **not recommended** because it increases the risk of hemorrhage (bleeding) in the vitreous space in the eye. If you have had laser photo-coagulation therapy because of your retinopathy, wait 3–6 months before starting or resuming your exercise program.

Peripheral neuropathy (this causes loss of sensation in the feet), avoid weight-bearing exercise because of the danger of injury to your feet. If the condition is mild, suitable footwear can give you enough protection, but alternative exercises such as swimming, cycling, rowing or arm exercises should be considered.

Getting advice on exercise

Exercise specialists such as physiotherapists, exercise physiologists and personal trainers can create an individualized program to suit your needs. Make sure a personal trainer is certified by the American College of Sports Medicine (ACSM)—this means they should be able to work with people who have prediabetes, diabetes or other health problems.

If you have type 1 diabetes

If you have type 1 diabetes, be extremely cautious about taking on sports where a hypoglycemic episode could be difficult to handle, such as:

- Auto racing
- Single-handed sailing
- Rock climbing
- Gliding
- Diving
- Hang gliding

Consider the possibility of hypos and dehydration when exercising, and think about how you can prevent them by:

▶ Planning your food and insulin intake before you begin exercising, and making the necessary adjustments according to your expected level of energy output.

How often should you exercise, and for how long?

For general health, we'd suggest you aim to do 30–60 minutes of exercise most days. If you prefer, you can break this into two or three sessions of 15 or 20 minutes. For weight loss, research suggests that you need to do 150–210 minutes of moderate-intensity exercise each week.

For maximum benefits, leave no more than two days between exercise sessions, because the effect of aerobic exercise on insulin sensitivity lasts only 24–72 hours, depending on the duration and intensity of what you do.

To increase your muscle strength and size, do some resistance exercises 2–3 times a week (not on consecutive days); to maintain strength, once a week is enough. Don't worry—you won't end up looking like a bodybuilder unless you spend many hours each day in the gym. But a little bit of extra muscle will help you achieve two important goals for people with prediabetes or diabetes. It will:

▶ Increase your metabolic rate, and
▶ Decrease your insulin resistance.

How intense should exercise be?

Lower-intensity exercise (exercise that doesn't get you to more than 50 percent of your maximum heart rate) is effective for weight loss. During light exercise, the body uses a larger percentage of fat than glucose (carbohydrates) as a fuel. If you haven't just eaten, the fat is drawn from your body's own stores. As the intensity increases, the body relies more on carbohydrates. A higher intensity (around 75 percent of your maximum heart rate) will be effective for increasing your fitness. For more specific advice on what exercise intensity is best for you, see an exercise specialist.

Measuring the Intensity of Exercise

THERE ARE TWO ways to do this:

- Monitoring your pulse (heart rate)
- The simple "talk test"

MONITORING YOUR PULSE

Measure your pulse rate with a pulsemeter or by using your wristwatch—this will give you the beats per minute. Then aim for 50–75 percent of your maximum heart rate. Your maximum heart rate is 220 minus your age. For example, if you are 50 years old, here's how you would calculate the number of beats per minute you need to achieve:

1. 50 percent of your maximum heart rate
   220—50 (age) = 170,
   170 x 50 ÷ 100 = 85 beats per minute
2. 75 percent of your maximum heart rate:
   220—50 (age) = 170
   170 x 75 ÷ 100 = 128 beats per minute
3. When you exercise, aim to keep your heart rate between 85 and 130 beats per minute.

TALK TEST

The "talk test" simply means exercising at a pace where you are breathing harder than usual but can still carry on a conversation comfortably.

When is the best time to exercise?

We're frequently asked this. The unspoken words behind this question are, "When will I burn up the most body fat?"

The best time to exercise is when you can best fit it in. Look for a fairly regular time slot most days. For a lot of people this ends up being first thing in the morning, before the other activities of the day interrupt. But the connection between your head and the pillow can be really strong. Lunchtime exercise sessions can be a great way of destressing from a hectic morning and boosting your energy levels in the afternoon. Even 15–20 minutes here can be a useful regular addition.

In the evening you might have more time available, but there are dangers. Do not sit down in front of the TV or your computer or watch a DVD until you've done your exercise. If you do, you're gone. Your energy levels are likely to be pretty low at this time, which is great for sleeping but not good for leaping off the couch. If you exercise strenuously, make sure you allow for some wind-down time before bed, or getting to sleep can be difficult.

The length of time you spend on one exercise session will vary depending on where you are. If you're just starting out on an exercise program, you might begin with bouts of 10 minutes. The aim should be to get up to 30 minutes a session. If you're exercising comfortably for 30 minutes and want to go even further, you may decide to increase this to 45 or 60 minutes.

∎

If you don't use it you lose it: a physically inactive adult can expect to lose 3–5 percent of muscle mass and strength per decade after the age of 40.

∎

TYPES OF EXERCISE

What you do is going to depend on how long you've been logged onto the couch. If your body talks back when you try to move it, high-impact activities aren't for you. Swimming, cycling or rowing might be better choices.

For optimal physical fitness, your exercise program ought to include two main types of exercise—aerobic exercise and strength or resistance exercise. Combining the two forms of exercise will have added benefits for diabetes management. Also, stretching, yoga, tai chi and Pilates-type exercises will increase your flexibility and balance, and increase your freedom of movement. They are also great for relaxation.

While exercise works through three different systems, as illustrated below, many forms of exercise work more than one system, and some work all three. Cycling, for example, is primarily an aerobic exercise, but also involves resistance training for the legs, as they have to push against a force. Yoga is usually thought of as primarily improving flexibility, yet holding the poses involves a good deal of strength training using your body weight as resistance.

Aerobic exercise such as walking, running, swimming or cycling gives your heart and lungs a good workout. So it's a great way to get some freshly oxygenated blood pumped through your blood vessels and boost your circulation. Aerobic exercises are also the most efficient way to burn fat. "Aerobic" means "with oxygen," so it is literally any activity that increases your heart rate and breathing.

Strength or resistance exercise

Strength or resistance exercises such as sit-ups, squats or using weights or resistance bands will shape and tone your muscles and improve your muscular strength and body composition (decreased fat and more muscle). This kind of exercise is making your muscles work against a resistance or weight. The resistance may be dumbbells, a resistance elastic band, or even your own body weight (as in squats).

Nearly all people who have diabetes can incorporate upper-body strength training with light weights and high repetitions: 1–3 sets working each of the major muscle groups with 8–10 repetitions in each set, for instance.

More strenuous strength training may be acceptable for young people who have diabetes, but it is not recommended for older people or those who have longstanding diabetes.

Strength Training Is *Not* for You if You Have:

- Long-term diabetes complications
- Unstable angina (heart pain)
- Uncontrolled hypertension (high blood pressure)
- Uncontrolled dysrhythmia (irregular heartbeat)
- Hypertrophic cardiomyopathy (swollen heart muscles), and/or
- Certain stages of retinopathy.

Benefits of strength training

A recent study (reported in the *Journal of the American Medical Association*) involving nearly 500 men followed for 12 years showed that the reduction in coronary heart disease risk associated with weight training was as good as that from aerobic activities such as running, rowing and walking.

The 3 Phases of a Typical Exercise Session

1. **Warming up (5 minutes):** this prepares your body for more strenuous activity and helps prevent injuries. Try gentle walking, cycling, swinging arms, etc.

2. **The activity phase:** this includes either aerobic and/or resistance exercises. This is the period of more intense aerobic exercise. Try brisk walking, cycling, dancing, stair climbing or even heavy gardening. This will pump up your heart rate and your breathing rate. You might then include some strengthening resistance exercises such as push-ups, lunges, or squats—with or without weights— and some for balance, such as side leg raising or standing on one foot for as long as you can.

3. **Cooling down (5 minutes):** this could include some stretching after your session. Try touching your toes, reaching for the sky, neck stretching. This keeps you flexible and decreases your chances of injury. It also dissipates the lactic acid that is formed by exercising muscles and gradually returns your body to its normal state. This prevents pooling of blood in the arms and legs, which could cause fainting.

Building up the aerobic activity phase from 15 minutes to 30–40 minutes will maximize the health benefits.

Strength training decreases both total and intra-abdominal (inside the tummy) body fat, and—very important—helps maintain lean body mass (which would usually be lost when this kind of training is included as part of a weight loss regimen). Very important, increased lean body mass is associated with improved insulin sensitivity. Resting metabolic rate is also related to levels of lean body mass. So if you do enough resistance training to increase your muscle mass, you will also get the added bonus of increasing your resting metabolic rate.

As well as the benefits for blood glucose levels, resistance exercise normalizes blood pressure in people with elevated (but not high) blood pressure. Strength training has traditionally not been recommended for people with high blood pressure, but a recent analysis of clinical trials has shown that people with high blood pressure that is treated will also benefit from strength training and that it can be safely done.

Another important finding for people with diabetes and prediabetes is that resistance training improves blood fats. When you look at all the benefits of resistance exercise, it's clear that it is a great all-around activity for people with diabetes.

And that's not all. Strength training also:

- Increases bone mineral density
- Reduces the risk for falls
- Reduces pain and improves functioning in osteoarthritis

Walking

ONE OF THE most popular forms of physical activity is simply going for a walk—whether it's around your house or garden, the neighborhood, the park, or perhaps along the beach. Walking is a surprisingly effective form of exercise for people with diabetes or those trying to prevent it.

A recent study reported in the American Diabetes Association's prestigious journal *Diabetes Care* provides convincing proof that regular walking can provide significant health benefits for very little cost. A group of nearly 200 people with type 2 diabetes were given physical activity counseling every 3 months for 2 years. Some took it more seriously than others. The researchers found that those walking 1–3 miles (2,400–6,400 steps) more than usual each day achieved the most benefits for their diabetes.

Measuring Your Steps

PEDOMETERS ARE SMALL electronic devices you wear on your belt. They measure how many miles or steps you do. First, measure how much you do during a typical day, then add the 2,400–6,400 steps and make that your goal. Remember, it's best to start out with realistic goals and work up to the more difficult ones slowly. Pedometers are sold in most sports and electronic stores, and cost $15–40.

EXERCISE, EATING AND YOUR BLOOD GLUCOSE LEVELS

If you don't take insulin or blood glucose–lowering medication and your blood glucose level (BGL) is normally well controlled, you shouldn't need to do extra checks or eat differently when you exercise.

If you take diabetes medication of the sulphonylurea type or meglitinide and you are not sure how your body will respond to exercise, or you are doing something out of the ordinary, plan on doing exercise 1–2 hours after eating a main meal.

If you have type 1, check your blood glucose level (BGL) before you start exercising. If it is above 270 mg/dL (15 mmol/L), check your blood or urine for ketones. Do not exercise if your blood glucose is higher than 270 mg/dL and you have ketones in your blood or your urine tests positively.

If your blood glucose level (BGL) is less than 100 mg/dL (5.5 mmol/L), 125 mg/dL (7 mmol/L) in children, and you take insulin, aim to eat 15–20 grams of carbohydrates 15–30 minutes before you exercise. Recheck your blood glucose levels again 30 minutes into the exercise to prevent a "hypo." Finally, check your blood glucose levels immediately after you have finished exercising (see chapter 18).

Generally, exercise will lower blood glucose levels, but it can have the opposite effect sometimes. Exercising muscles are hungry for glucose and will use up their own stores, then search the bloodstream for more. When blood glucose levels start to drop, the liver releases its stores, and if they run out, it can convert protein to glucose. This glucose can be quickly released into the blood. Sometimes, if you do really strenuous exercise, or you are a little unwell, your blood glucose levels can go high when you exercise, due to the release of stress hormones such as adrenaline. If you have enough insulin, they will drop again over time, as the muscles and liver replenish their glucose stores.

·18·
Exercise and
Type 1 Diabetes

*I*f you have type 1 diabetes, exercise adds some extra challenges when it comes to keeping your blood glucose levels on an even keel:

▶ If you have too much insulin before exercising, your blood glucose levels may drop too quickly, and your performance may deteriorate, or worse still, you may have a hypo, and

▶ If you don't have enough insulin, glucose uptake into exercising muscles may not be fast enough, so your performance will again be affected.

What's the solution? Increase your blood glucose monitoring, eat more carbohydrates and/or take less insulin. If you are planning on doing less than 30 minutes of exercise, and your blood glucose levels are less than 100 mg/dL (5.5 mmol/L), eating 15–20 grams of carbohydrates before you exercise is usually enough to keep you going at an optimal pace.

If you are planning on exercising for longer, you may need to reduce your insulin (usually the short-acting) by 10–30 percent as well.

Because everyone is different, we suggest you discuss your plans and needs with your diabetes management team so you can work out what is best for you. Once you get into a routine, you can usually plan things pretty well.

Exercise Tips

■ If you don't need to lose weight, increase your food intake to match your increased exercise. This is particularly important during strenuous activity, when you need to replace the energy you have burned. Always have some fast-acting carbohydrates on hand too.

■ Drink water before, during and after exercise. Water is the best form of fluid replacement. Unless you are performing extreme endurance sports, sports drinks are not necessary. A good habit to establish is to have a large glass (10–16 ounces) of water 15 minutes before exercise. Take another 8-ounce glass of water for every 15 minutes of exercise, and have another large glass when you have finished.

■ Exercise regularly, ideally at the same time each day.

■ Be consistent with exercise and meal times and insulin injections.

■ Plan on adjusting your dose of insulin according to what you are going to do. This is particularly relevant if you are overweight. Take care not to exaggerate the calories burned during exercise: to burn up just 1 slice of bread (70 calories, on average), you need to walk for about 20 minutes or jog for 10 minutes.

■ Avoid heavy exercise when your insulin action is at its peak.

■ Use your stomach rather than your limbs for injecting. Insulin injected into muscle will be absorbed very quickly and could lower your blood glucose too much. You may need an extra 15–20 grams of carbohydrates during bouts of vigorous exercise that last an hour or more.

■ If you are planning on doing a particular activity regularly (and we hope you are), it's a good idea to experiment with the activity around the same time of day on at least three occasions to see how your blood glucose levels respond. Test before, immediately after and then again 6–8 hours after exercising.

EXERCISE: GETTING STARTED AND KEEPING IT GOING

Depending on how much of a couch potato you've been, it's going to take time to get fit. Initially there'll be some discomfort or breathlessness and you'll just want to stop. In time, breathing will become easier and you'll develop a feeling of physical well-being. Finally, you'll attain psychological fitness—exhilaration, mental relaxation and real enjoyment of the physical effort. Here are some tips for when the going gets tough:

▶ Try something different. Don't do the same exercise every session: ride a bicycle one day, walk the next, and swim another day. This gives you variety in your routine and reduces the risk of injury by avoiding straining the same muscles all the time.

▶ Record what you do and monitor your progress: show it to the members of your diabetes management team so they know how hard you have been working.

▶ Set goals: setting specific goals for yourself and then evaluating how you are doing is a great way to keep on track. Remember to write them down so that they are more tangible. But be realistic, because unrealistic goals can work against you.

▶ If time is tight, make your exercise time productive: you could prop your newspaper up on your stationary bike, or park your treadmill in front of the TV so you can watch the news or make phone calls while you cycle/walk/jog.

▶ Get an exercise buddy: if someone is there waiting for you, you are far more likely to keep on track. If you can afford it, you could get a personal trainer.

▶ Reward yourself: a good way to keep your motivation high is to reward yourself when you accomplish a goal. Give yourself a new item of training gear, a book, a visit to the movies, a massage—anything healthy that will keep you motivated.

EXERCISING SAFELY

It is a good idea to do the following:

- Carry some quickly absorbed carbohydrates, such as a sweetened drink or gummy bears, and try to exercise with someone who knows you have diabetes, not alone.
- Have a contact—someone who knows where you are, or who exercises with you—or keep a phone with you.
- Wear an ID bracelet or necklace so that if something does happen while you are alone, EMTs will be able to help more quickly.
- Replace fluids.
- Look out for hypo symptoms during and up to 24 hours afterward.
- Protect your feet by wearing good-fitting shoes and cotton socks.

Stop!
- At the first sign of injury
- If you feel light-headed
- At the first hint of a hypo
- If you experience severe shortness of breath
- If you have any pain or pressure in your chest, or
- If you experience any loss of balance or dizziness.

Reducing the risk of hypos

If you take insulin and/or sulfonylurea medications such as chlor-propamide (Diabinese), gliclazide (Diamicron), tolbutamide (Rastinon), glibenclamide (Glimel, Euglucon, Daonil), glipizide (Minidiab) or glimepiride (Melizide), you are more likely to develop hypoglycemia or "have a hypo" when you are physically active—particularly for prolonged periods.

It can also be more difficult to recognize the symptoms of a hypo when you are physically active, because the usual warning signs—sweating, rapid heartbeat and shaking—can be easily confused with normal responses to exercise. This is why it is so important to monitor your blood glucose before, during and after activity.

If you do have a hypo when exercising, one carbohydrate exchange (approximately 15 grams) will raise your blood glucose levels rapidly.

What kind of carbohydrate is best when you are exercising?

For practical purposes, when you are doing less than 1½ hours of exercise at one time, the type of carbohydrate you eat does not really need to be different from what you eat on days when you are not exercising. It is only when you are exercising for more than 90 minutes at a time that it seems to make a significant difference.

Exercise, blood glucose and carbohydrate quantity

ACTIVITY AND AND DURATION	BLOOD SUGAR (MG/DL)	CARBOHYDRATE QUANTITY
Light (walking for 30 minutes)	< 110 > 110	1–2 exchanges generally nothing
Moderate (swimming, cycling, running, brisk walking, surfing for 1 hour)	110–180 180–270 > 270	1–2 exchanges generally nothing if unwell, do not exercise and check ketones
Strenuous (hockey, football, cycling, continuous swimming, running, endurance sports, hiking for 1 hour or more)	< 110 110–180 180–270 > 270	3 exchanges 2–3 exchanges 0–1 exchange if unwell, do not exercise and check ketones

Adapted from Caring for Diabetes in Children and Adolescents: A Parent's Manual

GI AND EXERCISE

As we explained in chapter 10, low-GI foods deliver a slower, more sustained release of glucose into the bloodstream, and high-GI foods cause a fast and high glucose response, which means that they will be more immediately available.

Research has shown that using the GI to choose your carbs when exercising is most effective if you're doing very strenuous exercise that lasts longer than 90 minutes, such as a marathon, triathlon, cross-country skiing, mountain climbing, or long gym workouts. However, the same principle applies to less strenuous activity.

Carbohydrate choices for strenuous and sustained (more than 90 minutes) physical activity

BEFORE AND AFTER ACTIVITY	LOW-GI FOODS
Before: to produce sustained blood glucose	pasta, yogurt, milk, apples, dried apricots,
After: to improve muscle glycogen repletion	heavy-grain breads, oatmeal, rolled oats, All-Bran, baked beans, fruit juice, Boost energy drink
DURING ACTIVITY	**HIGH-GI FOODS**
To maintain glucose for working muscles	sports drinks such as Gatorade and Powerade

STEP 3

Manage
Your Weight

No matter what type of diabetes you have, or even if you have prediabetes, excess body weight is going to make your blood glucose levels more difficult to control. Extra body fat, specifically, contributes to insulin resistance—the condition where your cells are "deaf" to the effect of insulin. Also, excess weight makes exercising difficult, increases your blood pressure and increases your chances of developing diabetic complications. So managing body weight is an issue for lots of people with diabetes.

·19·

How to Achieve Your Weight Loss Goals

*W*eight **"control" comes** easily for some. Without any real conscious effort, they maintain a fairly stable weight throughout their adult life, thanks mainly to good in-built regulatory control.

Weight management shouldn't be an issue for the human body. We are designed with a whole host of systems that regulate energy intake and expenditure in order to maintain a steady state. But something has gone wrong, and for many people, excess weight gain occurs.

So what do you do about it? Well, losing a little weight, or at least stabilizing it, is a priority. But as we said in chapter 6, you don't have to be "the biggest loser." Setting attainable weight loss goals is the key.

We are not talking about going on a traditional restrictive diet. The best way to achieve your weight loss goals (and maintain your new weight) is through changing your diet, including changing the way you eat, and increased physical activity. In **Part 3: Living with diabetes and prediabetes**, we have put together a series of eating plans for people with diabetes and prediabetes.

Along with making sure you move more, we focus on the following types of changes:

- Reducing how much you eat (but we promise you won't feel hungry)
- Cutting back on saturated fats and cholesterol
- Modifying your carbohydrate intake
- Eating more regularly
- Moderating your protein intake
- Eating more (yes, more) healthy foods like fruit and vegetables of all sorts except potatoes, and
- Cutting back on salt.

WHY RESTRICTIVE DIETS DON'T WORK

If you are overweight, chances are you have tried a number of diets over the years. At best, a restrictive diet will reduce your calorie intake (while you stick to it!); at worst it will change your body composition for the fatter. Why? When you lose weight through severely restricting your food intake, you lose some of your body's muscle mass. Over the years, this type of dieting will change your body composition to less muscle and proportionately more fat, making weight control increasingly difficult. Your body's engine will require less and less energy to keep it running. In fact, the majority of people who lose weight by "strict" dieting will regain it.

Restricting food also has adverse psychological consequences. Self-imposed dieting and starvation tend to result in:

- Eating binges when food is around
- A preoccupation with food and eating, and
- A heightened emotional response to food.

■

**Remember, most people don't fail to lose weight;
they fail to maintain the weight loss.**

■

WHAT WE KNOW ABOUT WEIGHT MANAGEMENT

There is no single approach to weight management that guarantees success (despite what the advertisements for the latest "miracle" weight loss program claim). There is no magic bullet. Being over-weight or obese is a complex condition with many causes—and sadly, a very low "cure" rate.

While research regularly gives us new insight into the complexities of "obesity genes," "appetite hormones" and neurotransmitters that affect eating behavior, what we know about weight management can actually be stated quite simply.

First of all, weight loss diets alone stand little chance of success. So what does help?

- ◗ Consuming low–energy density foods (fewer calories per bite)
- ◗ Exercise, especially for maintaining weight loss
- ◗ Modifying your behavior so that you become more aware of what you eat, why and when, and
- ◗ An intensive lifestyle change program that includes regular physical activity, reduced calorie intake, support and frequent contact with a health professional (such as a dietitian). As few as six biweek visits either face-to-face or in a group makes all the difference; it is good to know you are not alone.

■

How often you eat (one or two large meals or six small ones of equal energy density) makes little difference to the rate of weight loss.

■

We also know that not all foods are created equal. Research has shown that the type of food you give your body determines what it is going to burn and what it is going to store as body fat and that certain foods are more satisfying to the appetite than others. Low-GI foods (fruit and vegetables, low-GI cereal grains and products made from them, legumes, nuts and low-fat dairy foods) give you the edge. They fill you up and keep you satisfied for longer and they help you burn more body fat and less muscle.

UNDERSTANDING "ENERGY BALANCE"

Think of your body as a set of balance scales. On one side is the food you eat (energy in). On the other is the fuel you burn (energy out).

If you eat more food than your body burns, you will gain weight. Simple. Right? This is what's called the principle of energy balance. So to lose weight all you need to do is eat less or burn up more. Correct?

Well, not quite. If it were this easy there would be a lot fewer overweight people.

The belief that we have conscious control over our appetite (and therefore how much food we eat) and our energy expenditure (how active we are) is just not true. While we might seriously desire to be trim, taut and terrific, or sleek, willowy and slender, our body (and brain) has other ideas. You see, our body is designed for survival, so it has a host of built-in strategies just waiting to undo all our efforts at weight loss.

To give you an example, let's look more closely at energy expenditure. Most of the energy your body burns is used up for the following three key processes:

1. Your basal metabolism (energy needed just to keep you alive—heart beating, lungs expanding, that sort of thing)
2. The **digestion** and metabolism of the meals and snacks you eat and drink, and
3. Any spontaneous (involuntary) **physical activity**—what you do without thinking (fidgeting or wriggling or doodling or waving your hands as you talk).

On top of this add your voluntary energy usage for physical activity and exercise (we say more about this below).

Now in theory you could reduce your energy intake (how much food you eat) by a significant amount, say around a thousand calories a day, and lose about 2 pounds of weight a week without doing any extra exercise. But—and this is a very big but—your body will strongly oppose this. In fact, it simply responds to your eating less by reducing its energy spending in each of the three key processes:

▶ It reduces its basal metabolic rate, first in response to lower energy intake and then as a consequence of your smaller body size,

▶ It reduces the energy you use for digesting food (by about 10 percent), and

▶ It reduces the energy you use for spontaneous physical activity (the energy costs for the same physical activity decrease as a consequence of smaller body size).

So how do you get around the defenses your body puts up against your efforts to eat less and lose weight? First, it helps if you contribute to the energy deficit by increasing your energy expenditure as well (yes, you're getting the idea: this means doing more exercise).

EXERCISE FOR WEIGHT LOSS AND WEIGHT MAINTENANCE

How much exercise do you need to do to get weight off and keep it off?

Although it varies, the short answer is, more than you think. The best evidence comes from the United States National Weight Control Registry. This includes the data of approximately five thousand people who have lost an average of 65 pounds and maintained their weight loss for at least 1 year (the average of those on the register is 5 years). These people report doing the equivalent of approximately 7 hours per week of moderate intensity exercise. This means something close to really brisk walking for at least one hour a day, every day.

ENERGY IN—WHAT YOU ACTUALLY EAT

However, if you are obese, exercise alone is unlikely to be enough to bring about much weight loss (partly because extra physical activity is so difficult and is very easily counterbalanced). Most obese people have to reduce their energy intake as well.

There is not one ideal "diet" that will be right for everyone. Most weight loss diets are based on a particular nutrient composition, and the potential combinations are endless. Low-fat and low-carbohydrate diets have been popular choices in recent years and high-protein diets were the "last big thing."

If you accept that you have to create an energy deficit, the solution is really to find the easiest way to do this, a strategy that you can live with. And there are lots of strategies:

- ▶ **Strategy 1:** Most people don't find it easy simply to eat less of their favorite foods. But some types of foods can make it easier to eat less. Foods that are high in protein or low-GI carbohydrate are more satisfying and make you feel fuller for longer than fat-rich foods.
- ▶ **Strategy 2:** Don't eat less in terms of volume, but eat foods with a lower energy density (fewer calories per bite). Fruits and vegetables, for example, have very few calories, but because they are bulky and fibrous, they can be very filling. The same can be said about low-GI whole-grain and high-fiber cereals, which are more filling and less energy dense than their refined counterparts.
- ▶ **Strategy 3:** Focus on eating a low-fat diet to reduce your calorie intake without necessarily eating less. Because fat provides more calories per gram than any other nutrient, avoiding fats will automatically lower your calorie intake.

WILL WEIGHT LOSS CURE DIABETES?

You might have heard that if you lose weight, diabetes will go away. This can only be true if you are diagnosed in the very early prediabetes stages with impaired fasting glucose or impaired glucose tolerance.

If you have type 2 diabetes, losing weight has many benefits (it can reduce your insulin resistance and help you manage your blood glucose levels), but it can't make diabetes go away. Losing weight will also make it easier to exercise, and exercise will further help overcome insulin resistance.

There is no cure for type 2 diabetes yet. Once the beta cells that make insulin have burned themselves out with overuse, they don't come back to life. But if you catch the problem early enough and lessen the load on your pancreas, there may be enough life left in the remaining cells to cope. What this means is that if you are overweight, losing weight earlier is better than later. By losing weight you'll reduce insulin resistance and lessen the load on your beta cells, thus helping to preserve them.

The Importance of a Good Night's Sleep

UNITED STATES RESEARCHERS analyzing data of 18,000 adults in the National Health and Nutrition Examination Survey found a correlation between **body mass index (BMI)** and hours of sleep per night. Those who got less than 4 hours of sleep a night were 73 percent more likely to be obese than those who slept 7–9 hours a night. In a separate study of 924 adults, researchers determined that 2 hours less sleep per week amounted to an increase in BMI of 10.

They're still at a loss to explain how sleep helps our weight, but there are lots of theories. It may be related to lower production of the hormone leptin (a natural appetite suppressant) with sleep deprivation. In the meantime, it's a good reason to make sure you get enough shut-eye.

GET A GRIP ON HOW MUCH YOU'RE EATING ✶

For many people, one piece of the puzzle is how much to eat. Not just at each meal, but over the day. One of the "highly effective" habits of women and men who successfully maintain weight loss is self-monitoring—simply keeping a daily record of all the food you eat, the circumstances surrounding your eating and any strong emotions you felt at the time of eating. Why is this helpful? Because becoming more aware of your eating behavior lets you identify the triggers or cues that lead to inappropriate and excessive eating. Give it a try.

A typical food diary will include the following information.

- Foods and drinks consumed—type and amount
- Time eaten
- Place eaten

▶ Level of hunger, and
▶ Feelings.

How much is a "normal" serving?

Portion distortion is a relatively recent phenomenon, and it stems partly from the commercial food sector. In the Daily Food Guide in part 3, we've listed serving sizes and daily requirements for a range of foods (no "king" or "jumbo" or "super" or "one-third more" sized chocolate bars here!). We use household measures and weights, but since you won't generally be carrying a set of scales around with you, it helps to be able to judge your portions relative to common objects. Here's a guide.

1 tsp of margarine or butter	=	a marble
½ cup fruit, vegetables, pasta or rice	=	a small fist
3 oz cooked meat or chicken	=	a deck of cards or the palm of a small adult hand
2½ tbsp of a serving of food	=	a golf ball

IF YOU NEED TO LOSE WEIGHT, HOW MUCH SHOULD YOU AIM TO LOSE?

Setting attainable goals is extremely important. You can achieve significant health benefits by losing just 5 percent of your body weight if you were overweight or obese when you were first diagnosed with diabetes.

For some people, losing this amount (and maintaining the loss) is easy, though it needs some fairly major changes in eating habits. For others, losing even 10 pounds and maintaining that loss is very difficult. If this is the case for you, it might be more realistic to simply aim for no weight gain (because we all tend to get fatter as we get older).

Weight management has two different phases—losing weight and maintaining the weight loss. During the weight loss phase, a reasonable aim (unless you are very overweight) might be to lose 2–4 pounds a month over a period of about 3 months. After losing 10–12 pounds, your weight will probably plateau.

Maintaining your weight loss, give or take a pound or two, over the next 3-month period is crucial in terms of helping you consolidate your diet and exercise habits. Giving your body time to adjust to a lower weight takes the pressure off and increases your chances of maintaining your new weight.

If you succeed in losing 5–10 percent of your body weight but want to lose more, only try to do it after a period of weight maintenance. Using an alternating "weight loss/weight maintenance" strategy increases your chances of success.

What's a Good Rate of Weight Loss?

2–4 pounds a month

What Does It Take to Lose about 2 Pounds a Week?

In theory, to achieve weight loss of about 2 pounds a week you need to reduce your daily energy intake by about 1,360 calories a day—assuming you haven't increased your physical activity expenditure.

WHERE THE FAT IS AND WHY IT MATTERS

From a medical standpoint, the problems associated with obesity and being overweight are more closely related to **where** the excess fat is than to **how much** there is. Fat around your abdomen and upper body carries the biggest health risk. This is known as visceral fat (deep, intra-abdominal fat), in contrast to subcutaneous (just underneath the skin) fat. This visceral fat is a characteristic of insulin resistance, which may be part of the reason why people with diabetes have so much difficulty losing weight.

Today there are sophisticated imaging techniques, such as magnetic resonance imaging (MRI) and computed tomography (CT), that can pick visceral fat from subcutaneous fat very precisely.

But you don't need to go this far. Getting out the tape measure and measuring your waist circumference first thing in the morning is better than using scales. The scales can't tell the difference between water, fat and muscle loss. The tape measure will tell you all about *fat* loss.

Did you know?

▶ Weight loss is usually more difficult for women than men. One reason is that women's bodies have more fat and less muscle than men's, and muscle burns more calories than fat.

▶ One of the reasons why weight loss may be more difficult for people with diabetes is their "thrifty genes," which make their body very good at storing fat and reluctant to part with it.

▶ Some oral diabetes medications and insulins tend to cause weight gain or make it more difficult to lose weight.

▶ When it comes to weighty matters, your genes are one of the strongest influences on being overweight or obese: identical twins (who have the same genetic makeup), for example, nearly always have an identical BMI, and adopted children, when they grow up, have a BMI similar to their biological parents, rather than to their adoptive parents.

What's Your BMI?

YOUR BODY MASS index (BMI) is a measure of your weight in relation to your height. For most people, a BMI greater than 25 is classified as overweight, and above 30 as obese. (People of Asian origin should use a cutoff of 23.) To calculate your BMI, multiply your weight (in pounds) by 705 and divide it by your height (in inches) squared.

Example:
A woman who is 5 feet (160 inches) tall and weighs 155 pounds would calculate her BMI like this:

$$\frac{155 \times 705}{60 \times 60} = 30$$

But you don't have to do the math. There are some handy online BMI calculators. Try www.nhlbisupport.com/bmi

Your Good Girth Guide

THE IDEAL

Men: less than 37 inches

Women: less than 31½ inches

URGENT ACTION REQUIRED—

YOUR HEALTH RISKS ARE SUBSTANTIALLY INCREASED

Men: greater than 40 inches

Women: greater than 34½ inches

AMY

WHEN I CONSULTED dietitian Johanna Burani about my weight and my diabetes, I weighed in at 320 pounds and I am only 5'7" (giving me a scary BMI of 50)—yes, I had trouble walking, even getting out of bed! My doctor was not optimistic about what the future held unless things changed, as there's diabetes on both sides of the family. I really hoped there'd be a way to control it naturally. I am not a "pills" person, and was already taking blood pressure medication and was not happy about that at all.

I knew I simply had to straighten out my diet, and the big incentive was when my doctor told me I could come off glucophage if I lost weight and kept it off. I first started walking for 45 minutes in my lunch hour, and lost 36 pounds. But I always felt hungry and the temptation to grab a cake or donut or chocolate candies to snack on was constant, and all too often I gave in and raided my boss's candy dish in the afternoons. And all too soon the weight started coming back on.

So I decided to consult a dietitian. Johanna explained that she could probably "kill two birds with one stone"—that is, she could help me lose weight and control my blood glucose levels naturally! So we put together a game plan that I could stick to. Essentially, all I had to do was exchange my quickly digested carbs for more slowly digested ones. This meant I had to decrease the high-GI fruits and replace them with trickler fruits; breads had to be whole grain (with lots of grainy bits) and my evening meal would consist of smaller starch and protein portions with half my plate covered in vegetables.

Amazingly, Johanna said that this might be all I would have to do (as well as some exercise and drinking lots of water). I have to say I couldn't believe it; but it was virtually all I had to do! I signed up at a women's only gym near where I worked, doing both cardiac and resistance training workouts for 45 minutes most lunchtimes, and stuck to my low-GI "trickler" diet. In a little over a year I lost 118 pounds—and after the first 50 my doctor took me off blood pressure medication! My most recent bloodwork shows a 31 percent jump in my good (HDL) cholesterol; a 74 percent drop in triglycerides and a 26 percent drop in mean glucose levels. So I got my wish—no medication and a nice bonus—no joint pain. I also got back my life. I work out six days a week—I love my spinning classes. In fact I am thinking of becoming a spinning class instructor—part-time of course.

from *Good Carbs, Bad Carbs*, Johanna Burani
(reproduced with permission)

STEP 4

Don't Smoke.
If You Do, Quit

Smoking increases the risk of developing type 2 diabetes, as well as the complications of all types of diabetes. The more you smoke, the greater your risk. There are lots of options to help you kick the habit: nicotine patches, gums, medication, counseling, even hypnosis.

Be aware that nicotine patches may raise blood glucose levels in some people with diabetes. Talk to your doctor, diabetes educator or other members of your healthcare team for advice.

You may also wish to consider calling the Quit Line for help. Trained advisers can provide you with valuable advice and support.

800-QUIT-NOW (800-784-8669)

· 20 ·

Smoking and Diabetes Complications

S **moking damages and** constricts our blood vessels, decreasing the flow of blood throughout our body so that less oxygen is delivered to our vital organs and tissues. Smoking also raises blood glucose levels, making diabetes harder to manage. Finally, smoking increases our cholesterol and triglyceride levels.

So a smoker's risk of developing heart and blood vessel diseases such as stroke and peripheral vascular disease are substantially increased. For example, it has been estimated that people with diabetes who smoke have at least three times the risk of developing heart disease as a person with diabetes who's a nonsmoker, and they are much more likely to die if they do suffer a heart attack.

The damage to the blood vessels and circulation caused by smoking also leads to poor wound healing, which can lead to leg and foot infections, and then lead to amputation—95 percent of the people with diabetes who need amputations are smokers.

If you smoke and you have diabetes, you are also more likely to get nerve damage and kidney disease, and you'll get colds and respiratory infections more easily, and these cause fluctuation in blood glucose levels.

If all these problems are not a big enough incentive to stop, smoking can also increase the risk of impotence, which is a significant problem for men with diabetes even if they don't smoke!

■

Smoking just one cigarette reduces the body's ability to use insulin by 15 percent! Once you stop smoking, the insulin resistance does not start to improve until 10–12 hours later.

■

SMOKING AND FOOD

Smoking also influences dietary habits.

- ▶ Smokers tend to eat less fruit and vegetables than nonsmokers (and so they get less of the protective antioxidant plant compounds that these foods provide), and
- ▶ Smokers tend to eat more fat and more salt than nonsmokers.

These characteristics of the smoker's diet may be caused by a desire to seek strong food flavors, which could itself be because smoking blunts your ability to taste. There is only one piece of advice for anyone who smokes: quit.

THE BENEFITS OF QUITTING

When you quit smoking, your insulin resistance decreases, and you will have less chance of developing diabetes (if you have prediabetes), and of developing its common complications (such as kidney and nerve damage).

You may also find that you have lower blood glucose and HbA1c levels, lower total and LDL (bad) cholesterol and triglyceride levels and higher HDL (good) cholesterol levels. The combined effect will be a lower risk of having a heart attack or stroke.

Once you stop smoking, your insulin requirements may drop by up to 30 percent. So if you are taking diabetes medications or insulin it's very important to monitor your blood glucose levels more frequently when you first quit.

Because of the decrease in insulin resistance, many people with diabetes find their blood glucose levels are significantly lower after they quit. This may mean insulin or medication adjustments—see your doctor, diabetes educator or dietitian for further advice.

STEP 5

Limit Your Consumption of Alcohol

One of the things many people ask when first diagnosed with diabetes is, "Can I still have a drink?" In the past, the usual answer was no, because it was thought that the sugars in many alcoholic drinks could affect blood glucose levels, and alcohol contributes to weight gain. Alcohol is very high in calories, providing 7 calories per gram (an average drink has 10 grams of alcohol or more). In fact, it is the second most concentrated source of energy in the diet after fat, which provides 9 calories per gram.

We now know that there may be some benefits to enjoying an occasional glass of wine or beer if you have diabetes or prediabetes.

■

**Whatever your reason for having a drink,
the key message for everybody, whether you
have diabetes, prediabetes or neither,
is do it in moderation!**

■

• 21 •

Can I Still Have a Drink?

𝓘**f you are** trying to lose weight, it is best to think of alcohol as an indulgence, as "keep for a treat" fare. It may be enjoyable, but it doesn't provide any essential nutrients and it is high in calories.

If you have diabetes or prediabetes, it's important to limit your daily consumption of alcohol to no more than one standard drink if you are a woman and two standard drinks if you are a man. This is because alcohol contributes to weight gain, high triglycerides and high blood pressure, and therefore increases the risk of developing diabetes complications.

If you use insulin or are taking certain blood glucose–lowering medications, such as sulphonylureas or meglitinides, alcohol increases your risk of having a hypo for up to 24 hours after you have stopped drinking. This is because alcohol reduces glucose production by the liver and reduces the body's ability to release glucose into the blood. This may also make the hypo harder to treat than usual. Even a small amount of alcohol impairs your ability to detect a hypo, and if the people you're drinking with are drinking too they may not be any help—so beware.

ALCOHOL AND THE BODY

Alcohol affects your body in many different ways. In fact, excessive consumption is linked to over 60 different medical conditions—so far. Most of us know that excessive consumption can damage our brain and liver. What many don't know is that it can also damage your stomach and pancreas, and it increases the risk of developing heart disease, stroke, and breast, mouth and throat cancer. For men it has a particularly unfortunate effect on the sex organs, leading to "brewer's droop"—the inability to get and/or sustain an erection—despite its ability to increase sexual desire.

Alcohol is "fattening"—the body has no place to store alcohol, so it takes top priority as a source of fuel, sending other fuel sources (food) to storage. This means that if you drink a can of beer with a bag of chips, or have a glass of wine with cheese, your body will "burn" the alcohol first and most likely store the fat from the chips or cheese.

As we said, alcohol is just extra indulgence calories, and unfortunately, the "beer belly" is now on show in women as well as men. In fact, the latest research shows that more women (57 percent) than men (55 percent) have a high waist circumference—a classic sign of eating and drinking to excess.

HOW MUCH IS SAFE TO DRINK?

Enjoying a moderate amount of alcohol with food will have little effect on your blood glucose levels. Indeed, recent research from the University of Sydney suggests that a glass or two of wine with or before a meal may reduce glucose levels by 25 percent. But the amount and kind of carbohydrates you eat with the alcohol is much more important than the alcohol itself. This is because there's very little carbohydrate in most alcoholic drinks: on average, a 10-ounce glass of regular beer contains only 5 grams (or 1 teaspoon) of sugars; low-alcohol beer has 4 grams; a ½-cup glass of wine has a mere 2 grams; and a standard shot of spirits has less than 1 gram of sugars.

Moderate drinking is the amount that has been linked with the least risk and greatest benefits. The good news is that research indicates that in general, the level of alcohol consumption associated with the least risk for people with diabetes is the same as that for the rest of the adult population. That is, men are advised to drink no more than two standard drinks on any day, women no more than one, and both men and women should aim to have at least two alcohol-free days each week.

However, if you are overweight, have poorly managed blood glucose levels, high blood pressure, high triglycerides or other diabetic complications, your diabetes healthcare team may advise you to drink less or not to drink at all.

WHAT IS A STANDARD DRINK?

A standard drink is less than you think! Technically it's an amount that contains 10 grams of pure alcohol and is equal to:

- a can (12 ounces) of regular beer
- about 2 cans (22 ounces) of low-alcohol beer (less than 3 percent alcohol)
- half a glass (5 ounces) of wine
- a small glass (3 ounces) of fortified wine (sherry, port)
- a "nip" (1 ounce) of spirits

It's easy to underestimate the amount you drink, so if you want to stick to the guidelines, learn how much is in a standard drink of whatever types of alcoholic drink you like before you start drinking. Simple ways of doing this include:

- Checking the number of standard drinks listed on the label of the bottle, and
- Measuring out a standard drink with a measuring cup so you know exactly what it looks like.

When you do this, you will probably be surprised by how much your favorite glass actually holds. For example, most wine glasses, when full, can hold almost two standard drinks!

WHAT ABOUT MIXERS?

As we said, alcoholic drinks contain very little carbohydrate, so they have very little impact on blood glucose levels if they are drunk in moderation. However, many people like to mix alcohol with soft drinks, fruit punch drinks (such as Hi–C or Tang) or fruit juices, and standard varieties of all those are high in sugar. Though moderate amounts of added sugars will not necessarily cause blood glucose levels to rise rapidly, they do contribute to the overall glycemic load of your diet without giving you any vitamins, minerals or fiber. Therefore for many, it may be wiser to simply choose "diet" mixers instead of the "standard" varieties. The following list will help you understand why:

MIXER	CARBOHYDRATES IN ¾ CUP
Fruit-flavored soft drinks	26 g
Cola	22 g
Fruit punch drink (Hi–C or Tang)	19 g
Tonic water	18 g
Fruit juice	17 g
Tomato juice	9 g
Sugar-free fruit drink	3 g
Diet soda	0 g
Diet tonic water	0 g
Soda water	0 g
Water	0 g

Note that low-carb or low-sugar beers have no real advantage over regular beer in terms of your blood glucose levels, because regular beer has very little carbohydrate anyway. Also, low-carb beers are often higher in alcohol, which can increase the risk of hypoglycemia. Don't be fooled by the advertising.

WHAT ABOUT "ALCOPOPS?"

Many people now have premixed drinks (such as Smirnoff Ice) instead of the more traditional beer and wine. Unlike beer and wine, most premixed drinks *do* contain significant amounts of carbohydrates.

Most of the mixers that are used have an intermediate GI (less than 70), and in moderation, they are unlikely to cause hyperglycemia (high glucose readings). However, they do give you extra carbohydrates: most contain at least as much as you would find in a slice or two of bread, and some, such as Sparks, an alcoholic energy drink, contain a lot more. Take this into account when you plan your meals (and insulin doses, if you take insulin).

BRAND	VOLUME (OZ)	ENERGY (CAL)	ALCOHOL (G)	CARBOHYDRATES (G)
Bacardi Silver	12	220	14	35
Mike's Hard Lemonade	11.2	220	16.5	37.8
Seagram's Coolers	12	230	12	36
Smirnoff Ice	12	228	19.2	32
Sparks	16	350	20.5	4

HOW DOES ALCOHOL INTERACT WITH INSULIN OR BLOOD GLUCOSE–LOWERING MEDICATIONS?

Take extra care when drinking alcohol if you take these medications:

- Sulphonylureas (such as Amaryl, Diamicron, Minidiab, Daonil or Rastinon)
- Meglitinides (such as Novonorm), or
- Insulin.

The alcohol and the medication can interact and cause hypoglycemia (hypos). Speak to your doctor or pharmacist if you are not sure what type of medication you are taking.

What about other medications?

Loads of other medications react with alcohol, so if you are taking any, check with your doctor or pharmacist before drinking alcohol.

WHAT SHOULD I EAT WHEN I'M DRINKING?

It's a good idea to combine drinking alcohol with food. This will slow the rate of absorption of the alcohol, and thus reduce the degree of intoxication. Low-fat, low-GI carbohydrate foods are the least likely to make you store fat—they will release glucose slowly into the bloodstream, reducing the risk of both high and low blood glucose levels.

If you have been drinking during the afternoon or evening, we recommend a low-GI snack before going to bed to help maintain your blood glucose levels through the night. A piece of whole-grain toast, a glass of milk, a container of yogurt or pieces of fruit are good. This is particularly important if you take insulin.

If you take insulin, sulphonylureas or meglitinides, make sure you eat some carbohydrate foods (see ideas below) while you are drinking, to prevent hypos. If you are at a party and food is not available, try using juice, milk or a regular soft drink as sources of carbohydrates. Avoiding a hypo is more important in the short term than watching your carbohydrate intake!

SAVORY SNACKS	FRUITS
Any bread	Fruit platter
Rice crackers	Fresh fruit salad
Oven-baked pretzels	Dried fruit (dates, apricots, figs, etc.)
Microwaved popcorn	
Ryvita	
Vita-Wheat	
Premium crackers (97% fat free)	

WHO SHOULDN'T DRINK ALCOHOL?

If you have a fatty liver, high triglycerides, pancreatitis, advanced neuropathy or any form of liver disease you should not drink any alcohol.

Also, if you are pregnant, planning to have a baby or breastfeeding, we recommend you do not drink any alcohol.

Tips for drinking less

If you think you are drinking too much, try some of the following ideas to help reduce your alcohol intake:

- Drink some water or a diet soda before you drink any alcohol, so you are not thirsty when you start.
- Order a glass of wine and a glass of water at the same time.
- Sip your alcoholic drink slowly.
- Drink a nonalcoholic drink after every alcoholic drink (for example, water or a diet soft drink).
- Dilute alcohol (make a shandy by diluting your beer with low-calorie lemonade, or dilute your wine with club soda for instance), or
- Drink low-alcohol beer.

Taking Control

FOR INFORMATION, COUNSELING or other assistance to help moderate your alcohol intake, contact the alcohol and other drugs service in your area. By dialing the numbers below you can locate the alcohol and drugs center nearest you. These information centers are bound by confidentiality (they cannot tell anyone anything you tell them) and you don't have to give your name if you don't want to.

National Alcohol and Substance Abuse Information Center (NASAIC)
   800-784-6776
Substance Abuse & Mental Health Services Administration (SAMHSA)
   800-662-HELP (800-662-4357)

OH NO, I THINK I DRANK TOO MUCH . . .

Unfortunately, many people experience a hangover at least once in their lives. The aching head, parched mouth, burning stomach and general feeling of having been hit by a truck often lead to promises of "giving up the grog" . . . well, at least for a few days.

While there is no such thing as a cure for a hangover, there are a number of simple, inexpensive things that you can try to help you get through the day. The main symptoms of a hangover are thought to be due to lack of deep sleep, dehydration, irritation of the digestive tract, loss of B vitamins in the urine, and decreased blood glucose due to decreased glucose production by the liver. If you think about these individually, you can put together a "recipe" that should at least give you some temporary relief:

Step 1: Replace the fluid you lost. Electrolyte drinks such as Gatorade come in handy here—they help you absorb the fluid more quickly, and give you some carbohydrates.

Step 2: Take 2 Tylenol (not aspirin—it may irritate your stomach more) along with the fluids.

Step 3: Have a B multi-vitamin.

Step 4: If you find your blood glucose levels are dropping low, have some low-GI carbohydrates (reduced-fat milk or yogurt, or fresh fruit, for example). These foods will also give you some extra fluids, and help soothe your sore stomach.

Step 5: Avoid caffeinated beverages (coffee, tea, cola drinks and chocolate), because they make you go to the toilet more.

Step 6: Monitor your blood glucose more than usual to ensure you don't go hypo.

Mocktail, anyone?

Whatever your reason for not drinking alcohol, or reducing your alcohol intake, there are many low-alcohol or nonalcoholic alternatives that can help you enjoy the spirit of a social occasion without the side effects.

Very-low-alcohol beers and wines are available in most supermarkets. Low-alcohol beers contain roughly the same amount of carbohydrates as the alcoholic varieties and will have little effect on your blood glucose levels if you drink them in moderation.

Most nonalcoholic wines, on the other hand, are based on grape juice, and give you about 15 grams of carbohydrates per 3½-ounce serving. Like most juices, they probably won't cause your blood glucose levels to rise rapidly, but just because they are alcohol free, don't think you can drink them freely!

If you're after a fancy drink without alcoholic side effects, try a "mocktail"—an artistically presented blend of nonalcoholic beverages. There are lots of recipes for mocktails on the Internet. Here are some to try:

Sundowner
Glass: 7-ounce wine glass
Mixers: 3 ounces apple juice
2½ ounces sparkling water
Method: Build over ice and stir
Garnish: Sprig of mint
calories = 41; carbohydrates = 10.5 g; alcohol = 0 g

Virgin Mary
Glass: 10-ounce highball glass
Mixers: 7 ounces tomato juice
1 teaspoon chili sauce
Salt and pepper
1 tablespoon lemon juice
Method: Build over ice and stir
Garnish: Celery stalk
calories = 60; carbohydrates = 10 g; alcohol = 0 g

Shirley Temple
Glass: 10-ounce highball glass
Mixers: 1 tablespoon grenadine
Diet ginger ale or lemon-lime soda
Method: Build over ice
Garnish: Slice of orange with straw
calories = 38; carbohydrates = 9 g; alcohol = 0 g

PART 3

Living with Diabetes and Prediabetes

Managing
Prediabetes

"*J*ust a touch of the sugar" is how prediabetes is often described, which is why, not surprisingly, so many people think it's not such a big deal. But it is potentially a very big deal. If you have prediabetes, you're also more likely to have more of the risk factors for heart disease and stroke, including high blood pressure and high levels of LDL (bad) cholesterol, thanks to insulin resistance. And you are more likely to develop full-blown type 2 diabetes within 5–10 years.

As we explained in chapter 2, if you have prediabetes, it means your body doesn't handle blood glucose as well as it used to or should, but your blood glucose levels are not high enough yet to say that you have type 2 diabetes. It's a step toward type 2 diabetes and heart disease, but it's not necessarily a one-way ticket.

• 22 •

Living with Prediabetes

TRAN

I WAS BORN to Southeast Asian parents in the early 1960s. I work long hours as a chef in my own restaurant, which is also where I live—I just walk upstairs to go home. Having grown up in Australia, I have to confess that I enjoy pizza, French fries and cakes, but I still tend to eat more traditional Asian foods most of the time—steamed white rice, dumplings, stir-fried meats and vegetables. Although my work is unbelievably hectic and I am on my feet and active all the time, I don't do any "proper" exercise because my business has grown enormously in recent years and I am simply too busy. Being a chef, I tend to eat regularly throughout the day and evening. Although I don't look overweight by typical Australian middle-aged male standards, I have to confess that I have developed some bulge around the middle in recent years.

Recently I went to my local doctor after a particularly bad dose of the winter flu. As well as checking my mouth, throat and airways, my doctor checked my blood pressure, which was a little high. As I am over 45, he decided to send me off for a series of blood tests to check my cholesterol and glucose levels, as part of a routine medical checkup. When I went back to get the results, my doctor broke the news—my fasting blood glucose levels were higher than normal at 117 mg/dL, but not high enough to say that I had diabetes. I had what he called impaired fasting glucose, or what is now commonly known as prediabetes. He referred me immediately to a local dietitian, who carefully went through my diet with me and gave me lots of really practical information and advice on what to eat (and not eat) that fits in with being a chef and running a restaurant, and with my cultural background. If I can improve my diet, exercise more and lose a little weight, I have a very good chance of preventing type 2 diabetes. And that's my goal.

WHAT CAN YOU DO ABOUT PREDIABETES?

Plenty.

Lifestyle changes—moderate weight loss, healthy eating and regular physical activity—will go a long way. In fact three out of five people (as shown in the United States Diabetes Prevention Program) with prediabetes can keep it from developing into type 2 diabetes simply by adopting these lifestyle changes.

TAKING STEPS TO AVOID DIABETES

- Aim for moderate weight loss
- Lower your saturated fat intake
- Boost your omega-3 intake
- Lower the GI of your diet
- Increase your fiber intake, and
- Get regular physical activity.

Aim for moderate weight loss

For most people with prediabetes, the first priority has to be reducing body weight. You don't have to lose a lot of weight for it to help.

Research has shown that people with prediabetes who lose 5–10 percent of their body weight at diagnosis can prevent or delay the onset of type 2 diabetes.

Lower your saturated fat intake

We know that people who develop type 2 diabetes are more likely to have a high saturated fat intake. Saturated fat promotes insulin resistance, making it harder for insulin to do its job of regulating your blood glucose levels. To eat less saturated fat:

Use low-fat dairy products—Routinely purchase low-fat milk, cheese, pudding, ice cream and yogurt rather than their regular forms.

Choose your snack foods wisely—Don't buy chocolate bars, cookies, potato chips, granola bars, muffin, etc. See chapter 13 for healthy snack options.

Cook with the good oils—The healthier oils to use are olive, canola and mustard seed.

Take care when you are eating away from home—Give up the French fries and onion rings along with other deep-fried foods, pizza and burgers.

Eat lean meats.

Boost your omega-3 intake

While high fat intakes are associated with diabetes, there is one type of fat that's the exception—the very-long-chain omega-3 fatty acids. Dietary trials in animals and people have shown that increased omega-3 intake can improve insulin sensitivity and therefore could reduce diabetes risk.

Our bodies only make small amounts of these unique fatty acids, so we rely on dietary sources, especially fish and seafood, for them. Aim to include fish in your diet at least twice a week, such as an entrée of fresh fish *not* cooked in saturated fat, plus at least one sand-wich-sized serving of, say, canned salmon or tuna.

Which Fish Is Best?

OILY FISH, WHICH tend to have darker-colored flesh and a stronger flavor, are the richest source of omega-3 fats. Some examples are: her-ring, Atlantic salmon, smoked salmon, tuna, mackerel and sardines. Medium sources are: mullet, blue mussel, calamari, mackerel, oysters, herring, cod.

Canned fish such as salmon, sardines, mackerel and, to a lesser extent, tuna are all good sources of omega-3s; look for canned fish packed in water, canola oil, olive oil, or brine—and drain the fish well.

As well as eating these great sources of long-chain omega-3s, you can also increase your total omega-3 intake by eating short-chain omega-3s, which are found in canola oil and margarine, nuts and seeds (particularly walnuts and flaxseeds), and legumes such as baked beans and soybeans.

Lower the GI of your diet

Studies show that people who base their diet on carbohydrates with a low GI are the least likely to develop type 2 diabetes. Some studies have shown that simply changing the bread you eat can make a dif-ference. Here are some key ways to lower the GI of your diet:

- Choose low-GI breads such as grainy bread, sourdough, flaxseed bread, or a fruit loaf. See the table below for a range of brands on the market with a low GI. There are even low-GI white breads in your supermarket.
- Swap high-GI cereals such as cornflakes and Rice Krispies for less processed and higher-fiber cereals such as rolled oats, traditional (not instant) oatmeal and natural muesli. See the table below—there's plenty to choose from. Or make your own muesli (see our recipe on page 356).

- Limit cookies and bakery products and include fruit and low-fat milk or yogurt as low-GI snacks.
- Replace potato with new potato, sweet potato and corn.
- Include legumes (home-cooked or canned beans, chickpeas and lentils) in your diet regularly.

Your low-GI choice with breads and breakfast cereals

To get started on low-GI eating, replace some of those high-GI breads and breakfast cereals with low-GI carbs that will trickle fuel into your engine. Here's a list of the tested brands you will find in your local supermarket or shopping center.

BREADS	GI
Bakers Delight	
Hi Fiber, Lo GI white bread	52
Bürgen®	
Mixed Grain	52
Oat Bran and Honey bread	45
Rye bread	51
Soy and flaxseed bread	36
Wholewheat and Grain	43
Country Life	
Country Grain and Organic Rye	48
PerforMAX	38
Rye Hi-soy and flaxseed	42
Cripps	
9 Grain loaf	43
EnerGI	
White sandwich bread	54
President's Choice® Blue Menu®	
Multi-grain flax loaf	51
Tortillas, flax	53
Whole grain English muffins	51
Whole wheat soy loaf	45
Spelt	
Multigrain bread	54
Stonemill	
3 grain bread	55

Vogel's	
Original Mixed Grain	54
Rye with Sunflower	47
Seven Seed	50
Soy and flaxseed with Oats	49
Wonder	
White Low GI sandwich bread	54

BREAKFAST CEREALS AND BARS	**GI**
Bürgen®	
Fruit and Muesli	51
Rye Muesli	41
Soy-Flax Muesli	51
Kellogg	
All-Bran® Fruit 'n' Oats	39
All-Bran®	34
Frosted Flakes®	55
President's Choice® Blue Menu®	
Steel-cut oats	51
Purina	
Muesli, toasted	43

Increase your fiber intake

Higher fiber intakes are also associated with a lower incidence of type 2 diabetes. Specifically, higher intakes of whole-grain cereals and fruit and vegetables are recommended.

Get the benefit of whole grains (grains that are eaten in nature's packaging or close to it) with foods such as:

- Barley—try pearl barley in soup, or in recipes such as barley risotto or a barley salad
- Whole wheat or cracked wheat such as bulgur in tabbouleh
- Rolled oats for breakfast in oatmeal or muesli, and
- Whole-grain breads—the ones with chewy grains and seeds (low-GI versions are best).

If you don't eat much fruit or vegetables at the moment, aim for at least one piece of fruit and two servings of vegetables each day, then build up gradually by eating one extra piece of fruit and one extra serving of vegetables each week.

If you are already eating a lot of fruit and vegetables, increase your intake until you reach two servings of fruit and five servings of vegetables every day.

Get regular physical activity

All the studies that have proven that a healthy lifestyle can prevent the development of type 2 diabetes have included a comprehensive exercise program in their definition of a healthy lifestyle. You need 150–210 minutes of moderate level physical activity each week, which is of course around 30 minutes of activity each day. The kinds of activities that proved most useful to people with prediabetes included walking, jogging, cycling, swimming, dancing and ball games—activities that are suitable for most North Americans.

TYPE 2 DIABETES is increasing in young people, so encouraging your children to be more active is a very important part of reducing their risk of later developing prediabetes or diabetes. Turning off the TV and computer and getting kids outside to play may be one of the most health-promoting things you can do as a parent.

Physical activity has many benefits, including increasing your lean body mass (giving you more muscles) and decreasing your body fat stores, which lead to lower insulin resistance and better insulin sensitivity. You get these benefits with regular exercise even if you don't lose weight.

And being physically active is not just about playing sports. Make it part of your day: "Add physical activity to your daily routine. For example, walk or ride your bike to work or shopping, organize school activities around physical activity, walk the dog, exercise while you watch TV, park farther away from your destination, etc." urges the U.S.

Department of Health and Human Services, as do many countries around the world (see chapter 17 for ways you can activate your day).

Exercise Safely

1. If you have not been physically active for some time, and you are over 40, have a medical checkup with your doctor before you start any physical activity program.

2. Choose an activity or sport that suits your ability and a level that suits your skills and fitness level, and be prepared:

   - Wear appropriate, comfortable clothing and shoes at all times
   - Always start with a warm-up (such as stretching or jogging on the spot for a few minutes)
   - Never exercise too hard: you should be able to speak comfortably, breathing just a little more often than usual
   - Slow down gradually after any activity: don't just suddenly stop
   - Finish with some gentle stretching
   - Drink plenty of water during and after activity
   - Always protect yourself from the sun
   - Do not do any form of physical activity after consuming alcohol or if you are feeling unwell, and
   - If you feel pain or you get breathless, stop: go and see your doctor before continuing.

Q&A

I have heard that there are medications you can take to help prevent type 2 diabetes. Is that true?

A number of trials using medications that are commonly used to treat type 2 diabetes that have aimed to see if they can also prevent it. These trials have used metformin, glucobay and troglitizone (which is no longer available). All the trials showed that they could prevent, or at least delay type 2 diabetes from developing, in people with prediabetes.

However, the medications were not as effective as lifestyle changes at reducing progression, so they are not currently recommended as a prevention strategy.

I have heard that drinking alcohol reduces the risk of diabetes. Is that true?

Moderate alcohol intake has been related to improved insulin sensitivity and reduced risk of type 2 diabetes, but there is not enough evidence to recommend that you start drinking if you are currently not a drinker.

▪23▪

Prediabetes:
Your Daily Food Guide and Recipes

*W*ith prediabetes, the aim is to optimize your nutritional intake to minimize your risk of progression to diabetes and development of cardiovascular disease. On average*, your daily food intake should include the following foods.

YOUR DAILY FOOD GUIDE

- 5–6 servings breads, cereals and other starchy foods
- 2–3 servings fruit
- 2–3 servings milk products
- 2–3 servings meat or alternatives
- 2–3 servings fat-rich foods, and
- 5 or more servings vegetables.

* The daily food guide is based on the requirements of a 50–60-year-old, overweight adult who is otherwise well and active in all normal daily activities. The calorie content is in the range of 1400–2000 calories, with approximately 45–50 percent of energy from carbohydrates.

HOW DO YOU FIT THIS INTO A DAY?

To illustrate what this looks like in terms of actual foods, we've laid out a meal plan showing the above servings distributed over the meals of a day. Beverages are not included unless they make a significant nutrient contribution.

MEAL PLAN FOR AN ADULT WITH PREDIABETES	DAILY FOOD SERVINGS	EXAMPLE	OTHER IDEAS
Breakfast	1 serving bread, cereal or other starchy foods	⅓ cup crunchy muesli	toast, English muffins, raisin toast, oatmeal or low-GI breakfast cereal
	1 serving fruit	1 large fresh peach, diced	fruit, fresh or canned, juice or dried fruit
	1 serving milk product	1 cup fruit yogurt	milk and cereal, to drink
Lunch	2 servings bread	2 slices whole-grain bread	a bread roll, toast, whole-grain crackers, baked beans, pasta, noodles
	2 servings vegetable	1 sliced tomato, ½ cucumber, 3 slices beet and grated carrot	Salad veggies or soup are good ways to boost intake
	1 serving meat or alternative	About 3 ounces lean cooked roast beef	tuna, salmon, egg, mixed beans
	1 serving fat	1 teaspoon mayonnaise on the sandwich	soft margarine, nut spreads, avocado or salad dressing
	1 serving milk product	1 glass low-fat milk	Yogurt or other dairy dessert
Dinner	2 servings bread or other starchy food and 1 serving fat	1 potato and ¾ cup sweet potato baked with a little olive oil	rice, pasta or bread is important for your carbs
	3 servings vegetables	baked pumpkin, beans, peas and broccoli	at least 1½ cups non-starchy vegetables

MEAL PLAN FOR AN ADULT WITH PREDIABETES	DAILY FOOD SERVINGS	EXAMPLE	OTHER IDEAS
Dinner	1 serving meat or alternative	1 small drumstick and thigh of roast chicken (skin removed)	this protein component needs to be lean to keep saturated fat intake down
	1 serving fruit	1 cup fresh fruit salad	fruit salad, dried fruit or a small juice

A MENU AND RECIPES FOR A DAY

The menu for this day is based around recipes from food and wine commentator Peter Howard's latest book, *Delicious Living*. You'll find them on the following pages. The nutritional analysis of the day allows for the inclusion of a ½ a cup of skim milk for tea or coffee if desired.

Breakfast

Pancakes with fruit topping
TOTAL CARBOHYDRATE (G) 49

Snack

Container of low-fat fruit yogurt
TOTAL CARBOHYDRATE (G) 12

Lunch

A glass of tomato and vegetable juice (homemade or reduced-sodium commercial type)
Tuna Salad
An apple
TOTAL CARBOHYDRATE (G) 46

Dinner

Chicken, Wilted Spinach and Curried Chickpeas served with ½ cup rice and ½ cup servings of steamed zucchini and carrot
TOTAL CARBOHYDRATE (G) 42

Dessert

Orange Mango Custard with Mango and Almonds
TOTAL CARBOHYDRATE (G) 14

Nutritional analysis of this daily menu						
ENERGY (CAL)	PROTEIN (G)	FAT (G)	SATURATED FAT (G)	CARBOHYDRATE FAT (G)	FIBER (G)	SODIUM (MG)
1480	105	35	5	175	30	1600

For Canadian readers: This conversion chart applies to all of the following recipes, as well as those in chapters 25, 27, 29 and 31–34.

DRY MEASUREMENTS	
IMPERIAL	METRIC
½ oz	15 g
1 oz	30 g
1½ oz	45 g
2 oz	55 g
4 oz	125 g
5 oz	150 g
6½ oz	200 g
7 oz	225 g
8 oz	250 g
1 lb	500 g
2 lb	1 kg

TEMPERATURES	
FAHRENHEIT	CELSIUS
250°F	120°C
300°F	150°C
315°F	160°C
350°F	180°C
375°F	190°C
400°F	200°C
425°F	220°C
450°F	230°C
475°F	240°C

LIQUID MEASUREMENTS		
IMPERIAL	STANDARD CUPS	METRIC
1 fl oz	2 tbsp	30 mL
2 fl oz	¼ cup	60 mL
2¾ fl oz	⅓ cup	80 mL
4 fl oz	½ cup	125 mL
6 fl oz	¾ cup	185 mL
8 fl oz	1 cup	250 mL

PANCAKES

*P*eter Howard's pancakes are so versatile—sweet or savory. And for breakfast, you can make the choice. Avocado slices + pepper + cottage cheese makes a suitable lunch with salad on the side.

PREP TIME: 5 minutes ■ COOKING TIME: 10 minutes ■ SERVES: 6

---

2 cups self-rising whole-wheat flour

¼ tsp baking soda

1 egg

1½ tbsp psyllium husks

2 cups 2% milk

Fruit topping

2 large bananas

8 large strawberries

2½ tbsp pure floral honey, warmed

Savory topping

1 cup (8 oz) low-fat cottage cheese

1⅔ cups (10 oz) diced ripe tomatoes

black pepper

1. Whisk the flour and baking soda to aerate; add the egg and psyllium and then whisk in the flour to form the batter. Film spray a nonstick frying pan. Using 2 tablespoons of the batter for each pancake gives you 12 pancakes. Cook the pancakes over medium heat. Flip each one when bubbles are popping in the uncooked side. Keep warm to serve.

2. To serve, put 2 pancakes overlapping onto each large plate; spoon one-sixth of the cheese onto the overlap and top with a sixth of the diced tomatoes. Grind black pepper over and serve. For the fruit topping, dice the bananas and strawberries and stir gently and quickly. Spoon a sixth over each plate of pancakes and drizzle with honey.

PER SERVING
Energy (cal) 190 ■ Protein (g) 11 ■ Fat (g) 2 ■ Saturated fat (g) 1 ■
Carbohydrate (g) 30 ■ Fiber (g) 4 ■ Sodium (mg) 120

TUNA SALAD

A loaf of whole-grain bread, a can of tuna and a bag of ready-to-eat salad will see you eating a super-healthy lunch wherever you are.

PREP TIME: 5 mins ■ COOKING TIME: nil ■ SERVES: 1

½ x 6-oz can (approximately) tuna in spring water or flavoring of your choice

a few pieces of bagged, washed lettuce or other salad greens

10 cherry or grape tomatoes

½ cucumber, sliced

2 fresh mushrooms, thinly sliced

bottled marinated vegetables, such as roasted peppers, marinated mushrooms, grilled eggplant (optional)

2 tsp your favorite salad dressing

2 slices dense whole-grain bread

1. Lay the salad leaves over a plate, top with the tuna, tomatoes and other vegetables. Drizzle over 2 tsp dressing and enjoy with the bread.

PER SERVING
Energy (cal) 180 ■ Protein (g) 23 ■ Fat (g) 6 ■ Saturated fat (g) 1 Carbohydrate (g) 7 ■ Fiber (g) 5 ■ Sodium (mg) 240

CHICKEN, WILTED SPINACH AND CURRIED CHICKPEAS

PREP TIME: 15 mins ■ COOKING TIME: 45 min ■ SERVES: 4

4 x 4 oz skinless chicken breasts, cut into medallions

2 scallions, chopped

1 tbsp oil

½ medium white onion, finely chopped

½ medium carrot, finely chopped

2 tbsp Indian curry powder

1 15-oz can chickpeas, drained

2 cups water

8 cups baby spinach leaves

PER SERVING
Energy (cal) 310 ■
Protein (g) 33 ■ Fat (g) 14 ■
Saturated fat (g) 3 ■
Carbohydrate (g) 12 ■
Fiber (g) 6 ■ Sodium (mg) 262

1 Ensure all the fat is removed from the chicken medallions. Heat enough water to poach the chicken, add the chicken and scallions and simmer for 10 minutes. Turn off the heat until ready to use.

2 Heat the oil and lightly fry the onion and carrot pieces. Add the curry powder and stir. Add the drained chickpeas and stir to coat with the curry mixture. Pour in the 2 cups of water, bring to a boil, then reduce to a simmer and cook for 30 minutes. You may need more water, depending on the saucepan you use.

3 Reheat the poaching stock and simmer the chicken slices to cook through: 3–5 minutes. Do this in batches, depending on your pan size. Keep slices warm in a low oven (200°F) if you're doing it in batches.

4 In another saucepan bring ½ cup chicken poaching liquid to a boil. Tip in the spinach and stir to allow it to wilt/break down. Do not overcook or you will lose the color and nutritional value. Drain well and keep warm.

5 To serve, put equal amounts of chickpeas into the center of four deep plates. Top with spinach, then equal amounts of chicken slices. Spoon over some of the chicken poaching liquid and serve immediately, with good bread.

ORANGE MANGO CUSTARD WITH MANGO AND ALMONDS

PREP TIME: 20 mins ■ REFRIGERATION TIME: 2 hours ■ SERVES: 4 big servings

1 package sugar-free orange mango–flavored Jell-O

1 cup boiling water

1 cup cold water

2 egg whites

¾ cup light evaporated milk, chilled in a medium-sized bowl in the freezer for 1 hour before use

1 cup sliced mango

½ cup almond slivers, toasted

1 Put the Jell-O in a large bowl and stir in the 1 cup of boiling water. Stir well to dissolve the powder. Pour in the cold water and stir. Cool for a couple of minutes, then refrigerate for about an hour.

2 When the Jell-O is starting to set you'll notice it around the edges of the bowl. The larger the bowl, the quicker it will set. Whisk the egg whites with an electric beater. Once soft peaks form, refrigerate. Whisk the chilled evaporated milk in a chilled bowl. It will become thick, but not like whipped cream.

3 Put the Jell-O, egg whites and milk on the counter. Beat the gelatin with the electric beaters for 20 seconds, lower the beaters into the milk and pour in the Jell-O, with the beater on slow. Make sure the mixture is well combined. Fold in the egg whites and refrigerate, covered, for 45–60 minutes.

4 Serve decorated with equal amounts of mango slices and sprinkled with the almonds.

PER SERVING
Energy (cal) 185 ■ Protein (g) 12 ■ Fat (g) 9 ■ Saturated fat (g) 1 Carbohydrate (g) 13 ■ Fiber (g) 2 ■ Sodium (mg) 86

Managing
Type 2 Diabetes

$\mathcal{I}$f you have type 2 diabetes, your insulin does not work properly (insulin resistance) or you have a shortage of insulin. The aim of treatment is to help you make the best use of the insulin you have and to try to make it last as long as possible.

As we said in the introduction to this book, the most important thing you can do is to take control of your condition: get informed about what having diabetes means and what is recommended to manage diabetes and your health.

Because lifestyle factors contribute to type 2 diabetes, looking at the way you live (especially your diet and exercise habits) is the key to managing diabetes well.

•24•

Living with
Type 2 Diabetes

JOHN/GIANNI

MOST OF MY life I worked long hard hours in the mines, but I have been taking it easy ever since retiring at the age of 65. I was pretty fit when I was working, but 10 years on, most of my muscles have wasted away, and I have developed a pretty impressive beer gut—which surprised me, because I don't drink much. I have been feeling rundown and tired in recent years, I admit, and certainly seemed to pick up colds, flu and infections more easily than I used to. And my eyesight was getting bad. I thought it was just old age, but I decided to have a medical checkup anyway after one of my close friends had a heart attack. I just wanted to make sure everything was okay.

My local doctor checked my blood pressure, which was a little high, and sent me off for a series of blood tests to check my cholesterol and glucose levels. At my next appointment, he broke the news. I had type 2 diabetes, and my blood cholesterol was very high. At first I just couldn't believe it. What had I done to deserve this?

> My doctor referred me immediately to the local diabetes clinic, where the dietitian gave me some practical tips for healthy eating, and my diabetes educator taught me how to monitor my blood glucose levels. And she got me moving, too. I started walking. Within six months I felt the best I'd been in years—even my eyesight has improved. I joined the local diabetes group, too, and was really surprised to see how many people I knew there. I never even realized that they had diabetes.

For some people with type 2 diabetes, all they have to do to keep their blood glucose levels in the normal range is manage their weight, eat a healthy diet and be active. Others also need to take medication and some may need insulin.

The first thing you have to come to terms with when diagnosed with diabetes is that high blood glucose levels are probably not your only problem: you may also have high blood pressure, abnormal blood fats (high LDL [bad] cholesterol, low HDL [good] cholesterol and high triglycerides) and abdominal obesity (fat around the middle of your body). This is a potentially lethal health cocktail that increases your risk of developing major blood vessel diseases, especially heart disease, stroke and peripheral vascular disease (thrombosis), particularly of the lower limbs.

Second, it's highly likely that the way you have been living (diet and lack of exercise) contributed to your getting diabetes. So the first step for the majority of people with type 2 diabetes involves taking a good hard look at themselves and thinking about the changes they can make that will improve their blood glucose levels and blood fats and blood pressure, if they are higher than recommended.

For most people, the place to start is with what they eat.

YOU ARE WHAT YOU EAT

What changes do you need to make to your diet? Of course it varies, but these are the aspects to focus on:

▶ **Reduce how much you eat.** Key foods to reduce are those high in saturated fats and/or added sugars, and alcohol. This doesn't mean just downsizing your daily chocolate bar from king size to standard (although this would definitely help). It means saving the chocolate bar for very special occasions only.

▶ **Cut back on saturated fats and cholesterol.** This is absolutely essential for everyone with type 2 diabetes. You must get and keep your LDL (bad) cholesterol down. Don't obsessively avoid high-cholesterol eggs and shrimp. It's the saturated fats in those lamb chops and chocolate chip cookies that are having the greatest effect on your cholesterol levels. If you've been eating healthily and doing regular exercise for at least three months and your cholesterol levels still haven't improved, talk to your doctor about cholesterol-lowering medications. A practical intermediate step may be to try one of the reduced-fat margarines that have added phytosterols for a further three months. Provided you can eat the 4–5 teaspoons a day of margarine without gaining weight, these margarines can reduce your blood cholesterol levels by around 10 percent.

▶ **Modify your carbohydrate intake.** This means thinking about carb quality and quantity and getting familiar with the sources and amounts of carbohydrate in your diet. There's no point buying the "99 percent fat-free" product if it packs in 120 grams of high-GI carbs per serving. For carb quality, make sure that you are eating the low-GI ones as much as possible. As for quantity, 50–60 grams of carbohydrates at any one sitting is a good average. Replacing some carbohydrates in your diet with monounsaturated fat can reduce your post-meal blood glucose levels and lower your triglycerides, but you have to be careful with this. Too much added fat may lead to weight gain. Talk to your dietitian about the proportion of fat to carbohydrates that's right for you.

▶ **Eat more regularly.** Whether you want to eat three meals a day or small meals plus snacks is up to you. However, if you use insulin or take medication that stimulates insulin production from your pancreas, it will be helpful if you can maintain some consistency in the times you eat your meals and the amount of carbohydrates you eat at those meals. A regime of multiple insulin injections usually gives you more flexibility in your food intake.

▶ **Moderate your protein intake.** Protein won't increase your blood glucose level (BGL) and is valuable for satisfying appetite. The usual recommended protein intake is 15–20 percent of your total energy intake. Most North Americans already eat this according to the latest National Health and Nutrition Examination Study (NHANES), so there is no need to eat any more. There is currently no evidence that high-protein, low-carbohydrate diets are safe or even effective in the long term for managing type 2 diabetes. People with kidney disease (about 1 in 3 people with diabetes) should avoid a high protein intake, because research shows that a more moderate intake helps preserve kidney function.

▶ **Eat more of the healthy foods (such as fruit and vegetables).** You see, it isn't all about cutting back. Most people don't eat anywhere near enough of these foods. Fresh, dried and canned fruits are all suitable, and you can eat as much as you like of most nonstarchy vegetables (leafy greens, carrots, tomatoes, onions, etc.).

▶ **Cut back on salt.** Chances are you've got high blood pressure too. Reducing your sodium intake by not adding salt to food when cooking or at the table, and choosing reduced-sodium or low-salt foods at the supermarket, is a great start. If you think you have done this but your blood pressure is still high, you might need medication as well. See your doctor for further advice.

YOUR HEALTHY TYPE 2 DIABETES DIET CHECKLIST

▶ Use poly- and/or monounsaturated margarines and spreads instead of butter and butter blends.
▶ Use olive and/or canola oils in cooking and for salads.
▶ Don't drink more than 1–2 standard alcoholic drinks a day.
▶ Eat more than 3 cups of vegetables every day (this includes soups).
▶ Eat more than 2 pieces (200 grams) of fruit every day.
▶ Include legumes (canned or dried peas, beans or lentils) in your diet at least twice a week.
▶ Eat fish (4 ounces or more) at least twice a week.

- Include low-fat dairy products (or calcium-enriched alternatives) in your diet daily and generally avoid whole milk and other full-fat types.
- Eat whole-grain and high-fiber cereals, breads and grains daily—look for the low-GI ones.
- Eat lean red meat or poultry in moderately-sized (less than 5 ounces) portions regularly.
- Drink 6–8 glasses of water, or other low-calorie beverages, every day. Drinking more water won't lower your blood glucose levels, but high blood glucose means you should drink more water to avoid dehydration.

ROSE

MY HUSBAND HAD a major stroke in 2004, and was diagnosed with type 2 diabetes, as well. His blood glucose has been like a roller coaster no matter how carefully I monitored his diet, until we accidentally happened upon *The Low GI Diet Revolution* at our local bookstore.

For the past three weeks we have followed your 7 days of menus religiously, and my husband's blood glucose has been holding so well it is unbelievable. The calorie and carb levels of your menu plans appear to be absolutely perfectly calibrated, as he cannot exercise because he is paralyzed.

It is nothing short of a miracle. In just three short weeks there's been a remarkable turnaround in his blood glucose and in the way he feels. His blood glucose has been right on target every day and he has lost 6 pounds! It's wonderful to see him feeling so well.

Now he has asked if I could come up with 7 more days of menus so that he doesn't eat the same thing every week!

Did you know that as you age, you are at greater risk of dehydration as your sensitivity to thirst and your kidney function decline?

EXERCISE

The other aspect of your lifestyle to modify is exercise—because lack of it probably contributed to your getting diabetes. How much? You need to do at least 30–45 minutes, 3–5 days a week, or accumulate at least 150 minutes (that's 2½ hours) of exercise per week. And here's the pay-off for that 2½ hours exercise a week. It will:

- Improve your blood glucose levels
- Decrease your insulin resistance, and
- Reduce your risk of heart and blood vessel disease—which is the number one cause of death in people with diabetes.

What sort of exercise? The most beneficial forms of exercise are aerobic (walking) and resistance (weight lifting) exercise. Now before you scoff at the image of a geriatric Mr. or Mrs. Bodybuilder, you would be wise to heed the fact that older muscles are just as responsive to strength training as younger muscles. If you don't do something to maintain your muscles, they will shrink as you age. In fact a decrease in lean muscle mass and increase in body fat is the most common nutritional scenario in older people. It is never too late to get a set of light dumbbells and start training. Talk to your exercise specialist about a program that will suit you, not strain you.

For elderly people, one of the most important benefits of exercise is that it helps you stay mobile and independent. It will reduce the muscle wastage and frailty that make it difficult for you to care for yourself. You can rebuild weakened muscles and improve your balance to reduce the risk of falls and fractures. Exercise can even help maintain mental sharpness. Studies have shown that physical training improves mental function in elderly people with dementia.

Finally, it's worth noting that exercise can be a valuable mood enhancer in times of stress. People who are physically active are far less likely to be depressed, tense, confused, anxious and stressed out.

MEDICATION

The number of medications available for managing type 2 diabetes has increased in recent years. When your blood glucose levels can no longer be managed just through healthy eating and regular physical activity, your doctor can prescribe one or more different types of medications—oral hypoglycemic agents (they work to lower your blood glucose levels).

A common type of drug used is from the class known as sulphony-lureas (the actual medication is sold under a number of different brand names). These stimulate your pancreas to make more insulin. Like injected insulin, they can sometimes cause your blood glucose levels to go too low (hypoglycemia) and they can also increase your body weight.

Biguanides are a type of medication that lower blood glucose levels and increase your body's sensitivity to insulin, so that your insulin works better. The only biguanide available in the United States and Canada today is metformin.

Another class of medications delays carbohydrate digestion from your gut by preventing your digestive juices (specifically a digestive enzyme called alpha-glucosidase) from working properly. Glucobay is a common example of this kind of medication. A little bit like low-GI carbohydrates, it lowers your blood glucose levels after meals. Unfortunately, side effects such as flatulence and diarrhea are common with this type of drug.

A newer class of blood glucose–lowering drugs are the thiazo-lidinediones. These improve your blood glucose levels by decreasing insulin resistance and decreasing the liver's production of glucose. Examples are rosiglitazone (marketed as Avandia) and pioglitazone (marketed as Actos). These medications can cause weight gain, but usually the body tolerates them well, and they don't cause hypos.

The latest class of blood glucose–lowering medications are the meglitinides. Brand names include Prandin and Starlix. Like sulpho-nylureas, they lower blood glucose levels by stimulating your pancreas to release more insulin; they are not chemically related to the sulphonylureas, though. They start working quickly and don't last long, so a pill is taken before each meal to stimulate immediate insulin release. This is pretty much what your body would normally do in response to a meal. Because of this, they offer greater flexibility than some of the other medications, and are particularly useful for people with erratic or irregular eating patterns, such as shift workers. Like insulin and sulphonylureas, they can cause hypoglycemia (low blood glucose or a "hypo"). Side effects, other than low blood glucose level (BGL) are unusual, but can include stomach upsets.

DO YOU HAVE TO USE INSULIN
IF YOU HAVE TYPE 2 DIABETES?

It's not inevitable. But after you have had diabetes for many years, your pancreas may no longer be able to produce enough insulin to overcome your insulin resistance, even if you have a healthy lifestyle and are taking all the currently available medication at your maximum tolerated dose. This happens in about 50 percent of people within 10 years of being diagnosed, but it can happen more quickly—particularly if you have not been able to manage your blood glucose levels well for some time. Why? Because high blood glucose levels are toxic to the insulin-producing beta cells: having high blood glucose levels for long periods of time will kill off beta cells, speeding up the need for insulin injections.

Modern insulins are very similar to what your body produces naturally, and you will be surprised at how much your blood glucose levels improve once you start using them. "But I can't bear the thought of injecting myself," you say. Don't worry—modern needles are so fine that they are relatively painless. In fact you will probably feel less than when you prick yourself with the lancet device you use to test your blood glucose levels.

Like some of the pills prescribed for lowering your blood glucose, insulin increases the risk of having a hypo. Also, your improved blood glucose levels means less glucose is being lost in your urine, so the food you eat is used much more effectively. An unfortunate consequence of this may be weight gain. This is not a sign of failure. It may actually be a sign that your blood glucose levels are being better managed. If you do put on weight, talk to your diabetes team to see how you can reduce your food intake and/or insulin injections.

IT'S VERY IMPORTANT not to think that insulin therapy means you're a failure—research has shown that for many people, there comes a time when they have no choice but to have insulin injections, regardless of how well they have looked after themselves.

ANY POSSIBILITY OF PREGNANCY?

If you're a woman with type 2 diabetes and you're planning a pregnancy (or even if you're not planning it), you ought to talk to a doctor about what you need to do *before* you become pregnant (or talk about contraception). It is essential that your blood glucose levels be well managed before conception, to reduce the chance of miscarriage, deformities and other complications. A dietary supplement of folate (5 mg per day) is also recommended, and your doctor may want you to stop or change your diabetes medications. So make sure you see your doctor before you conceive for a complete diabetes health review (see also chapter 28).

Q&A

Why is my blood glucose level (BGL) higher in the morning than when I go to bed at night? I swear I don't eat anything during the night.

A higher blood glucose level (BGL) (above 110 mg/dL) when you get up in the morning is a very common feature of type 2 diabetes and, understandably, a puzzle to many who experience it.

Part of the reason for it is what's described as the "dawn phenomenon." This is a normal physiological process: certain hormones in your body set to work to raise your blood glucose levels before you wake up. The hormones stimulate glucose production and release from your liver and inhibit glucose use by your body. The result is an increase in your blood glucose levels, ensuring that you have a supply of fuel ready for your wakening body's needs.

Other possible causes are more likely if you are taking insulin. If the insulin you took at night is running out by the morning, this could mean your blood glucose levels will be high when you wake up.

Should I be taking a vitamin supplement?

When first diagnosed, your blood glucose levels may have been high for some time, which means you may be deficient in a number of vitamins and minerals, because many are either lost in the urine, or you need more of them because of the diabetes. The most common problems are with the vitamins E, B_6, folate, B_{12}, and the minerals calcium, zinc, magnesium and possibly **chromium**.

After a few months, when your blood glucose levels have returned to normal (or close to it) through healthy eating, regular physical activity and appropriate medication, your vitamin and mineral needs will return to normal too.

However, some people—some elderly people, plus pregnant and lactating women, strict vegetarians and those on a severely restricted diet (for example, someone with severe food allergies or intolerances)—may benefit from specific vitamin and/or mineral supplements. Sometimes people taking the medication metformin develop a B_{12} deficiency, so a B_{12} supplement may be necessary.

Whatever the case, it's best to talk about which vitamin and mineral supplements you need, if any, with your dietitian or doctor. Most of the rest of us, who are able to eat a wide range of nutritious foods, don't need to worry about supplements—it's just not necessary.

It is important to note that nutrient balance is controlled by your body, so you should always be cautious about taking large doses of any vitamin or mineral supplement. Research has proven conclusively that megadoses of certain vitamins and minerals can cause imbalances in other vitamins or minerals, or even be toxic.

Vitamin and Mineral Deficiencies

TRUE VITAMIN AND mineral deficiencies are associated with poor wound healing, bruising, anemia, increased risk of infections, cognitive (mental) impairment, neurological disorders, stroke and some cancers. If you are getting less than the optimum intake of nutrients, you may not have the classic symptoms of deficiency, but there could still be subtle effects.

Are there any foods I can eat to improve my cholesterol levels?

Foods that will improve your cholesterol levels by lowering the bad (LDL) cholesterol and raising the good (HDL) cholesterol include those rich in polyunsaturated and monounsaturated oils (sunflower, safflower, canola and olive, nuts and seeds), plant sterol–enriched margarines, soy protein (soy beverages, tofu, soybeans) and foods that are low GI and high in soluble fibers.

Foods high in soluble fibers include legumes (lentils, peas and beans), whole grains such as barley, oats, and fruits and vegetables. A recently published study has found that including a combination of these high-fiber foods in your diet can be as effective at lowering LDL cholesterol as the new generation of cholesterol-lowering drugs known as statins (Lipitor, Zocor, Crestor, Vytorin, Pravachol, Lescol).

Some foods help your cholesterol profile by raising levels of the HDL cholesterol. Omega-3 fatty acids—found in fish, soybean oil, avocados and walnuts—raise HDL levels and even have blood-thinning and antiarrhythmic properties that help maintain normal heart rhythm and reduce your risk of heart problems.

Some studies have shown that moderate consumption of alcohol (1–2 drinks per day) also leads to increased levels of HDL. However, because of the other health risks associated with alcohol consumption, doctors recommend that nondrinkers don't start drinking.

Some experts suspect that high blood levels of the amino acid homocysteine may promote atherosclerosis (hardening and narrowing of the arteries). Increasing your intake of folic acid, vitamin B_6 and vitamin B_{12} can help reduce levels of homocysteine. Natural sources of these vitamins include leafy greens, legumes, whole grains, lean meats and nuts.

My doctor says I have a fatty liver. What can I do about this?

A fatty liver that develops in the absence of alcohol consumption is a metabolic abnormality that is associated with insulin resistance. In this condition, fat infiltrates the liver causing inflammation, damage and subsequent scarring inside the liver. It's similar to the changes in the liver of an alcoholic, but it can occur in people who don't drink at all. The advanced stage of fatty liver disease is known as NASH (nonalcoholic steatohepatitis). As many as 75 percent of people with type 2 diabetes have fatty liver disease, but it's often undiagnosed. It only occasionally causes symptoms such as fatigue, feeling vaguely unwell and discomfort in the upper right abdomen. What should you do about it? Management of fatty liver includes:

- Losing weight *gradually*. Rapid weight loss (by a very low-calorie diet) can speed up the movement/accumulation of fat into the liver

 ▶ Improving blood glucose levels
 ▶ Following a low-GI diet
 ▶ Avoiding all alcohol, and
 ▶ Lowering blood fats with a diet low in saturated fat and
   appropriate medication.

The use of diabetic medications that reduce insulin resistance is
also being studied as part of treatment.

I've heard that coffee is good for diabetes. Is that true?

There are studies both for and against coffee in relation to diabetes. Occasional coffee drinking may actually decrease insulin
sensitivity, but drinking coffee or other high-caffeine foods or beverages on a regular basis does not appear to have any detrimental
effects on people with diabetes in the long run. The body seems to
adapt to the caffeine so that it no longer has any negative effects.

Coffee (regular and decaffeinated) contains lots of antioxidants
and magnesium that may improve insulin sensitivity. A study of the
dietary habits of more than 125,000 people in the United States
over 20 years found that men who drank more than six cups of caffeinated coffee a day reduced their chances of getting type 2 diabetes by more than 50 percent compared with men in the study
who didn't drink coffee.

Among the women, those who drank six or more cups a day
reduced their risk of type 2 diabetes by nearly 30 percent. These
effects could not be accounted for by lifestyle factors such as smoking, exercise or obesity. Decaffeinated coffee was also beneficial,
but it had less effect than regular coffee.

Type 2 Diabetes:
Your Daily Food Guide and Recipes

*A*s an adult with type 2 diabetes, you have similar nutritional requirements to someone without diabetes, but meeting those requirements might hopefully have taken on a higher priority for you now. On average*, your daily food intake should include the following foods:

YOUR DAILY FOOD GUIDE

▶ 5–6 servings breads and cereals and other starchy foods
▶ 2–3 servings fruits
▶ 2–3 servings of milk products
▶ 1–2 servings meat and alternatives
▶ 2–3 servings fat-rich foods, and
▶ 5 or more servings vegetables.

*The daily food guide is based on a 60-year-old, overweight adult who is active in usual daily living. The calorie content will range from

1,300 to 1,900 calories with approximately 50 percent energy from carbohydrates.

HOW DO YOU FIT THIS INTO A DAY?

Here's an example of how you could fit this food into a day. Beverages are not included except where they make a significant nutrient contribution.

Meal plan for an adult with type 2 diabetes	Daily food servings	Example	Other ideas
Breakfast	1 serving bread, cereal or other starchy food with ½ serving fats	1 slice soy-linseed toast spread with margarine	toast, oatmeal, muesli, rice
	1 serving fruit	topped with sliced banana	a glass of juice, a tablespoon of raisins, an apple
	1 serving milk products	and a skim milk coffee	milk or yogurt on cereal, or a glass of milk to drink
Lunch	2 servings bread, cereal or other starchy food	a seeded bread roll	rice, pasta, potato, or bread
	2 servings vegetables	a handful of lettuce, 1 sliced tomato, ½ small cucumber and 2 sliced mushrooms	any combination of vegetables or salad
	1 serving fat-rich food	¼ avocado	margarine, mayonnaise or even a handful of nuts
	1 serving fruit	2 large fresh apricots	any piece of fresh fruit, a bowl of fruit salad, or a cup of canned fruit
Dinner	2 servings other starchy foods and ½ serving fat-rich food	4 baby new potatoes with parsley and a teaspoon of margarine	noodles, rice, sweet corn, lentils
	1 serving meat or alternative	3½ ounce beef steak	fish, cheese, chicken, tofu

Meal plan for an adult with type 2 diabetes	Daily food servings	Example	Other ideas
Dinner	3 servings vegetables	1½ cups steamed seasonal vegetables dressed with a teaspoon of lemon juice	3 cups of salad vegetables
	1 serving milk products	8-ounce lite peach yogurt	a cup of cocoa, a container of yogurt or some ice cream

A MENU AND RECIPES FOR THE DAY

The menu for this day is based on 3 nutritious meals with a sweet treat at the end of the day. The nutritional analysis of the day allows for ½ cup of skim milk for tea or coffee if desired.

Breakfast
Hot Breakfast for One
and an orange
TOTAL CARBOHYDRATE (G) 40

Lunch
Sweet Potato and Lentil Bake
with a green salad, oil and vinegar dressing
and a glass of low-fat, calcium-enriched milk or a skim milk coffee
TOTAL CARBOHYDRATE (G) 40

Dinner
Crisp Whiting Fillet, Sweet Potato and Turnip Cake and Green Beans
TOTAL CARBOHYDRATE (G) 20

Dessert
Chocolate Walnut Dessert Cake
with a dollop of natural yogurt
TOTAL CARBOHYDRATE (G) 30

Nutritional analysis of this daily menu

ENERGY (CAL)	PROTEIN (G)	FAT (G)	SATURATED (G)	CARBOHYDRATE FAT (G)	FIBER (G)	SODIUM (MG)
1550	105	60	15	135	30	1600

HOT BREAKFAST FOR ONE

PREP TIME: 5 mins ■ COOKING TIME: 7 mins ■ SERVES: 1

cooking spray oil

1⅓ cup fresh mushrooms, trimmed and sliced

few sprigs parsley, leaves chopped

freshly ground black pepper

1 tsp canola margarine

2 omega-3-enriched eggs, beaten with 3 tbsp low-fat milk

pepper and salt to taste

1 slice whole-grain bread, toasted

½ cup reduced-sodium baked beans

1. Heat a small frying pan over medium heat and spray with cooking oil. Add the mushroom slices and cook, stirring occasionally, for 5 minutes, or until done to your liking. Mix in chopped parsley and pepper, then remove to a warm plate. Cover to keep warm.

2. Return the frying pan to the heat and add the margarine. Once it's melted, pour in the beaten eggs and reduce heat to low. Cook for 1 minute, until eggs are just beginning to firm around the edges. Stir over low heat with a wooden spoon for 1 minute more, until cooked.

3. Serve the eggs on top of the toast, alongside the mushrooms, with the warmed baked beans spooned over.

PER SERVING
Energy (cal) 390 ■ Protein (g) 26 ■ Fat (g) 15 ■ Saturated fat (g) 4
Carbohydrate (g) 30 ■ Fiber (g) 12 ■ Sodium (mg) 438

SWEET POTATO AND LENTIL BAKE

PREP TIME: 20 mins ■ COOKING TIME: 45 mins ■ SERVES: 4

1-lb sweet potato, peeled, halved lengthwise and sliced thinly

2 tsp olive oil

1 medium onion, chopped

3 cloves garlic, crushed

1 tsp chopped fresh rosemary

14-oz can diced tomatoes

14-oz can brown lentils, drained

¼ cup drained and chopped roasted red peppers or ¼ fresh red pepper

2½ tbsp chopped fresh parsley

⅓ cup frozen peas

freshly ground black pepper

1 cup grated, reduced-fat pizza cheese

1. Preheat oven to 350°F. Boil, steam or microwave sweet potato until cooked. Set aside to cool.

2. Meanwhile, in a large nonstick frying pan, heat the oil and cook onion, garlic and rosemary until soft, about 3–4 minutes. Add the tomatoes, bring to a boil, then reduce the heat and simmer for 5 minutes. Mix in the lentils, red peppers, parsley and peas. Season to taste with freshly ground black pepper and cook for 2 minutes, or until the mixture is just heated through.

3. In a 6-cup baking dish, spoon in half the lentil sauce, then layer with half the sweet potato and half the cheese. Add the remaining lentil sauce, then the remaining sweet potato. Sprinkle the remaining cheese over the top. Bake for 30–35 minutes, or until cheese has melted and top is lightly golden.

PER SERVING
Energy (cal) 260 ■ Protein (g) 16 ■ Fat (g) 9 ■ Saturated fat (g) 5
Carbohydrate (g) 27 ■ Fiber (g) 7 ■ Sodium (mg) 480

CRISP WHITING FILLET, SWEET POTATO AND TURNIP CAKE AND GREEN BEANS

*P*eter Howard's sweet potato and turnip cake is a beauty in that it is excellent served cold or at room temperature. It can be used under a can of salmon for lunch with some salad on the side.

PREP TIME: 20 minutes ■ COOKING TIME: 80 minutes ■ SERVES: 4

---

21 ounce whiting fillets

1 egg white, lightly whipped

1 cup rye flour

The cake

½ medium-sized onion, finely diced

2 cups (9 oz) Swede turnip, peeled and grated

1½ cups (7 oz) white sweet potato, peeled and grated

½ tsp allspice

½ tsp dried chili flakes

1 egg

2½ tbsp whole-wheat self-rising flour

spray canola oil

1¾ cup (7 oz) green beans, topped and tailed

4 lemon quarters

1. Preheat the oven to 350°F.
2. Trim the whiting fillets (if necessary) and refrigerate until ready to use.
3. Make the cake by combining all ingredients well. Line a baking dish (8" square × 2" deep) with parchment paper. Spray with a film of oil and spoon in the mixture. Pat it down with your hand, spray it with a film of oil and bake for 60 minutes.
4. Pat the fish dry, then dip in egg white and then into the flour. Shake off excess flour and put onto a lightly oiled, parchment paper-lined tray. Spray with some oil and bake until browned and crisped (around 15 minutes).
5. Boil the beans until done to your liking. Drain and keep warm for serving.
6. Let the cake rest for 10 minutes, then invert the baking dish and remove the cake. Cut it into 4 equal squares and then into triangles. Put the fish fillets on top of the cake, put the beans and lemon quarter on the side.

PER SERVING
Energy (cal) 345 ■ Protein (g) 40 ■ Fat (g) 4 ■ Saturated fat (g) 1
Carbohydrate (g) 32 ■ Fiber (g) 8 ■ Sodium (mg) 175

CHOCOLATE WALNUT DESSERT CAKE

PREP TIME: 30 mins ■ **COOKING TIME:** 45 mins ■ **SERVES:** 10

1½ cup walnuts

⅓ cup plain unbleached flour, sifted

1 tsp baking powder

3 eggs, separated

½ cup superfine sugar

2 oz dark chocolate, finely chopped

1 cup dates, chopped

natural yogurt, to serve

1. Preheat the oven to 325°F and grease and line the base and sides of 7- or 8-inch round cake pan.

2. In a food processor, grind the walnuts, using the pulse button, until just ground. In a bowl, combine the walnuts, flour and baking powder.

3. Beat the egg yolks and sugar with an electric mixer until thick and pale. Fold in the flour mixture, then the chocolate and dates. The mixture will be very thick.

4. In another bowl, beat the egg whites until firm peaks form. Fold carefully into the cake mix.

5. Spoon the mixture into the cake pan and bake for 40–45 minutes, or until a skewer inserted in the center of the cake comes out clean. Set the cake in the pan on a wire rack to cool for 10 minutes, then turn out and leave to cool completely on the wire rack.

6. Serve with a dollop of natural yogurt.

PER SERVING
Energy (cal) 270 ■ Protein (g) 7 ■ Fat (g) 17 ■ Saturated fat (g) 3 Carbohydrate (g) 22 ■ Fiber (g) 3 ■ Sodium (mg) 62

· 26 ·

Type 2 Diabetes
in Children

MICHAEL

MICHAEL WAS BORN in Australia to Chinese parents. He was very overweight, carrying a hefty 225 pounds on his 5'10" frame. His mother took him to see the family doctor because he had symptoms such as constant thirst, excessive urination and lethargy. The doctor found he had fasting blood glucose of 350 mg/dL (the normal range is 65–110). Further tests revealed that Michael's **glycosylated hemoglobin** was 9.6 percent (the normal range is 4.0–6.0) and his liver function tests were way up, suggesting he had either fatty liver or hepatitis. The raised insulin levels (suggestive of insulin resistance) confirmed a diagnosis that his doctor didn't expect. Michael had type 2 diabetes. He was only 16 years old.

---

*I*n the past, when a child was diagnosed with diabetes, the typical symptoms of weight loss, dehydration and thirst made it easy to classify as type 1, juvenile onset or insulin-dependent diabetes. In recent years a new picture has emerged:

- Instead of being thin this child is fat, and
- Instead of his or her body not making insulin, it is making lots of insulin.

Michael's story is typical of a health problem that is sweeping the world—type 2 diabetes in children. In North America, up to half of children newly diagnosed with diabetes have type 2. Twenty years ago it was almost unheard of in this age group.

If you are a young person with type 2 diabetes (or if you have a child with type 2), this chapter will tell you what to do about it.

And if you have type 2 diabetes, your children are also at risk for this disease; this chapter will also show you the types of diet and lifestyle changes which will reduce their risk.

YOUNG PEOPLE WITH DIABETES—A NEW EPIDEMIC

There is currently no cure for diabetes. It's for life. Not only that, but children with type 2 diabetes face the same risk of complications as adults with type 2—heart attack, stroke, impotence, blindness, kidney disease. But not when they are old or retired. Children who develop type 2 diabetes will be facing these health problems at the peak of their adult life, when their working and earning capacity is greatest and when they have their own young families to educate and care for. For the individual, the implications are terrible; for the health system, the burden is overwhelming.

For obese children and teenagers, the diagnosis of type 2 diabetes is really just the final straw, because their fatness has an impact on them every day of their lives. It's no fun being fat in a world that equates attractiveness and intelligence with body shape. Maintaining high self-esteem can be very difficult for fat children. Just getting through each day is of much greater concern to them than the high blood pressure, orthopedic problems and high blood fats which commonly precede the diagnosis of type 2 diabetes.

■

**Obese children, in particular older children, are
very likely to become obese adults.**

■

WHICH BABIES AND CHILDREN ARE MOST AT RISK?

We don't know the precise cause of type 2 diabetes (even in adults), but we believe a combination of behavior and environment can trigger the condition in someone who is genetically susceptible.

In North America, most children diagnosed with type 2 diabetes are in the ethnic groups that have a high susceptibility to type 2 diabetes—Native Americans, Hispanics, Pacific Islanders, African Americans, children from the Indian subcontinent and from Asia.

A genetic susceptibility can also come about through a strong family history of type 2 diabetes. For example, we know it's highly likely that a child with type 2 diabetes will have at least one parent or grandparent with type 2 diabetes.

Type 1 diabetes is still the most common form of diabetes in children. But researchers are predicting that in the next decade, we will see type 2 become the dominant form in many ethnic groups. In Japan, for example, it already accounts for 80 percent of all newly diagnosed childhood diabetes.

We know that risk of type 2 diabetes can begin before a baby is born. A pregnant woman's nutritional and health status influences her unborn baby's metabolic characteristics. Exactly how this works is complex, but it is thought to relate to overnutrition or undernutrition.

Scientists have identified a relationship between birth weight and type 2 diabetes: both low (under 5½ pounds) and high (over 9 pounds) birth weight increase the risk of type 2 diabetes in young people. Also, if a mother has gestational diabetes mellitus, her child is more likely to develop type 2 diabetes.

The effect of nutrition on a baby's risk of developing type 2 diabetes later on continues after the baby is born: breastfeeding for the first six months of life is a major protective factor. Breastfeeding may reduce the risk of the baby's consuming excessive calories, as it is associated with lower weight for length (or height). Special fats in breast milk are also thought to improve insulin sensitivity. Babies who are underweight at birth but gain weight rapidly in childhood seem to have the greatest risk of becoming obese and developing glucose intolerance in adulthood.

The link between type 2 diabetes in children and obesity is very strong—around 80 percent of children with type 2 are obese. So it's no surprise to find that the increasing incidence of type 2 in young people parallels the increasing incidence of overweight and obesity.

Overall, approximately 30 percent of children in the United States are overweight and 15 percent are obese. Even more worrying is the prevalence rate—it has more than doubled in the past 20 years.

Why are we only now starting to see a type 2 diabetes epidemic in children and adolescents? Because developing type 2 diabetes lags several years behind becoming overweight or obese. Given the current obesity rates among kids, it is almost inevitable that there will be an epidemic of type 2 diabetes if we don't start doing something about it now.

A major contributor to childhood obesity is lack of physical activity—nowhere near enough exercise, being driven instead of walking, watching TV or sitting in front of computer screens instead of running around and playing. And we also know that less physically active kids are more insulin resistant—another major risk factor for developing type 2.

HOW IS IT DIAGNOSED?

Type 2 diabetes in young people, just as in adults, usually develops over several years, and there may not be any easily recognizable symptoms. Children with type 2 diabetes are usually overweight or obese and have a strong family history of type 2 diabetes. There are a couple of things to watch for:

▶ They are very likely to have acanthosis nigricans, a dark pigmentation of the skin around the neck, which is a marker of insulin resistance, and
▶ Girls are also more likely to have polycystic ovarian syndrome (PCOS).

Just about all the symptoms indicative of type 1 diabetes can occur in a child with type 2 diabetes so diagnosis can be difficult. Blood tests confirming the absence of antibodies against the insulin-producing cells are necessary.

HOW IS IT TREATED?

Managing type 2 in kids is a family affair, and there are some (possibly major) diet and lifestyle changes the whole family is going to have to make. The good news is that these changes are good for everyone's health and well-being.

Who Is Responsible for What?

- Parents are responsible for choosing *when, where* and *what* is available to eat, and
- Children are responsible for choosing *how much* and *even whether* they eat.

Type 2 diabetes can be managed successfully through a combination of regular physical activity, healthy eating and, for some young people, medication, including insulin. The aim is to:

- Normalize blood glucose levels
- Reduce blood fats (cholesterol and triglycerides) and blood pressure, and
- Prevent the progression or development of complications.

One of the key ways to achieve these goals is by managing weight: intake of energy from food has to decrease, and output of energy (physical activity) has to increase.

Whether or not medication is needed depends on how high the blood glucose levels are—particularly when first diagnosed. Insulin injections are usually the first choice, because most of the oral blood glucose–lowering medications have not yet been properly tested in young people. However, metformin is prescribed in some countries, along with insulin. Once the blood glucose levels have come down, you may be able to come off insulin.

HELEN

(mother of a boy who developed type 2 diabetes at age 13)

WE DON'T KNOW the neighbors so the children don't play in the street. I don't think it's safe for them to go to the park on their own. And I certainly don't have time to take them—what with going to work, then cooking, shopping and cleaning—I'm exhausted as it is! They love the TV and PlayStation games and there are lots of good things on the Internet for them. So they don't spend much time outside anymore. It's too far to walk to school so I usually drive them and sports are optional at their school so they spend more time in the library.

Physical Activity

Increasing energy output through physical activity is absolutely essential to managing type 2 diabetes—in adults and children. If you want to see results in terms of fat loss, extra physical activity will bring about improvements more quickly than diet alone, making it a great motivational tool. Also, regular exercise can improve self-esteem, and reduce depression and anxiety.

As is true for adults with type 2 diabetes, a minimum of 30 minutes of some kind of physical activity, most days of the week, is essential. At least double that to lose weight!

Parents: when looking at your lifestyle, think about how you can reduce sedentary behavior and increase planned and incidental activity for everybody.

FAMILY BUSINESS—HOW THE WHOLE FAMILY CAN GET MOVING AND EAT BETTER

Limit screen time

Did you know that 5 hours a week sitting passively instead of moving amounts to more than 2 pounds of body fat not burned off every month? In most families, getting kids to be more active usually starts with limiting screen time—TV, computers, PlayStations, DVDs, movies, etc. An Australian study found that children who watched TV for more than 2 hours per day were more likely to consume high energy snacks and drinks and less likely to participate in organized sports. Currently the average number of "viewing hours" a day is about 4½.

■

If you want to get your kids more active, you have to be more active yourself.

■

Activating your child's day

Parental activity is a strong predictor of a child's activity, so start by taking a long hard look at your own lifestyle and figuring out how you could all move more.

Physical Activity and Insulin

PHYSICAL ACTIVITY USUALLY lowers blood glucose levels because the muscles use more glucose as energy and the body becomes more sensitive to insulin. If you are having insulin injections for your diabetes, you may need to eat extra carbs or reduce the amount of insulin you use (talk to your doctor, dietitian or diabetes educator about this) and test your blood glucose level (BGL) before getting active. While you are doing your physical activity, you may need to be supervised, and you should carry a hypo kit. And remember, a hypo can occur up to 24 hours after you've been active.

It's not hard to increase incidental activity. Get the whole family involved in helping with household tasks (including setting and clearing the table, doing the dishes, making their own beds, cleaning rooms and ironing their own clothes once they are old enough), and family activities (including shopping, sweeping the yard, mowing the lawn and walking the dog).

Planned activity can mean participating in organized sports such as tennis, soccer, baseball, basketball, football, hockey, T-ball, Little League, etc. If your children are not really into organized sports and prefer something individual that they can do at their own pace, there are plenty of other options, such as riding a bike, taking a swim, going for a walk, dancing or a martial art.

Whatever they choose, make sure they enjoy it. If they don't, try something else.

A HEALTHIER FAMILY DIET ✶

There are many approaches to managing the diet of a child with type 2 diabetes. They range from weighed and measured calorie-controlled plans to guided, progressive habit changes such as eating more fruit and limiting the number of snacks. We suggest you and your child see a registered dietitian to discuss and plan the right approach for you— this needs to be someone you are both comfortable talking to and working with over the long haul.

Whatever you do, it helps if the whole family eats the same way. This way you are all in it together and the child with diabetes is supported. Also, it makes meal preparation much easier. The whole family will benefit in terms of health and fitness. What's more, it's very likely that someone else in the family has diabetes too.

The daily food guide in chapter 27 will give you an idea of what's involved and how to get started.

■

**Quick-fix weight loss plans are not a good idea
for children because of children's nutritional
requirements and because type 2 diabetes
is a lifelong condition.**

■

Five of the best

Here are five proven strategies for achieving a healthier household diet:

- Have regular family meals
- Serve a variety of healthy foods and snacks
- Be a good role model by eating healthily yourself
- Involve kids in the process of food choice and preparation, and
- Avoid battles over food.

Have regular family meals

Family meals are a comforting ritual for children and a great way to end the day. Children like the routine and parents get a chance to catch up with what's been going on in everyone's lives. Research suggests other benefits too. Children who take part in regular family meals are also:

- More likely to eat fruits, vegetables and whole grains
- Less likely to snack on unhealthy foods, and
- Less likely to smoke, use marijuana, or drink alcohol.

Independent teenagers may turn up their noses at the prospect of a family meal. But despite what they say, they often do value parental guidance (not interference), so use meal times as a chance to reconnect in a relaxed way. Get to know their friends by inviting them over to dinner, too. Or get some help in the kitchen by involving them in planning and preparation.

What counts as a family meal? Any time you and your family sit down around the table and eat together—whether it's take-out food or a home-cooked meal. Maybe this means you have to eat a little later because you wait until someone gets home from work, or perhaps you set aside breakfast on the weekend as a leisurely family affair. Whenever it is, strive for healthy food (deliciously prepared, of course) and a happy, harmonious atmosphere (without TV).

Serve a variety of healthy foods and snacks

Children, especially younger ones, eat mostly what you have in the pantry, fridge and freezer. That's why it's important (and relatively easy) to control the supply lines—the foods that you serve for meals and have on hand for snacks. Here are some basic guidelines:

- Limit drinks such as fruit juice, fruit punch drinks and soft drinks to once a day: offer water and plain, low-fat milk instead
- Include a low-GI food with each meal: studies have shown that this can have a profound effect on lowering both fasting and overall 24-hour glucose profiles
- Don't put any limits on fruits and vegetables: instead, work on including some at each meal and snack
- Make eating fresh fruit easy by washing, peeling or slicing and presenting it attractively without any competition (like cookies)
- Serve lean meats, fish and poultry rather than sausages and chicken nuggets and include other good sources of protein, such as eggs and nuts
- Limit fat intake by using low-fat dairy products and avoiding deep-fried foods, and
- Avoid packaged snacks (chips, cheesy crackers, cereal and muffin bars) as much as possible: low-fat varieties are not filling and not a good alternative. But don't completely ban your children's favorite snacks—make them one of the "keep for a treat" foods.

■

What's a treat food? It's a food kept for a very special occasion. It's not an every day or even every second day food. Perhaps once a week?

■

Snacks

Children need regular meals and snacks (around 5–6 occasions of eating per day). Young children generally can't meet their energy needs for growth and activity with just three meals. For older children, snacks make up half to a third of their energy intake, so it is important that the snacks you offer contribute as much in terms of nutrients as they do in energy.

If you are on the go or if you find portion control helpful, prepackaged single-serving snacks can be useful. Granola bars, yogurt drinks, yogurt and granola mixes, nut bars, dried fruit and nut mixes, dried fruit bars, packs of cheese slices all fall into this category. But if it comes in a package, read the label carefully and compare brands. Here are some ideas for healthy, portable snacks:

- Fruit-filled cookies (such as Fig Newtons)
- A low-fat flavored milk
- A granola bar
- Fresh fruit, cut up
- Low-fat yogurt
- Handfuls of raw vegetables—carrot sticks, fresh green beans, celery pieces, cucumber, mini tomatoes, bell pepper strips, radishes
- A matchbox-sized piece of cheese
- A handful of dried apple rings
- A small bottle of a yogurt drink
- A cup of vegetable or pumpkin soup with toast fingers
- A slice of fruit toast
- A small cup of fruit salad
- Breakfast cereal and milk
- Dried apricots, raisins and almonds (½ cup)
- Whole-grain crackers with spread.

Why snack?
- Because you're hungry
- To prevent lows and maintain your blood glucose levels between meals
- To pick up an extra serving of fruit or dairy
- To lower the glycemic load of your entrées (by reducing their size)
- To prevent excessive hunger and subsequent overindulgence, and
- To overcome a midafternoon slump in energy levels.

Be a good role model by eating healthily yourself
Dieting is a not a normal way of eating. If you have a controlling and restrictive approach to food, try not to pass it on to your children; get some help yourself. Here's what you should do:

▶ Eat the foods you would like your children to eat, and
▶ Don't classify foods as "good" or "bad" or forbid certain foods.

Instead, teach your kids that all foods can be eaten—some every day, others sometimes. Avoid using food—for example, dessert—as a reward.

Withholding a child's favorite food can make them feel powerless, and is likely to increase their desire for it.

Pushing a child to eat everything on their plate with the temptation of a treat afterwards can condition them to overeat—this is a shame, because they have an excellent built-in ability to sense when they are full.

Involve kids in the process of food choice and preparation

Teach them how to cook. Grow some vegetables: little cherry tomatoes, strawberries or lettuce can easily be grown in pots, and they taste delicious. Take the kids to a farm or orchard when it's picking season. Let them select a new fruit or vegetable to try in the grocery store. Have them shop for food with you (sometimes). Get to know local shopkeepers—at the butcher's, bakery or deli—or the farmers and other purveyors at your local farmers' market. If you're a regular, many will be only too pleased to give a little one a taste of something.

Give Your Taste Buds Time to Adjust

MAKING GRADUAL CHANGES is more successful than making extreme changes overnight. Your taste for fat, for instance, will diminish as you decrease the amount of fat in your food.

It takes about six weeks for your taste buds to adapt to new tastes, so give yourself time.

After a few months on low-fat milk you'll find whole milk way too creamy—it will be too rich for your new palate.

Avoid battles over food

Children are naturally "neophobic"—which means being afraid of new things—so it is normal for them to refuse new foods. Vegetables included! Some people believe this is a protective instinct, but it can be excruciatingly frustrating to parents.

You can work on overcoming this tendency by exposing them often to whatever is the new food, so that pretty soon it is no longer new and unfamiliar. You have to be persistent. Offer a new food 5–10 times in small amounts, without pressuring the child to eat it, and gradually you should see some acceptance. Praise any efforts at tasting new foods.

•27•

Daily Food Guide and Recipes for Children with Type 2 Diabetes

*G*ood nutrition is essential in youth to optimize growth and development. With type 2 diabetes there is the added need to aim for a diet that minimizes the risk of progression or development of complications like blood vessel disease. On average* the daily diet should include something along these lines:

YOUR DAILY FOOD GUIDE

▶ 8–12 servings breads, cereals and other starchy foods
▶ 2–4 servings fruit
▶ 2–3 servings milk products
▶ 2 servings meat or alternatives
▶ 2–4 servings fat-rich foods
▶ 5 or more servings vegetables.

*The daily food guide is designed to meet the nutrient requirements of an overweight teenager (14–18 years) who is active in all daily living and does some regular moderate exercise. It provides 1,550–2,000 calories with approximately 50 percent energy coming from carbohydrate.

How do you fit this into a day?

Here is an example of how these daily food needs can be fitted into a day.

Meal plan for a young person with type 2 diabetes	Daily food servings	Example	Other ideas
Breakfast	4 servings bread, cereal or other starchy food and 2 fat sources	4 slices grain toast with margarine	English muffins, homemade pancakes or muffins
	1 serving fruit juice	a small orange	fresh or dried fruit
	½ serving meat or alternative	2 slices processed cheese	an egg, lean bacon
Midmorning	1 serving fruit	an apple	
Lunch	4 servings bread, cereal or other starchy food	2 slices toast and 1 cup baked beans	bread, rolls, pasta, rice noodles
	1 serving vegetable plus 1 fat serving	½ cup coleslaw	cherry tomatoes, carrot sticks, cucumber
	1 serving milk product	a glass of low-fat milk	yogurt, flavored milk, dairy dessert
	½ serving meat or alternative	an omega-3-rich egg	ham, cheese, canned fish
Midafternoon	1 serving milk product	a container of yogurt	milk, low-fat ice cream
	1 serving fruit	a small banana	
Dinner	4 servings bread, cereal or other starchy food	1 ear of corn and 1 cup mashed potato	legumes, pasta, rice, sweet potato
	1 serving meat or alternative	2–3 trimmed lamb cutlets	chicken, fish, lean ground beef
	4 servings vegetables	2 cups mixed vegetables	any mixture of low-starch veggies
	1 serving fruit	½ cup canned fruit	fresh fruit salad or fruit pops

A YOUNG PERSON WITH TYPE 2 DIABETES— A MENU AND RECIPES FOR THE DAY

Breakfast

Banana and Honey on Toast
A glass of low-fat milk
TOTAL CARBOHYDRATE (G) 58

Lunch

Vegetable Soup with Crunchy Bread Bits
and an apple
TOTAL CARBOHYDRATE (G) 47

Snack

Creamy Corn Dip with Vegetable Sticks and Crispy Dippers
TOTAL CARBOHYDRATE (G) 16

Dinner

Honey Soy Chicken with Asian Slaw
with ½ cup of noodles
TOTAL CARBOHYDRATE (G) 30

Dessert

Apricot and Yogurt Parfait
TOTAL CARBOHYDRATE (G) 20

Nutritional analysis of this daily menu						
ENERGY (CAL)	PROTEIN (G)	FAT (G)	SATURATED FAT (G)	CARBOHYDRATE FAT (G)	FIBER (G)	SODIUM (MG)
1675	90	50	15	175	30	1900

BANANA AND HONEY ON TOAST

PREP TIME: 5 mins ■ COOKING TIME: 2 mins ■ SERVES: 1

2 slices low-GI bread, preferably whole grain

1 small banana

1 tsp pure floral honey

1. Toast the bread.
2. Peel the banana and cut it into thin slices on the diagonal. Lay slices over the warm toast.
3. Drizzle each slice with honey.

PER SERVING
Energy (cal) 265 ■ Protein (g) 8 ■ Fat (g) 3 ■ Saturated fat (g) <1 Carbohydrate (g) 48 ■ Fiber (g) 6 ■ Sodium (mg) 300

VEGETABLE SOUP WITH CRUNCHY BREAD BITS

PREP TIME: 15 mins ■ COOKING TIME: 45 mins ■ SERVES: 4

½ cup split red or green lentils

1½ tbsp olive oil

1 brown onion, peeled and finely chopped

1 clove garlic, crushed or 1 tsp minced garlic

1 large stick celery, finely chopped

2 carrots, chopped into small dice

½ tsp ground cumin

½ tsp paprika

½ tsp ground chili (optional)

2 zucchini, roughly chopped

½ x 28-oz can diced tomatoes in tomato juice

3 cups chicken or vegetable stock

1. Place the lentils in a small bowl and cover with water. Set aside.
2. Heat a large saucepan over medium heat and add oil, then onion, garlic, celery and carrot. Stir over a low heat for 3–5 minutes, until onion is softened.
3. Add the spices to the pan and stir for a minute, then add the drained lentils, zucchini, tomato and stock.
4. Cover and simmer gently for 30–40 minutes, until lentils are soft. Puree with a blender, food processor or food mill, if desired. Serve topped with Crunchy Bread Bits (recipe follows).

PER SERVING
Energy (cal) 245 ■ Protein (g) 10 ■ Fat (g) 7 ■ Saturated fat (g) 1 Carbohydrate (g) 30 ■ Fiber (g) 9 ■ Sodium (mg) 600

CRUNCHY BREAD BITS

PREP TIME: 5 mins ■ COOKING TIME: 10 mins ■ SERVES: 4 (as a garnish)

4 slices low-GI bread

1½ tbsp canola oil

1. Trim the crusts from the bread and cut each piece into small squares.
2. Heat a nonstick frying pan over medium heat and add canola oil. Stir in the bread bits and toss with a wooden spoon every minute or so to crisp and brown all over.
3. Tip onto paper towel and allow to cool before using. They can be kept in an airtight container for 2 days.

CREAMY CORN DIP
WITH VEGETABLE STICKS

PREP TIME: 5 mins ■ COOKING TIME: nil ■ SERVES: 6

1⅛ cup (9 oz) low-fat cottage cheese

5 oz corn relish

2 sticks celery

1 large carrot

1 cucumber

1. Combine the cottage cheese and corn relish in a bowl.
2. Cut the vegetables into finger-sized strips and serve alongside the dip, with Crispy Dippers (recipe follows).

PER SERVING
Energy (cal) 110 ■ Protein (g) 8 ■ Fat (g) 2 ■ Saturated fat (g) 1 Carbohydrate (g) 14 ■
Fiber (g) 2 ■ Sodium (mg) 330

CRISPY DIPPERS

PREP TIME: 5 mins ■ **COOKING TIME:** 10 mins ■ **SERVES:** 4

2 tsp ground cumin

1 tsp dried oregano

½ tsp chili powder (optional)

1½ tbsp sesame seeds

1 tsp salt

1 tsp crushed garlic

olive oil

2 pieces wrap or lavash bread

1. Preheat the oven to 350°F.
2. Mix all the spices, sesame seeds, salt and garlic in a small bowl with enough oil to make a paste.
3. Using a spatula, spread one side of each piece of the bread with the mixture.
4. With a sharp knife, cut each piece of bread into 12 rectangles (3 cuts one way, and 4 cuts the other).
5. Arrange the pieces in a single layer on a baking tray lined with parchment paper. Bake in a moderate oven for 6–8 minutes, or until browned and crisp.
6. Remove from oven and cool on a wire rack. Store in an airtight container.

HONEY SOY CHICKEN WITH ASIAN SLAW

PREP TIME: 25 mins ■ COOKING TIME: 30–40 mins ■ SERVES: 4

1½ tbsp honey

1½ tbsp reduced-sodium soy
  sauce

juice of ½ lemon

1 clove or 1 tsp garlic, crushed

1 tsp grated fresh ginger

½ tsp sesame oil (optional)

½ tsp minced chili (optional)

8 small or 4 large (about 28 oz)
  chicken drumsticks, skin
  removed

1 Combine all the ingredients in a large shallow glass or ceramic dish, adding the chicken last and turning to coat it in the mixture. Set aside for 20 minutes or so while you make the Asian Slaw (or refrigerate overnight).

2 Preheat oven to 390°F. Line a baking tray with parchment paper or aluminum foil. Place the chicken legs on the tray, reserving the marinade. Bake in the hot oven for 10 minutes. Turn, baste with marinade and cook another 10 minutes. Repeat until cooked through (30–40 minutes total, depending on size of drumsticks).

> **PER SERVING**
> Energy (cal) 525 ■ Protein (g) 45 ■ Fat (g) 30 ■ Saturated fat (g) 6
> Carbohydrate (g) 12 ■ Fiber (g) 5 ■ Sodium (mg) 550

ASIAN SLAW

¼ Chinese cabbage, washed,
  trimmed and finely shredded

1 bunch bok choy, washed,
  trimmed and finely shredded

1 large carrot, coarsely grated

3 shallots, trimmed and finely
  chopped

Dressing

⅓ cup olive oil

⅓ cup white wine vinegar

1½ tbsp brown sugar

1½ tbsp chili sauce

1 tsp reduced-sodium soy sauce

1. Place the prepared vegetables in a large salad bowl. Pour over the dressing and toss to combine.

2. Serve the chicken drumsticks with a pile of slaw alongside.

APRICOT AND YOGURT PARFAIT

PREP TIME: 10 mins ■ COOKING TIME: nil ■ SERVES: 4

2 x 16-oz can whole apricots, drained

2 tsp superfine sugar

2½ cups plain low-fat yogurt

3½ tbsp pure maple syrup, or to taste*

1 tsp cinnamon sugar

*plain yogurt varies in tartness, so taste at 2 tbsp and then at 1–2 tsp more

1. Remove pits from apricots and chop apricots. Mix in sugar.
2. In another bowl, whisk yogurt with maple syrup.
3. Serve in 4 drinking glasses (1 cup capacity each). In each glass, place ¼ of apricot mix, then ¼ of yogurt mix, then sprinkle the top with cinnamon sugar. Chill until ready to serve.

PER SERVING
Energy (cal) 122 ■ Protein (g) 7 ■ Fat (g) 2 ■ Saturated fat (g) 1
Carbohydrate (g) 20 ■ Fiber (g) 2 ■ Sodium (mg) 83

Pregnancy, Birth, Breastfeeding and Diabetes

$\mathcal{A}$ woman with diabetes has just as much chance of a healthy baby as anyone else these days, if her diabetes is well controlled before and during pregnancy and her general health is good. So, if you have diabetes, want to have a baby and are trying to make it happen, make sure you're in as good health as you can be. If you don't want to get pregnant, take precautions to make sure it doesn't happen. Unplanned pregnancy with poorly managed diabetes can cause a lot of heartbreak to all involved.

·28·

Diabetes During Pregnancy, Birth and Breastfeeding

*I*n this chapter we cover some of the steps you need to take as you prepare for pregnancy. We focus on the nutritional needs of pregnancy for you and your baby, and on how you can best meet these while managing your diabetes and controlling your blood glucose. We also give you the answers to the questions we are most often asked about pregnancy and diabetes.

If you don't have diabetes before you get pregnant but develop it during pregnancy (gestational diabetes), the section on your diet during pregnancy may be the most useful.

PLANNING FOR PREGNANCY

Your blood glucose levels need to be as good as you can possibly get them *before you conceive*. This is because the first eight weeks (often before you know you are pregnant) is a critical time for your baby's development. It is when the major organs are formed, and optimal blood glucose management is vital. So make some appointments before you start trying for a baby.

■

Optimal diabetes management for pregnancy means HbA1c less than 1 percent above the reference range (generally less than 7 percent).

■

Who should you see before you get pregnant?

Your doctor or diabetes specialist: to discuss what you can do to improve your blood glucose levels and whether any of your medications will need to be changed.

If you have type 1 diabetes, using an insulin pump is one of the options you may want to consider to improve your blood glucose levels before you become pregnant.

If you have type 2 diabetes and you take medication to manage your blood glucose levels, your doctor or diabetes specialist will usually advise you to use insulin from early pregnancy. They will also check your vitamin B_{12} levels if you've been taking metformin.

Talk to your doctor about any other medications you take, including blood pressure and cholesterol medications. Sometimes you have to change medications or stop taking some while you're pregnant.

Some diabetic complications, such as retinopathy and nephropathy, can be made worse by pregnancy. Your doctor will want you to have an eye check (including examination of the retina). If you need laser therapy, do it before you become pregnant. Your kidneys will need to be checked too, and your doctor will also check for major blood vessel disease. In some cases, sadly, the doctor may even advise against trying for a baby.

Your diabetes educator and dietitian: to discuss your diet and exercise program and make sure you know how to deal with morning sickness, hypos and sick days.

As you already know, a major part of good diabetes management is eating healthily. If you begin your pregnancy well nourished, what you eat during pregnancy is not so critical. However, if you've been eating poorly before you get pregnant, a healthy diet during pregnancy is very important to the health of your baby. In chapter 29, you'll find our daily food guide for you and your baby during pregnancy and lactation.

You'll also be advised to take 5 mg of folic acid (folate) a day, from at least one month before conception and throughout the first three months, to prevent neural tube defects.

Stop!

IF YOU SMOKE, quit before conception. Smoking harms the development of your baby. If you want help with quitting, call the Quit Line:

800-QUIT-NOW (800-784-8669)

If you drink, give it up. Alcohol increases the risk of miscarriage and birth defects.

If you use recreational drugs, stop. Like alcohol, these substances increase the risk of miscarriage and birth defects.

YOU AND YOUR TEAM

Managing your diabetes well during your pregnancy means working with a team of health professionals, which may include:

▶ Diabetes specialist/endocrinologist
▶ Dietitian
▶ Obstetrician
▶ Midwife
▶ Diabetes educator

Diabetes and pregnancy clinics at large hospitals generally have all these professionals.

YOUR DIET DURING PREGNANCY

There are some wonderful changes that occur in your body during pregnancy (and some not so wonderful) to create the most favorable environment for the development of your baby. One of these changes relates to how your body absorbs nutrients. The recommended dietary intakes (RDI) for almost all nutrients are increased in pregnancy, and it is clear that your absorption of nutrients increases noticeably when you're pregnant (and breastfeeding) to meet these demands. This in part is thanks to progesterone, a hormone secreted by the placenta: it slows down your digestive tract, giving more time for nutrient absorption. (Incidentally, the slowing down of the digestive tract also contributes to constipation—that's the not so wonderful part.)

The key to providing these important nutrients is the food you eat. As long as you have had a nutritious diet before pregnancy and continue with it during pregnancy, you should be able to meet the recommended nutrient needs without a supplement. There are two possible exceptions—folate and iron.

To help ensure that your diet gives you all the nutrients you need, these are some general guidelines:

- Eat as wide a variety of nutritious foods as possible
- Limit fatty foods, especially those high in saturated fat
- Limit foods and drinks containing large amounts of refined or added sugar or starch with low nutritive value such as soda, candy, chips and other packaged snacks, and
- Avoid alcohol.

See chapter 29 for details of the amounts and types of foods recommended.

COPING WITH MORNING SICKNESS

The biggest influence on your diet when you are first pregnant is probably whether or not you get morning sickness—and if you do, how badly. "Morning" is a bit of a misnomer, as it can happen any time of day (or even last all day). Being tired seems to make it worse. Symptoms can range from periodic mild nausea to constant nausea and vomiting (such as hyperemesis). If you have type 1 diabetes and you get morning sickness, you must always take your insulin, but you may need to lower your dose.

Unfortunately, no one has yet come up with the ideal solution as to what's best to eat to help morning sickness. The following ideas may be useful:

- Aim to eat small amounts of carbohydrate-based foods or drinks frequently over the day. An empty stomach can make you feel worse
- Keep your fluids up, particularly if you're vomiting. If you are unable to eat and your blood glucose levels are less than 270 mg/dL, sip on flat lemonade, a sports drink (like Gatorade), fruit juice or fruit pops. If your blood glucose level (BGL) is greater than 270 mg/dL, sip on low-calorie fluids. If plain water makes you throw up, try crushed ice
- If mornings are a problem, try something first thing, before getting out of bed, such as plain water crackers or dry toast. A box of crackers by the bed can be handy
- Salty foods are sometimes better tolerated, so nibble guilt-lessly on pretzels, potato chips or salty crackers if they are the only food that stays down
- Fatty foods make some women feel worse, but for others it's what they feel like, so try different things and see what suits you best
- Ginger has antinausea properties, so ginger tea, ginger ale or supplements can be helpful, and
- You'll probably be aware that smells can really set some women off, so let those around you know if you want to avoid perfumes, bad breath or the smell of certain foods.

THE VALUE OF FOLATE

Folate (also known as folic acid) is a vitamin that is essential for the normal development of your baby in early pregnancy. Having enough folate in your diet will minimize the risk of neural tube defect (problems with the brain and spine, the most common of which is spina bifida).

You can get folate from green leafy vegetables (spinach, brussels sprouts, broccoli), legumes (chickpeas, soybeans, lentils), whole-grain breads, fortified cereals, and fruits and vegetables.

Your folate requirements are increased in pregnancy, partly because your body has greater nutrient requirements, and partly because estrogen and progesterone interfere with the body's normal folate metabolism. All women are advised to take a folate supplement during pregnancy.

Women with diabetes have an increased risk of having a baby with a neural tube defect, so they are advised to take a daily folate supplement of 5 mg for at least one month before and the first three months after conception.

Listeriosis and Pregnancy

Listeriosis is an illness caused by eating food contaminated with the bacteria *Listeria monocytogenes*. It is rare, and symptoms can be very mild, but the consequences for a pregnant woman can be very serious and the illness can be fatal to an unborn baby. Listeriosis causes inflammation of the brain and spinal cord (meningoencephalitis) and/or infects the blood (septicemia) in unborn and newborn babies.

How can it be prevented?

It is relatively easy to make food safe to eat:

- Freshly prepared food is safe because the bacteria has not had a chance to grow.
- Freshly cooked food is safe because listeria is destroyed during normal cooking.
- Wash raw fruit and vegetables thoroughly before you eat them.

To guard against listeriosis, don't eat:

- Perishable food (such as salad or meat) that has been prepared more than 12 hours earlier, because listeria can grow on these foods, even in the refrigerator
- Refrigerated ready-to-eat food that has not been freshly cooked or prepared: this includes cold meats, salads, soft cheeses and pâté
- Raw meats, raw seafood and unpasteurized milk.

WEIGHT CHANGE

Weight change varies considerably between women during pregnancy. The average weight gain is 25–30 pounds, but you may gain more or less than this and it could still be normal for you. Your baby's birth weight will not necessarily be a reflection of your weight change either. You could gain very little weight and still have a healthy-sized baby.

It is not a good idea to deliberately restrict your food intake in order to limit your weight gain during pregnancy.

A typical weight gain timeline during pregnancy is 2–4 pounds during the first trimester, then a steady average gain of 2–4 pounds a month for the next six months.

MANAGING YOUR BLOOD GLUCOSE LEVELS

This can present a challenge—to you, and to your diabetes team. We don't really know exactly why pregnancy affects blood glucose levels so powerfully, but one cause is a hormone called placental lactogen, which increases insulin resistance by up to 50 percent. This makes it more difficult for the mother's body to take up glucose, which means higher blood glucose levels.

JENNY

(who had gestational diabetes for her second and third pregnancies and developed type 2 diabetes 10 years later)

WITH GESTATIONAL DIABETES you're doing everything for a reason. You're not just doing it for yourself. For me that made it easier to deal with. I knew that the better I kept my blood sugars the easier it would be to get the baby out.

The most important part of your diet to monitor is carbohydrates, because they have the greatest effect on your blood glucose. You need to be clear about which foods are sources of carbohydrates and how they affect your blood glucose levels. You also need to know the low-GI foods that can help you manage your blood glucose levels better. If you take insulin, make sure you know how your insulin dose relates to the amount of carbohydrate you eat and how long your insulin lasts—you may need more snacks.

Home blood glucose monitoring will give you invaluable information on the impact of food on your blood glucose levels—we encourage all women whose pregnancy is complicated by diabetes to do this. Recommended testing times will vary, but many women test four times a day, including in the morning after an overnight fast and two hours after big meals. If you are having insulin injections, it's a good idea to test before meals as well. Make sure you check the results of your monitoring with a health professional regularly. Together you can plan adjustments to your insulin (if you take it) and diet to improve your blood glucose levels.

Here are the key guidelines to help you manage your blood glucose levels.

Eat regularly

While you will need to adjust your meal pattern and timing to your lifestyle and the results of your blood glucose monitoring, eating 3 moderately-sized meals and 2–4 snacks is generally recommended. This has a number of advantages. Eating regular meals and snacks can help you avoid getting overly hungry and then being tempted to "pig out." And if you have type 1 or type 2 diabetes, regular eating times will also make adjusting your insulin easier and help you avoid hypos. A bedtime snack can be particularly helpful to prevent ketosis overnight and avoid hypoglycemia.

Choose low-GI forms of carbohydrates

It is preferable to eat carbs with a low GI. Although there has been very little published work on the use of the GI in pregnancy, a huge body of evidence demonstrates the benefits of low-GI foods in reducing postprandial (after meals) glycemia.

If you can change your staple carbohydrate foods from high-GI to low-GI types, you are likely to see great benefits. We've seen many women who say a change from high-GI white bread to a specific low-GI grain bread keeps their blood glucose levels down and is more filling—and this makes it easier to go easy on the amount of carbohydrates!

ANNETTE

(28 years old, delivered a healthy baby boy)

IF I ATE HIGH-GI white bread, that was it! Bingo! My sugar was high. As long as I had that soy-linseed bread my blood glucose levels were fine and I wasn't as hungry.

Keep a check on how much carbohydrate you eat

Your dietitian will help you work out your carbohydrate requirements for pregnancy and will teach you how to monitor the amount you eat. Your carbohydrate intake generally shouldn't be any less than 40–45 percent of your total daily calorie level (which equates to about 175 grams of carbohydrates per day), but the amount will depend on your usual eating pattern and food preferences.

Hormonal changes in pregnancy (specifically, increasing levels of cortisol and growth hormone) mean that your body will tend to handle carbohydrates less well in the morning, so it could be a good idea to eat fewer carbs then. If high blood glucose levels are a problem after breakfast, talk to your dietitian about reducing your carbohydrates at this meal (to as little as 15–30 grams). You may need to add extra protein foods such as meat, cheese, egg, or fish to satisfy your appetite.

JANINE

I WAS REALLY upset when they told me I had gestational diabetes . . . but it has just been the best thing really. I've learned so much about food and I know how to eat healthily . . . the whole family's changed and we'll stay on the diet . . . I don't want to get diabetes later on, but doing all this now makes me feel like I could handle it.

YOUR BABY AND BLOOD GLUCOSE

Glucose crosses freely from your blood into the baby through the placenta. Your baby makes its own insulin, from about 15 weeks, to handle this glucose. If your blood glucose level (BGL) is high, higher levels of glucose will be transferred to your baby. This stimulates your baby's pancreas to make extra insulin. The extra insulin makes your baby grow bigger and fatter than normal, which presents complications for labor and delivery. It is also believed to have an adverse effect on the baby's later health—obesity and diabetes are more common in children born to women with diabetes.

Q&A

When I have a hypo, does my baby have one too?

No. When your blood glucose is low, it doesn't affect your baby the way it affects you. Babies can maintain their blood glucose by releasing glucose from their liver if there isn't enough glucose coming through the placenta.

Does the insulin I take affect my baby?

Insulin that you take by injection, or insulin that your own body produces, does not cross the placenta. However, insulin that you take has an indirect effect on your baby because of its effect on your blood glucose levels. That's why it's so important to manage your blood glucose levels with insulin really carefully.

If your blood glucose levels go too high, your baby may grow bigger and fatter than normal, and the risk of developing a range of birth defects increases. If they go too low, you and your baby are at risk of accidents, injury, even unconsciousness or death.

Will my baby be born with diabetes?

No. If you have type 1 diabetes the chance of your baby's developing type 1 diabetes is 1.25–2.5 percent; it is actually greater (up to 5 percent) if the baby's father has type 1 diabetes. (If neither parent has diabetes, there is 0.1 percent chance that the baby will develop type 1 diabetes.) However, if your blood glucose levels are not managed well during pregnancy, your baby may be at increased risk of becoming overweight and obese and developing type 2 diabetes later in life.

Breastfeeding is believed to offer some protection against type 1 diabetes: rates of type 1 diabetes are lower when breastfeeding rates are higher. It has also been suggested that early exposure to cow's-milk protein (in infant formula) is involved in the development of type 1 diabetes in infants who have a family history of the condition, but more research is needed to determine whether or not this is a significant problem.

Is It Safe?

IS IT SAFE to drink coffee during pregnancy?

Coffee is a source of caffeine, a stimulant that speeds up your heartbeat, dilates your blood vessels and relaxes smooth muscles. It is definitely harmful in large doses, but moderate consumption (300 mg a day, equivalent to three cups of coffee) is unlikely to pose any significant risk.

Caffeine does, however, interfere with iron absorption. A review of the effects of caffeine consumption on newborn babies showed that if their mother drank more than three cups of coffee a day during pregnancy and the early months of breastfeeding, her breast milk contained one-third less iron than that of mothers who didn't drink coffee.

Approximate caffeine content of beverages

A cup of instant coffee	50 mg
Standard cappuccino	100 mg
A cup of tea made with teabag	45 mg
12-ounce cola soft drink	40 mg
A cup of hot chocolate	5 mg

WHAT TO EXPECT AFTER DELIVERY

What to expect if you have type 1 diabetes

Your blood glucose levels will be lower after delivery, so you will need to take less insulin and be prepared for hypos, especially in the first week. This is the case whether you breastfeed or not, but is more so if you are breastfeeding. Your insulin requirements will remain lower than they were before pregnancy over the next few months but will gradually increase if you are not breastfeeding. You will need to monitor your blood glucose carefully, and restabilize your levels with adjustment of your insulin doses.

What to expect if you have type 2 diabetes

Your blood glucose levels will fall after delivery, and if you took insulin during your pregnancy, you may not need it now. You may well be able to keep your blood glucose levels down just through your diet, especially if you are breastfeeding. If you need medication to manage your blood glucose levels, insulin is recommended—other diabetes medications are okay, but be aware that some, such as metformin, can be passed through to your baby through breast milk.

What to expect if you have gestational diabetes

Your blood glucose levels will be checked for 24 hours after delivery to see whether or not they have returned to normal levels. Your doctor will arrange for you to have an oral glucose tolerance test (GTT) 6–12 weeks after the birth to make sure your blood glucose levels remain normal. In the meantime, focus on healthy eating, weight management and regular physical activity: this will reduce your risk of developing type 2 diabetes in the future. Annual checks of your blood glucose through a doctor are recommended.

BREASTFEEDING

Breastfeeding is recommended for all babies for their first 12 months, and as their sole food for their first 6 months. Breast milk is a unique and perfect gift that only a mother can give to her baby. Whether or not you intend to breastfeed, your breasts are prepared for lactation during pregnancy, and breastfeeding will help you manage your blood glucose levels and will improve your long-term health. When you breastfeed, the fat stores laid down in pregnancy are mobilized, which opens the door to weight loss. This weight loss does not affect your milk volume or content.

To be successful with breastfeeding, try to breastfeed as soon as possible after birth—definitely within the first 4 hours. Prolactin, a hormone produced by your body in response to suckling, initiates your milk production. Early and frequent feeding will improve your prolactin production and help you establish breastfeeding. If it isn't possible to have your baby with you all the time, expressing milk by hand or pump will also help increase your prolactin levels. For women with type 1 diabetes, the time for milk to "come in" (normally about day 3 after the birth) may be delayed for 24–48 hours due to lower prolactin secretion, but if you stick with it, it will happen!

Your blood glucose levels may fall rapidly during and after breastfeeding. If you have type 1 diabetes, you will need about 25 percent less insulin than your prepregnancy dose. Once breastfeeding is established and your insulin dose is adjusted, the way to prevent hypos is to eat more, not keep dropping your insulin dose.

A blood glucose test before feeding will give you an indication of whether or not your insulin dose is correct—and an idea of how much carbohydrate you might need for a snack. It's important to get it right: not enough insulin may inhibit milk production, and too much causes hypos, which stimulate the release of adrenaline, which in turn inhibits milk production.

If My Blood Sugar Is High, Will My Breast Milk Be Higher in Sugar, Too?

NO. YOUR BLOOD glucose concentration does not affect the glucose concentration of your breast milk.

Don't worry if you feel hungry all the time. Like all new mothers, you do need to eat more when you are breastfeeding: 400 extra calories per day is recommended. For a typical woman, this means eating about 25 percent more food than usual. You'll probably find that your appetite will increase. Your carbohydrate requirements may vary according to your baby's feeding pattern. When your baby is feeding a lot, you may need to increase your carbohydrates; and maybe you'll need to cut down if your baby is unwell or if she/he is feeding less.

What Foods Should You Avoid While Breastfeeding?

IN GENERAL THERE are no foods that a breastfeeding mother shouldn't eat, but you should certainly be careful with caffeine and alcohol. We recommend eating a wide variety of foods, to increase your chances of getting all the nutrients your body needs. This will also introduce your baby to a greater range of flavors, which may improve his/her acceptance of foods later.

People may tell you to avoid strongly flavored food such as garlic, or "gassy" vegetables such as cauliflower, but there is actually no good evidence to support this. In fact, studies show babies prefer milk after their mother has consumed some flavors like garlic, and of course there are many women around the world who eat these things every day and have happily breastfed babies.

If you have a family history of food allergy, be careful about your diet and avoid known allergens when pregnant and breastfeeding.

Caffeine is excreted into breast milk and will peak 1 hour after you have drunk anything containing it. If you have your caffeine drinks after a breastfeed rather than before, the caffeine concentration in your breast milk will be lower. Newborns metabolize caffeine very slowly, which means caffeine can accumulate in a baby if the mother is consuming caffeine regularly. Occasional caffeine consumption is believed to have little effect on breastfed babies, but it is advisable to limit your caffeine intake to less than 300 mg per day (see the Is it Safe? box on page 289).

Alcohol consumption should be minimized while you are breastfeeding, especially during the first 3 months. It does enter breast milk, and appears at levels about equal to the levels in the mother's bloodstream. Studies have shown that within 30 minutes of drinking 1 standard drink, there are changes to the smell of breast milk and it will have a mildly sedative effect on a baby. In the first few weeks of life, babies cannot detoxify alcohol at the same rate an adult can, so the effect of alcohol is likely to be greater on your baby. If you do drink alcohol, try not to breastfeed for 2–3 hours afterward.

Is your baby getting enough milk?

As long as you put your baby to the breast on demand, rather than trying to stick to a rigid feeding schedule, your body will make enough milk to meet the demand. How much milk you make is largely determined by your baby and how often your baby feeds.

The composition of the milk depends in part on what you are eating and in part on your body's overall nutritional stores. If your diet is low in vitamin C, for example, the vitamin C content of your breast milk will fall. An extra glass of fruit juice or 1 or more servings of fresh fruit will meet the extra vitamin C requirement.

Diet tips while breastfeeding

▶ Snack before or while feeding: keep a glass of milk or fruit juice handy.
▶ Drink at least 2 liters of fluids a day, and
▶ Test your blood glucose levels after you feed your baby, especially during the night, to prevent nocturnal hypos, and consider a reduction in long-acting insulin if they do occur.

See chapter 29 for details of what and how much to eat.

▪ 29 ▪

Diabetes During Pregnancy and Breastfeeding:
Your Daily Food Guide and Recipes

*D*uring pregnancy there is a small increase in energy requirements during the second and third trimesters of pregnancy, but you don't have to eat for two. Only about 290 calories per day extra are required—two extra servings of fruit plus an extra meat or alternative serving, for example. It is important that the extra calories come from nutrient-rich foods. If you are eating the suggested minimum daily servings of each food group, your appetite is your best guide to whether you are eating enough, unless you are gaining too much weight.

YOUR DAILY FOOD GUIDE DURING PREGNANCY

▶ 6–10 servings breads, cereals and other starchy foods
▶ 2–3 servings fruits
▶ 2 servings milk products
▶ 3 servings meat and alternatives

▶ 3 servings fat-rich foods
▶ 5–6 servings vegetables

The daily food guide provides between 1,800–2,300 calories, with 40–50 percent of energy from carbohydrates. At the lower calorie level, iron (15 milligrams) and folate (500 micrograms) contents are less than the recommended daily intake (RDI) for pregnancy (27 milligrams and 600 micrograms, respectively), so a supplement is recommended. At the higher calorie level the iron content meets the average requirement but a supplement would still be a good idea if you are not eating iron-fortified foods.

HOW DO YOU FIT THIS INTO A DAY?

This sample meal plan illustrates one way of distributing the recommended servings of foods over the day. For a meal plan that is individualized to your needs, we suggest you consult a dietitian.

Meal plan for pregnancy	DAILY FOOD SERVINGS	EXAMPLE	OTHER IDEAS
Breakfast	2 servings bread, cereal or other starchy food	1½ cups muesli with ½ cup All-Bran	toast, granola, oatmeal or a low-GI cereal
	1 serving milk product	1 cup low-fat milk	milk or yogurt for cereal
Snack	2 servings bread, cereal or other starchy food with 1 serving fat-rich food	2 slices grain toast topped with 2 teaspoons margarine	whole-grain crackers with avocado
Lunch	2 servings bread, cereal or other starchy food + 1 serving fat	2 fresh medium corn cobs with 1 teaspoon margarine	2 thick slices of grain bread
	1 serving fruit	⅓ cantaloupe	diced apple
	1 serving meat or alternative	6-ounce can tuna	2 ounces cheddar cheese
	2 servings vegetables + 1 serving fats	2 cups chopped mixed salad vegetables with 1 tablespoon dressing	lettuce, celery, walnuts and mayonnaise

Meal plan for pregnancy	DAILY FOOD SERVINGS	EXAMPLE	OTHER IDEAS
Snack	1 serving vegetables + 1 serving fruit	1 large glass fresh squeezed carrot and apple juice	commercial boxed fruit and vegetable juice
Dinner	2 servings bread, cereal or other starchy food	1 cup Asian noodles	rice, chickpeas
	2 servings meat or alternative	7 ounces lean beef strips	chicken, fish
	3 servings vegetables + ½ serving fat-rich food	stir-fried mix of broccoli, onion, peppers, snow peas, baby corn	at least 1½ cups cooked vegetables
Snack/dessert	1 serving milk product	1 cup low-fat fruit yogurt	milk, low-fat ice cream
	1 serving fruit	½ cup diced peach and pear	any fresh, dried or canned fruit

WHAT IF I'M BREASTFEEDING

During lactation you need to eat more from most food groups, except meat and alternatives because your iron needs are not as high as they are during pregnancy. An average* guide should include the following:

- 8–10 servings breads, cereals and other starchy foods
- 4–5 servings fruits
- 2 servings milk products
- 2 servings meat and alternatives
- 3 servings fat-rich foods
- 6+ servings vegetables

*The daily food guide provides 1,980–2,200 calories, with 50 percent of energy coming from carbohydrates. It meets the RDI for all the nutrients we have food composition data on.

HOW DO YOU FIT THIS INTO A DAY?

It might look like a lot of food—let your appetite guide you with quantities if you are in doubt.

Meal plan for breastfeeding	Daily food servings	Example
Breakfast	4 servings bread, cereals or other starchy foods	2 slices thick-cut grain bread
	1 serving vegetables	pan-fried tomato, mushroom and onion
	1 serving meat or alternative	2 omega-3-rich eggs
	1 serving fruit	a small apple juice
Snack	1 serving fruit with 2 servings fat-rich foods	2 ounces mixed dried fruit and nuts
Lunch	3 servings bread, cereal or other starchy foods	one round of Lebanese flat bread
	½ serving meat or alternative	a couple of thin slices of cooked chicken or beef
	3 servings vegetables	tomato, onion, lettuce
	1 serving milk product	a glass of low-fat milk
Snack	1 serving milk product with 1 serving fruit	1 cup of mixed berries with 1 cup of vanilla yogurt
Dinner	½ serving meat or alternative	1 ounce grated parmesan cheese
	2 servings other starchy foods	1 cup of cooked pasta
	3 servings vegetables	1½ cups tomato and vegetable pasta sauce
	1 serving fruit	handful of black grapes
Snack/dessert	1 serving bread or cereal 1 serving fat-rich food	a slice of raisin toast topped with margarine
	1 serving fruit	a couple of fresh plums

A MENU AND RECIPES FOR THE DAY
FOR A PREGNANT WOMAN WITH DIABETES

Breakfast

Cheese, Corn and Mushroom Muffin
and ¾ cup fresh orange juice
TOTAL CARBOHYDRATE (G) 45

Snack

Dried Fruit and Nut Mix
TOTAL CARBOHYDRATE (G) 30

Lunch

Roast Beef on Rye with Baby Spinach and Horseradish Cream
TOTAL CARBOHYDRATE (G) 40

Snack

1 glass low-fat milk
and 2 slices raisin toast
TOTAL CARBOHYDRATE (G) 45

Dinner

Atlantic Salmon with Citrus Sauce
with 1 cup mashed sweet potato
steamed broccoli, zucchini and carrot
TOTAL CARBOHYDRATE (G) 45

Dessert

Fruit Salad with Low-Fat French Vanilla Yogurt
TOTAL CARBOHYDRATE (G) 38

ENERGY (CAL)	PROTEIN (G)	FAT (G)	SATURATED FAT (G)	CARBOHYDRATE (G)	FIBER (G)	SODIUM (MG)
2365	130	75	20	275	45	2000

Nutritional analysis of this daily menu

CHEESE, CORN AND MUSHROOM MUFFIN

PREP TIME: 5 mins ■ COOKING TIME: 5 mins ■ SERVES: 1

1 whole-grain English muffin

3 tbsp creamed corn

3 small fresh mushrooms, thinly sliced

2 oz reduced-fat cheddar cheese, thinly sliced or grated

1. Split the English muffin in half and toast or grill lightly.

2. Spread the cut half of each muffin with creamed corn and top with mushroom slices. Place under a broiler for 2 minutes, until the mushroom slices begin to soften.

3. Remove from the broiler. Top with the cheese and return to the broiler for 1 minute to melt the cheese. Serve immediately.

PER SERVING
Energy (cal) 335 ■ Protein (g) 24 ■ Fat (g) 13 ■ Saturated fat (g) 8
Carbohydrate (g) 30 ■ Fiber (g) 6 ■ Sodium (mg) 750

DRIED FRUIT AND NUT MIX

PREP TIME: 5 mins ■ COOKING TIME: none ■ SERVES: 2

10 dried apple rings

6 dried apricot halves

20 almonds

10 walnut halves

1½ tbsp raisins

1. Combine all ingredients in a small airtight container and carry as a portable snack.

PER SERVING
Energy (cal) 305 ■ Protein (g) 6 ■ Fat (g) 17 ■ Saturated fat (g) 1
Carbohydrate (g) 30 ■ Fiber (g) 6 ■ Sodium (mg) 9

ROAST BEEF ON RYE WITH BABY SPINACH AND HORSERADISH CREAM

PREP TIME: 5 mins ■ COOKING TIME: none ■ SERVES: 1

2 slices dark rye bread

1 tsp canola margarine (reduced sodium)

2 oz lean roast beef, thinly sliced

1 tsp horseradish cream

½ small tomato, thinly sliced (optional)

handful of baby spinach leaves

black pepper

1. Lightly spread the bread with the margarine and top one slice with the roast beef.

2. Spread the horseradish cream over the beef and top with slices of tomato then the spinach leaves. Grind some pepper over the spinach, then top with the other slice of bread.

PER SERVING
Energy (cal) 360 ■ Protein (g) 25 ■ Fat (g) 9 ■ Saturated fat (g) 3
Carbohydrate (g) 40 ■ Fiber (g) 7 ■ Sodium (mg) 660

ATLANTIC SALMON WITH CITRUS SAUCE

*I*t's hard to beat Atlantic salmon as a source of omega-3 fats.

PREP TIME: 10 minutes ■ **COOKING TIME:** 10 minutes ■ **SERVES:** 2

---

1 tsp olive oil

2 Atlantic salmon cutlets (about 14 oz in total)

2 tsp canola-based margarine

finely grated rind or zest of 1 lemon

2½ tbsp lemon juice

1 shallot, finely chopped or 1½ tbsp finely chopped fresh chives

1½ tbsp finely chopped fresh parsley

black pepper

1. Heat a frying pan (or grill) over medium heat and oil lightly. Add the salmon and cook about 3 minutes each side, until beginning to brown. Turn once only. Transfer to a plate and cover to keep warm.

2. Add the margarine to the frying pan (or a separate small pan), followed by the lemon rind, juice and herbs. Stir over low heat until combined.

3. Serve the salmon drizzled with the lemon and herbs, and grind a little pepper over it.

PER SERVING
Energy (cal) 340 ■ Protein (g) 40 ■ Fat (g) 20 ■ Saturated fat (g) 4
Carbohydrate (g) 1 ■ Fiber (g) 0 ■ Sodium (mg) 134

FRUIT SALAD WITH LOW-FAT FRENCH VANILLA YOGURT

PREP TIME: 10 mins ■ **COOKING TIME:** none ■ **SERVES:** 2

---

1 small apple, cored and cubed

1 small pear, cored and cubed

1 small orange or mandarin, peeled and cut into segments

1 small bunch of grapes

½ cup strawberries, hulled and chopped

1¼ cups low-fat French vanilla yogurt

1. Mix all fruits in one large bowl, then divide into 2 serving bowls.
2. Add equal amounts of yogurt to each bowl and serve chilled.

PER SERVING
Energy (cal) 215 ■ Protein (g) 10 ■ Fat (g) 1 ■ Saturated fat (g) 0 Carbohydrate (g) 40 ■ Fiber (g) 6 ■ Sodium (mg) 120

Managing
Type 1 Diabetes

$\mathcal{T}$ype 1 diabetes is one of the most common childhood diseases. At the moment, half the people with type 1 diabetes are diagnosed before they are 16 years old. Ways of managing type 1 diabetes vary slightly depending on age. For children and teenagers, for example, who are still growing and developing, it is absolutely essential that you do everything possible to achieve and maintain optimal blood glucose levels. Poorly managed diabetes, particularly before puberty, can mean that children don't reach their full growth potential—this isn't an area where you get the chance to go back and try again.

In adulthood, the focus shifts slightly to maintaining good health and preventing the common complications of diabetes. This is also the time when people choose a life partner, settle down and have children of their own. If you are a woman, good health and optimal blood glucose are vital when you want to start your own family.

• 30 •

Living with
Type 1 Diabetes

KYLIE

WHEN KYLIE WAS 6, she was always thirsty and going to the toilet, and she felt very lethargic and had no energy. She had also lost a lot of weight, despite eating what seemed to her mom huge amounts of food. Her mom and dad were very concerned and took her to see their family doctor, who immediately arranged for Kylie to be admitted to the local children's hospital for some tests. In the hospital, the doctors checked her blood glucose level (BGL) and found it was very high—465 mg/dL (25.7 mmol/L) (the usual range is 70–110 mg/dL.

Kylie had type 1 diabetes.

In this chapter we cover the general nutritional guidelines for managing type 1 diabetes. Chapters 31–34 cover the specifics of type 1 diabetes for infants and toddlers, school-age children, teenagers and adults.

As we have done in the rest of this book, we are talking here to the individual with diabetes, but we know that many of our readers will be parents with toddlers or young children with diabetes. Obviously, parents must be involved in all aspects of a toddler's or young child's diabetes management, but as children get older, it's a good idea for them to get more involved in their diabetes management routines.

YOUNG PEOPLE WITH DIABETES

Generally, children and adolescents who have diabetes have the same basic nutritional requirements as children and adolescents who don't have diabetes—remember, what's good for someone with diabetes is good for the whole family.

Nutrition for Young People with Type 1 Diabetes

YOU NEED TO eat essentially the same foods that everybody needs for long-term health and well-being:

- Plenty of vegetables, legumes (such as beans, peas and lentils) and fruits
- Plenty of cereals, including breads, rice, pasta and noodles, preferably whole grain and those with a low GI
- Moderate amounts of lean meat, fish, poultry and/or alternatives such as legumes, nuts, seeds, and
- Dairy foods such as milks, yogurts, cheeses and/or alternatives (soy milk, for example)—choose reduced-fat varieties whenever you can.

You need to cut back on foods that are:

- High in total and saturated fat
- High in salt, and/or
- High in added refined sugars and starches.

Here are two key tips for parents:

▶ Don't single out the child with diabetes and make them eat radically different foods from the rest of the family, and
▶ Try to get the whole family to eat similar foods—it will benefit everyone.

If you have diabetes, the ultimate aim for eating a healthy diet is to make sure that your food gives you:

▶ Enough energy (calories), protein, fats, carbohydrates, vitamins and minerals for normal growth and physical development, but not so much that you gain too much weight, and
▶ The right quantity and quality of carbohydrates so that you can keep your blood glucose levels near the recommended range (65–110 mg/dL) without having too many episodes of severe hypoglycemia and/or prolonged hyperglycemia.

One of the biggest challenges for you and your family is keeping your blood glucose levels within the recommended range, without too many episodes of hypoglycemia or hyperglycemia, while you are still growing and developing. This is no mean feat. It requires a combination of individualized meal planning, food selection, blood glucose self-monitoring, flexible insulin regimens and ongoing diabetes education and support.

Ideally, you and your family will have access to a diabetes management team similar to the one we talked about in chapter 5—and in particular, a registered dietitian.

Your dietitian will talk to you and your parents and make suggestions based on the foods you usually eat. You can of course review this as you grow or become more active. Your endocrinologist and diabetes educator will work out with you and your parents which insulin type, dose and frequency will suit your lifestyle and your preferred eating habits. When they set up these kinds of routines, your diabetes management team will look at all sorts of factors to make sure that they will work for you and your family.

First, they will talk about your whole family's eating habits. Often these are related to your cultural and religious background. For example, families from a Mediterranean background may usually eat meals with pasta, olive oil, lean meats (but perhaps not pork) and legumes, and families from an Asian background may usually eat rice, noodles, soy-bean products and seafood. No one is going to try to make you and your family eat food you don't want to eat.

Another important thing your team will talk about is when you and your family normally have meals together (if you do!), and when your meal breaks are at school or at work. With parents working longer hours and travel times to and from school and work in major capital cities increasing, breakfast may be very early in the morning and dinner relatively late in the evening. Your insulin regimen has to take all this into account; some people have to find some time during the day for snacks and other meal breaks. This may be necessary in schools and workplaces where break times are highly regimented.

How active you are is the third factor your team will take into account, because it can vary considerably from day to day. Some days you may have physical education classes at school, sports training or competitions after school or other after-school or work activities (such as dancing or martial arts sports); other days you may spend more time studying, having coaching, playing with friends or watching TV. Your diabetes management plan has to take all this into account.

COUNTING YOUR CARBS—WHAT'S THE BEST WAY?

Most people who have type 1 diabetes need to eat similar amounts of carbohydrate-containing foods, at regular times, each day. While the days of matching your foods to a rigid insulin regime are long gone, it is still important to maintain a regular eating pattern.

Exchanges: Beginning in the 1950s, people with type 1 were taught to use the American Diabetes Association's Carbohydrate Exchange lists, where all items contained approximately 15 grams of carbohydrate per serving, or the European Carbohydrate Portions List, with 10 grams of carbohydrate per serving. These lists focused on the major food groups that had similar macronutrient (carbohydrates, fat and protein) levels, and the theory was that the foods within any particular group were interchangeable because they would have the same impact on your blood glucose levels. Although the GI has proved that this assumption is not correct, many people still like to use the basic principles of exchanges or portions to estimate the amount of carbohydrates they need to eat at each meal to match the amount of insulin they are taking. Few people, however, stick to these exchange lists as strictly as people did in the past.

Measuring Your Blood Glucose

SOME PEOPLE MEASURE their blood glucose levels 2 hours after a meal to see whether their blood glucose level (BGL) is less than 180 mg/dL. If you check yours and it's not, you may need to eat more of the low-GI carbohydrates and less of the high-GI varieties, less total carbohydrate, or have more short or rapid-acting insulin. If you are not sure what's best for you, talk to your dietitian and doctor.

DAFNE (Dose Adjustment For Normal Eating): The DAFNE program, which was developed in the United Kingdom, uses 10-gram carbohydrate portions because they are easier to use in making your insulin calculations. But one of the fundamental differences with the DAFNE program (compared with the old exchanges) is that you adjust the insulin to match the food you are eating, rather than adjusting your food to match your insulin. Because labeling on packaged foods today is also so much better than it was 50 years ago, you don't need to be as dependent on an exchange list—you can work out the amount of carbohydrates in your favorite food yourself simply by looking at the nutrition information panel.

What about sugar? You don't need to completely avoid table sugar, but if you or the family cook or add it to foods, remember that each teaspoon adds 5 grams of carbohydrate. So if you have more than one or two, you may need to eat less of another carbohydrate-containing food or have more insulin, or both. While they're not absolutely necessary, nonnutritive sweeteners such as Splenda and Nutrasweet can add sweetness without the extra carbohydrates or calories. They can be particularly useful when you need to use more than half a cup of sugar—that way refined sugars won't displace healthier choices, or add to your waistline.

CARB QUANTITY: YOUR OPTIONS

1. Working out how many exchanges or portions there are in a serving of food

The nutrition panel on food packages lists the amount of total carbohydrate in a serving of that food and the number of servings per container. If you eat the amount that the manufacturer defines as a serving, you can use that value; otherwise, you need to adjust the carbohydrate amount accordingly. For example, if you eat two servings, multiply the total carbohydrate amount by 2.

To work out the number of exchanges, you divide the amount of carbohydrate per serving by 15; to work out portions, divide it by 10.

Example of how to calculate exchanges/portions:

NUTRITIONAL INFORMATION	
Serving size:	14 g (approx. 2 breadsticks)
Servings:	about 9
Carb Amount/Serving:	7.4 g

This is the nutrition information from a package of breadsticks.

The manufacturer has provided information on a serving size of 14 grams (2 breadsticks). There are 18 breadsticks in the package. If you eat half the package (9 breadsticks), your serving size is 9 ÷ 2 × 7.4 grams = 33 grams of carbs.

So your half-package serving of 9 breadsticks contains 33 grams of carbs. Dividing this by 15 gives you about 2 exchanges.

2. Counting carbs

Instead of converting the grams of total carbohydrate in a food into exchanges or portions, today many people simply count carbs in grams. This works well if you use an insulin pump—pumps have much more precise control over the amount of insulin delivered in a bolus, so you can match it more precisely to the amount you have eaten.

REALITY CHECK. Don't get too carried away thinking that by counting every gram of carbohydrates you eat and every 0.05 of a unit of insulin you take your blood glucose levels will be perfect. It just doesn't happen like this. It's a fact of life that even the most processed of foods never contain exactly the same amount of carbohydrates in a serving as the label says.

How does this happen? Well, what's printed on the label is actually an average amount of carbohydrates per serving for that food. There are small and completely natural variations in the amount of carbohydrates in food depending on where it is grown and the actual crop variety (different wheats and rices, for example, can have a different carb quantity and quality). Manufacturing and processing techniques produce small variations, too. This, along with the small differences you introduce each time you prepare yourself a "serving," all adds up. So you can see how easily a 10–20 percent variation in the carbohydrate content of a food from what is printed on a food label can happen. It's not illegal either: food regulators such as the United States Food and Drug Administration (FDA) recognize the natural variability of foods and allow for this when they make the labeling regulations.

Another reason your blood glucose levels won't be as perfect as planned is that following highly prescriptive meal plans based on exact amounts of carbohydrates to suit your insulin dose is no longer recommended. Why? First, most people found these plans impossible to stick to for the long term, and second, they found their quality of life really suffered because enjoying any kind of social event involving food was impossible. Research over the years (such as the Diabetes Control and Complications Trial [DCCT] in the United States and the Dose Adjustment for Normalized Eating in the United Kingdom) has clearly shown that it's usually better to adjust the insulin to match the amount of carbohydrate eaten.

TYPICAL INSULIN REGIMES

There are lots of different insulin regimens used to manage type 1 diabetes. However, there are three main types that are used by the vast majority of people, plus one less common method that is rapidly growing in popularity throughout the world. They are:

- ▶ Twice-daily injections
- ▶ Three injections a day
- ▶ Multiple daily injections, and
- ▶ Insulin pump therapy.

Twice-daily injections

This is the most common regimen used by young children (3 out of 5) because it is the simplest. It usually involves a combination of short or rapid-acting and intermediate-acting insulins injected twice daily, usually before breakfast and before the evening meal.

If you follow this regimen you need to make sure that your daily meal plan consists of three main meals and three smaller snacks a day based on carbohydrate-containing foods. Try not to miss meals and snacks or delay them too long—hypoglycemia may occur.

Three injections a day

Many older children and teenagers use this approach, when a twice-daily regimen is no longer adequate. A mixture of short or rapid-acting and intermediate-acting insulins is given before breakfast, short or rapid-acting insulin is given before the afternoon snack or main evening meal and intermediate-acting insulin is given in the evening.

If you follow this regimen you usually need to have three main meals and three smaller snacks a day based on carbohydrate-containing foods.

Multiple daily injections

This is the preferred regimen for older adolescents and adults—the Diabetes Control and Complications Trial clearly showed that it achieved the best blood glucose levels, and reduced the risk of diabetic complications the most. It usually involves a total of four injections a day, with short or rapid-acting insulin taken before each main meal and intermediate- or long-acting insulin taken before bed. This regimen gives you more flexibility in meal timing and in the quantity of carbohydrate eaten at meals, and is usually better suited to the lifestyle of older adolescents and adults.

If you follow this regimen, the suggested meal plan is three main meals and an evening snack based on carbohydrate-containing foods. Morning and afternoon snacks are not necessary but you can have them if you want to.

Insulin pump therapy

Insulin pump therapy provides a continuous infusion of a small volume of insulin into the body, and additional insulin bolus doses can be administered by the click of a button for each carbohydrate-containing meal or snack you eat. As you can imagine, it gives you far more flexibility in relation to what and when you eat than injection regimes do. Overall, research has found that insulin pump therapy improves average blood glucose levels slightly more than a multiple daily injection regimen, and most people feel it improves their quality of life.

If you are using insulin pump therapy you can delay or miss meals and snacks and vary their carbohydrate content to suit your needs, with the insulin bolus easily adjusted to fit in.

Did you know?

The quality of insulin pumps has improved dramatically over the past decade.

With most United States health insurance companies covering the purchase cost and ongoing supplies, insulin pump therapy is a viable option for many people with type 1 diabetes in North America.

In Canada, most group health insurance policies provide assistance with the expense of pumps and supplies—you can contact the Canadian Diabetes Association to find programs that helps subsidize the costs of insulin pump therapy.

> WE KNOW THAT how much insulin you take before you eat affects what your blood glucose does afterward—depending on the quantity and quality of the carbs in the meal or snack. Your best option is to adjust your premeal insulin doses according to how much carbohydrate you intend eating for your meal or snack.
>
> If you aren't confident enough to adjust your own insulin doses and prefer to keep them fixed, it is very important to be consistent in the amount of carbohydrates you eat every day.

· 31 ·

Type 1:
Infants and Toddlers
(Plus Daily Food Guide and Recipes)

INFANTS

$\mathcal{D}$**iabetes is pretty** rare in infants under the age of 6 months, but it does occur: around 2 in 100,000 cases. Or to put it another way, less than 1 percent of all people with diabetes are diagnosed in the first year of life. However, when it does occur, it can be pretty scary—very much an unwanted complication in what for many new parents is already a pretty stressful period.

Breast or bottle?

Breastfeeding is recommended by the World Health Organization for the first 2 years of life and for as long as mother and child wish to continue after that. Ideally, breast milk should be the only food for the first 6 months of life. This is important for all infants, whether they have diabetes or not.

If you decide not to breastfeed, use an appropriate infant formula—there are many to choose from, but most are suitable; ask your dietitian if you are not sure.

Regular breast or bottle feedings approximately every 3 hours will help maintain blood glucose levels in infants with diabetes.

What about solids?

Early introduction of solids is not recommended. You can introduce them from about 6 months, beginning with small amounts of rice cereal, then vegetables, then fruits. At this stage, don't be concerned about getting your baby to eat a certain quantity of carbohydrate-containing food at a particular time. Simply let them get to know and enjoy the taste and texture of foods; let them rely more on breast milk or formula for their essential carbohydrates.

WHAT ARE THE OPTIMAL BLOOD GLUCOSE LEVELS FOR BABIES, TODDLERS AND PRESCHOOLERS?

Blood glucose targets for infants and young children are 90–215 mg/dL before a meal and 125–215 mg/dL at bedtime. This range gives them protection from hyperglycemia and reduces the risk of severe hypoglycemia.

These blood glucose levels are slightly higher than you might expect. This is because infants and young children cannot recognize the symptoms of low blood glucose, and repeated episodes of severe hypoglycemia in infants and young children can lead to mild intellectual or learning impairment later in life.

WHAT ABOUT HYPOS?

Even with careful management, your baby will probably have a hypo occasionally. Of course the baby will not be able tell you about it, so you need to become attuned to the typical signs, such as: a particular cry; becoming pale or cranky; sweating or trembling; developing a bluish tinge to fingers or lips; or increased clumsiness.

If you see any of these signs, it's time to check your baby's blood glucose levels. If you cannot do it right away, treat your baby as if he or she is having a hypo anyway—it's safer than waiting. Brain and nervous system development requires a constant supply of glucose, so preventing low blood glucose levels in infants is a very high priority.

What is the best way to treat a baby's hypo?

Because babies are small, it usually doesn't take much carbohydrate to bring their blood glucose level (BGL) up. For a mild hypo, a breast or bottle feed may be enough (and is probably the most comforting for baby). For a more severe hypo, give glucose syrup on a dummy or a small soft spoon, followed by a breast or bottle feed. Your diabetes team might also give you instructions on using **glucagon** (an injection)—this would be necessary only if blood glucose levels fall very low and baby is unable to feed.

TODDLERS

While diabetes is more common in toddlers than in infants, it's still less than 10 percent of all cases that are diagnosed before the age of 5 years.

Obviously, it is very necessary for you as parents to be involved in all aspects of your child's diabetes management at this early age, but gradually encouraging and helping your child participate in general diabetes management routines is recommended as they get older.

To decrease anxiety for you both, it's often helpful to invent games to play around the diabetes procedures. Perhaps you can encourage your toddler "to practice" on one of their favorite teddy bears or dolls.

Use lots of praise, plenty of hugs and kisses, hand stamps and stickers and tiny toys—all positive nonfood reinforcements—rather than scolding or threats of punishment if they refuse various aspects of their diabetes management.

Normal developments such as teething, growth spurts and immunization are all factors which may upset your toddler's eating and physical activity patterns and therefore raise blood glucose levels for a few days at a time.

Getting children to eat is probably one of the biggest issues at this age for all parents. In general, toddlers tend to eat erratically and have pretty unpredictable activity levels. And their appetite tends to fluctuate throughout the day depending on how active they are. So they have to regulate their own food intake, which means set meal plans of three meals and three snacks a day for toddlers are usually impractical—they're generally not recommended. Instead, most toddlers will "graze" on small amounts of food throughout the day.

Tantrums, food fads and food refusal are not uncommon at this age and stage. It may also look to you as if they are eating less. Don't worry too much—they need less because their growth rate has slowed down, compared with the rate in their first year. The best thing you can do is offer as big a variety of foods as you can so that your toddler develops an appreciation of different food tastes and textures, with an emphasis on finger foods.

Signs of a Healthy Infant or Toddler with Diabetes

- Normal growth in height and weight
- Achieving all the developmental milestones, such as rolling over, sitting up, crawling, standing, walking, and talking, at about the expected age
- No signs of high blood glucose levels, such as overly wet diapers or unusual thirst
- Good energy levels
- Few mild hypos, and no severe ones
- No ketones in the urine or blood
- Blood glucose levels that are not often less than 90 mg/dL
- Blood glucose levels that are not over 215 mg/dL for long periods of time, and
- Being happy and secure.

When it comes to carbohydrate-containing foods, only offer one or two substitute foods for those refused and be careful not to substitute "junk food" for more nutritious carbohydrate foods. Don't force-feed your child; it can encourage negative food-related behaviors that can be hard to change in later life.

Also, it is important to monitor their blood glucose levels regularly if you feel they have not eaten enough carbohydrate foods to avoid hypos.

What is the best way to treat a hypo in a toddler?

You could continue using glucose syrup if you've used it when they were younger. Otherwise, use something that is not too tempting for them, such as Lucozade, to raise blood glucose levels rapidly. You don't want to make hypos something they want, so make sure you don't use candy or chocolate as a treatment!

DAILY FOOD GUIDE
TODDLER

▶ 3 servings bread, cereals and other starchy foods
▶ 1–2 servings fruit
▶ 2 servings of milk products
▶ ½–1 serving meat and alternatives
▶ ½–1 serving fat-rich foods
▶ 2–3 servings vegetables

Meal plan for a toddler with Type 1 diabetes	Daily food servings	Example
Breakfast	1 serving bread, cereal or other starchy food + ½ serving fruit	¾ cup oatmeal with ½ small banana
	½ serving milk product	½ cup whole milk
Snack	½ serving fruit	½ sliced apple
	1 serving of milk	1 cup milk
Lunch	1 serving bread, cereal or other starchy food with ½ fat serving	1 slice bread, spread with margarine
	1 serving vegetable	1 small cup of cherry tomatoes, carrot sticks, cucumber rings
	½ serving meat or alternative	1-oz piece of reduced-fat hard cheese
Snack	½ serving bread, cereal or other starchy food	½ slice toast with margarine
Dinner	½ serving bread, cereal or other starchy food	⅓ cup sweet potato
	1 serving vegetables	½ cup diced peas and carrot
	½ serving meat or alternative	2½ ounces cooked boneless white fish
	½ serving milk product	½ cup whole milk

TYPE 1 TODDLER
A MENU AND RECIPES FOR THE DAY

Breakfast

Muesli with Milk and Banana
TOTAL CARBOHYDRATE (G) 47

Lunch

Runny Egg with Toast Strips
TOTAL CARBOHYDRATE (G) 25

Dinner

Spaghetti Bolognese
with vegetable finger sticks
TOTAL CARBOHYDRATE (G) 25

Dessert

Pear and Apricot Yogurt
TOTAL CARBOHYDRATE (G) 17

Nutritional analysis of this daily menu

ENERGY (CAL)	PROTEIN (G)	FAT (G)	SATURATED FAT (G)	CARBOHYDRATE (G)	FIBER (G)	SODIUM (MG)
840	35	30	10	112	10	600

MUESLI WITH MILK
AND BANANA

PREP TIME: 5 minutes ▪ COOKING TIME: none ▪ SERVES: 1

¼ cup Muesli

1 cup whole milk

½ small banana

1 tsp honey

1. Place Muesli in bowl, add milk, and warm in microwave for 30 seconds if desired. Slice banana on top and drizzle honey over.

PER SERVING
Energy (cal) 312 ▪ Protein (g) 12 ▪ Fat (g) 11 ▪ Saturated fat (g) 5
Carbohydrate (g) 47 ▪ Fiber (g) 5 ▪ Sodium (mg) 98

RUNNY EGG WITH TOAST STRIPS

PREP TIME: 5 mins ▪ COOKING TIME: 5 mins ▪ SERVES: 1

2 slices low-GI bread

2 tsp canola margarine (reduced sodium)

1 omega-3-rich egg

1. Fill a small saucepan with water (enough to cover the egg) and bring to a boil. Carefully add the egg and boil for 4 minutes. Drain and cool under running water.

2. Toast bread and spread with margarine. Cut toast into strips and serve with egg.

PER SERVING
Energy (cal) 330 ▪ Protein (g) 13 ▪ Fat (g) 15 ▪ Saturated fat (g) 3
Carbohydrate (g) 33 ▪ Fiber (g) 3 ▪ Sodium (mg) 420

SPAGHETTI BOLOGNESE

This makes a larger amount, so you can freeze the leftover portions.

PREP TIME: 5 minutes ■ **COOKING TIME: 15 minutes** ■ **SERVES: 5**

1½ tbsp canola oil
½ white onion, chopped finely
⅓ lb lean ground beef
3½ tbsp tomato paste
2½ tbsp finely grated sweet potato
⅓ cup water
½ teaspoon dried oregano

PER SERVING
Energy (cal) 280 ■
Protein (g) 12 ■ Fat (g) 7 ■
Saturated fat (g) 1
Carbohydrate (g) 38 ■
Fiber (g) 3 ■ Sodium (mg) 110

1. In a small saucepan, heat oil. Add onion and cook on a low heat for 3–4 minutes, or until soft, stirring often.
2. Add meat and cook until brown, stirring to break up lumps.
3. Add tomato paste and sweet potato, and stir to combine.
4. Add water and oregano and cook on low heat for 10 minutes.
5. When cool, divide sauce into 5 portions and freeze those you don't need now in labeled sealed containers or ziplock bags. Thaw in refrigerator when needed.
6. Meanwhile, cook pasta according to directions on package.
7. Drain pasta and mix in sauce.

PEAR AND APRICOT YOGURT

PREP TIME: 3 mins ■ **COOKING TIME: 1 min** ■ **SERVES: 1–2**

---

1 medium pear, peeled and diced
2½ tbsp diced dried apricot
2½ tbsp water
2½ tbsp plain or vanilla yogurt

1. Combine the pear, diced apricot and water in a small bowl and microwave for 1 minute to soften the fruit.
2. When cool, stir in the yogurt.

PER SERVING
Energy (cal) 85 ■ Protein (g) 2 ■ Fat (g) 1 ■ Saturated fat (g) 1
Carbohydrate (g) 17 ■ Fiber (g) 3 ■ Sodium (mg) 17

▪32▪

Type 1:
School-Age Children
(Plus Daily Food Guide and Recipes)

*F*or reasons we do not yet understand, the first peak in the occurrence of type 1 diabetes occurs around the time children start school. This can be a hard time for parents, because for perhaps the first time, children will be spending most of their day away from home and their parents' watchful eyes.

By the time they are old enough to go to school, children are usually becoming more independent, and they will be able to take on some aspects of their diabetes care themselves. Always let children set the pace, but you can gradually start teaching them to measure their own blood glucose levels, draw up and inject insulin, and simple ways of counting carbohydrates—usually by using carbohydrate exchanges or portions.

However, children cannot be expected to understand their diabetes treatment fully until late childhood and early adolescence, so you need to put some care into supporting them at school and making sure adults check that their insulin doses are accurate and are all given.

As children grow and get more active, their energy (calories) needs constantly increase. In boys and girls from 6 to 12 years of age, average weight gain is about 5½–6½ pounds per year, and that's fueled by their energy intake, which nearly doubles during this time. Frequent reviews of meal plans with your child's dietitian are going to be essential—perhaps every time you have to buy new shoes!

At this age, children have much more regular eating patterns. However, when they get to school, there's going to be playground peer pressure. They may want to:

- Eat the same kinds and amounts of food as their friends
- Swap foods with their friends, and
- Buy foods at the school cafeteria or corner store.

FOOD

Review the school cafeteria menu with them the first few times to help them identify the more suitable choices.

Breakfast

As most people know, breakfast is one of the most important meals of the day. And children with diabetes are no different. There is no need to be too rigid with what you suggest. Besides the standard cereal or toast, you can try a liquid breakfast (commercial or homemade smoothie) or a container of yogurt and piece of fruit.

School lunch

Now is also the time to start involving children in food preparation, which can include putting together lunch for school. Allow some give and take—if they want to eat the same thing at school every day, let them. Remember, you can offer variety at other times of the day.

Snacks

Because they want to spend as much of their breaks playing, many children need food that is full of nutrients, but quick and easy to eat. Power-packed snack foods include:

▶ Sandwiches made with low-GI white or multigrain bread
▶ Most fresh fruits
▶ Dried fruit and nut mix (check your school's policy on nuts)
▶ Breakfast and granola bars
▶ Fruit-filled cookies, and
▶ Yogurt and milk.

Generally, try to keep meal times the same as the other kids. However, in some schools recess is relatively late, and an extra snack may be necessary just before starting school each day.

Most active children are very hungry after school. Bulky foods such as noodles, grainy bread, fruits and vegetables are good snack choices to fill them up and keep them going until dinner.

PARENTS
THERE'S NO NEED TO BE A PARTY POOPER

This bit is for moms and dads: it's about how to plan for treats and special occasions. Children don't have to give up party food or birthday cake because they have diabetes. For children, fitting in with everyone else is generally their top priority, but you have a right to have your concerns heard as well. Talk about the occasion beforehand, using "I" statements to express your concerns, and invite your child to help you find a solution that works for you both. This approach is more likely to keep you both happy—and it's much better than if you set the rules by laying down the law. This isn't the same as letting them go for their life without any guidance. You both need to plan for those extra treats. Here are a few basic rules to follow:

Find out

▶ What kind of food will be served
▶ When will the kids eat, and
▶ What other activities are planned.

Work out

▶ How the food "fits in" with your child's normal meal times and the time their insulin peaks
▶ Whether you need to split a meal or snack to accommodate the time food will be served
▶ If a reduction in insulin is necessary (for example, if the event will include lots of exercise) or whether extra insulin might be needed (for example, if they're going to the movies or having a sleepover with popcorn, chocolate and ice cream), and
▶ If your child is open to the idea, put together some healthier or at least more familiar snacks for them to eat at the party (plus enough to share).

Go

▶ Get to the event on time or ahead of time if you want to run through anything (such as hypo symptoms) with the party organizer
▶ Leave a contact number, and
▶ Equip your child with hypo treatment.

Top tip

Taking the edge off children's appetite with a sandwich beforehand can mean they'll eat less party junk. Kids won't naturally overeat, even if what's on offer is very tempting.

PHYSICAL ACTIVITIES

Children need to get involved with a range of physical activities they enjoy, because then they will be more likely to continue to be physically active throughout their life. It is important to check blood glucose levels before, during and after physical activities to work out the effect of a particular activity on their blood glucose levels. This is something that you, a teacher, the coach, or the child can do.

If blood glucose levels are consistently low, it may be necessary to increase the amount of low-GI carbohydrates eaten before an event to prevent low blood glucose. Alternatively, a decrease in insulin may be helpful—this can be worked out with your diabetes management team.

It is important to be aware that blood glucose levels can go low many hours after an activity—up to 24 hours in some cases—so increased carbohydrates may be necessary after the first few events until you work out what the typical pattern is.

WHAT ARE OPTIMAL BLOOD GLUCOSE LEVELS FOR SCHOOL-AGE CHILDREN?

Blood glucose targets for school-aged children are 75–180 mg/dL before a meal and 125–215 mg/dL at bedtime. This range gives adequate protection from hyperglycemia while reducing the risk of severe hypoglycemia.

WHAT TO DO ABOUT HYPOS IN SCHOOL-AGE CHILDREN

We would encourage school-age children to carry "hypo food" with them at all times. Make them a hypo pack for school and sports. It can include:

- A juice box or fruit bar to treat the hypo, and
- A box of raisins or small package of cookies for follow-up.

YOUNG CHILD (4–8 YEARS) DAILY FOOD GUIDE

- 5–7 servings breads, cereals and other starchy foods
- 2–3 servings fruit
- 2 servings milk products

▶ 1–2 servings meat and alternatives
▶ 2–3 servings fat-rich foods
▶ 3 or more servings vegetables

This food guide is based on the nutritional requirement of active 4–8 year olds. It provides between 1250–1620 calories with 50 percent energy from carbohydrates.

Meal plan for a young child (4–8 years) with type 1 diabetes	Daily food servings	Example
Breakfast	1 serving bread, cereal or other starchy food	1 cup oatmeal with ½ small banana
	½ serving milk product	yogurt
Snack	1 serving fruit + ½ serving milk	1 apple, ½ cup flavored milk
Lunch	2 servings bread, cereal or other starchy food plus 1 serving fat rich food	2 slices bread with margarine
	1 serving vegetable	1 small cup cherry tomatoes
	½ serving meat or alternative	1 small skinless chicken leg
	1 serving fruit	a small bunch of grapes
Snack	1 serving bread, cereal or other starchy food	1 slice bread with margarine
Dinner	1 serving bread, cereal or other starchy food	½ cup noodles
	2 servings vegetables	1 cup stir-fry vegetables
	½ serving meat or alternative	1½ ounces stir-fry pork
	1 fat serving	oil for stir-frying
	1 serving milk product	1 cup low-fat milk

TYPE 1: YOUNG CHILD—
A MENU AND RECIPES FOR THE DAY

Breakfast

Oatmeal with Raisins and Honey

TOTAL CARBOHYDRATE (G) 40

Lunch

Salad Plate

with a slice of whole wheat bread

TOTAL CARBOHYDRATE (G) 30

Dinner

Vegetable Slice

TOTAL CARBOHYDRATE (G) 20

Dessert

Banana and Pudding

TOTAL CARBOHYDRATE (G) 25

Nutritional analysis of this daily menu						
ENERGY (CAL)	PROTEIN (G)	FAT (G)	SATURATED FAT (G)	CARBOHYDRATE (G)	FIBER (G)	SODIUM (MG)
840	40	20	6	120	14	900

OATMEAL WITH RAISINS AND HONEY

PREP TIME: 2 mins ■ COOKING TIME: 5 mins ■ SERVES: 1

⅓ cup traditional rolled oats

⅔ cup low-fat, calcium-fortified milk

2 heaping tsp raisins

1 tsp honey

1. Place milk in a small saucepan and heat over medium heat for 1–2 minutes, until hot. Stir in oats and cook, stirring occasionally for 2–3 minutes, until soft.

2. Add raisins and stir for another minute.

3 Serve in a warm bowl. Drizzle on honey.

PER SERVING

Energy (cal) 225 ■ Protein (g) 10 ■ Fat (g) 3 ■ Saturated fat (g) <1
Carbohydrate (g) 38 ■ Fiber (g) 2 ■ Sodium (mg) 95

SALAD PLATE

*Al*most any combination of fruits, vegetables or cold leftovers can be colorfully presented in small pieces for toddlers to help themselves to.

PREP TIME: 5 mins ■ COOKING TIME: none ■ SERVES: 1

¼ cup cooked small-shape pasta

1 hard boiled egg, cut into 4, or ⅓ cup (2 oz) chopped, skinless cooked chicken or meat

2–3 cherry tomatoes

½ small carrot, cut into sticks

1½ tbsp corn kernels or baked beans

½ small apple, thinly sliced

1 Arrange the ingredients in small piles on a plate or in a shallow dish.

PER SERVING

Energy (cal) 180 ■ Protein (g) 10 ■ Fat (g) 5 ■ Saturated fat (g) 1 Carbohydrate (g) 22
■ Fiber (g) 5 ■ Sodium (mg) 125

VEGETABLE SLICE

*T*his is a terrific recipe for kids (to make and eat!). It combines vegetables, ham and corn into one easy dish that can be eaten hot, warm or cold. It's great for picnics too.

PREP TIME: 30 mins ■ **COOKING TIME:** 40 mins ■ **SERVES:** 6

---

4 omega-3-rich eggs

1 x 16-oz can sweet corn kernels, reduced sodium, drained

2 slices (2 oz) leg ham, diced

½ cup reduced-fat grated tasty cheese

2 zucchini

2 carrots

1 onion

½ cup whole wheat self-rising flour

1. Preheat the oven to 300°F.

2. Lightly beat the eggs together in a large mixing bowl. Add the drained sweet corn kernels, diced ham and cheese.

3. Grate the zucchini, carrots and onion (this is easiest in a food processor) and add to the other ingredients in the bowl. Add the flour. Stir thoroughly to combine.

4. Spoon the mixture into a large greased lasagna dish and press down to flatten the top. Bake for 40 minutes, or until browned and set.

PER SERVING
Energy (cal) 200 ■ Protein (g) 12 ■ Fat (g) 7 ■ Saturated fat (g) 3 Carbohydrate (g) 19 ■ Fiber (g) 4 ■ Sodium (mg) 455

BANANA AND PUDDING

PREP TIME: 5 mins ■ COOKING TIME: 5 mins ■ SERVES: 2

1 cup reduced-fat milk

1½ tbsp pudding powder

2 tsp sugar

1 banana, sliced

1. Blend the pudding powder and sugar with a little of the milk in a microwave-safe bowl. Stir in the rest of the milk. Cook in the microwave for 1 minute. Stir. Cook for a further 30 seconds, until pudding boils and thickens.
2. Divide the banana into 2 dessert bowls and top with the pudding.

PER SERVING
Energy (cal) 145 ■ Protein (g) 6 ■ Fat (g) 2 ■ Saturated fat (g) 1
Carbohydrate (g) 26 ■ Fiber (g) 1 ■ Sodium (mg) 65

SCHOOLCHILD (9–13 YEARS) DAILY FOOD GUIDE

- 7–9 servings breads, cereals and other starchy foods
- 2–4 servings fruit
- 2–3 servings of milk products
- 1–2 servings meat and alternatives
- 2–3 servings fat-rich foods
- 4 or more servings vegetables

This food guide is based on the nutrient requirements of an active 9 to 13-year-old. The energy value ranges from 1,450 to 2,150 calories, with 50 percent of energy from carbohydrates.

Meal plan for a schoolchild (9–13 years) with type 1 diabetes	Daily food servings	Example
Breakfast	1 serving bread, cereal or other starchy + ½ serving milk product	¾ cup cooked oatmeal with low-fat milk
	1 serving fruit	½ cup apple juice
Snack	1 serving bread, cereal or other starchy servings + 1 serving vegetables	4 whole wheat crackers and 1 raw carrot
Lunch	2 servings bread + 1 serving fat	2 slices low-GI bread with margarine
	½ serving meat or alternative + 1 serving vegetable	1 slice of chicken breast with cucumber and lettuce
	1 serving fruit	1 apple
Snack	1 serving bread or other starchy food + 1 serving fat	1 English muffin with margarine and honey
Dinner	2 servings bread or other starchy food	1 mini corn cob + ½ cup mashed potato
	2 servings vegetables	½ cup carrot and ½ cup peas
	1 serving meat or alternative	1 lean ground meat patty
Snack	1 serving milk product	1 cup chocolate milk

A MENU AND RECIPES FOR THE DAY

Breakfast
High-Fiber Cereal and Raisins
TOTAL CARBOHYDRATE (G) 40

Snack
Lunch Box crackers and cheese
TOTAL CARBOHYDRATE (G) 15

Lunch
Lunch Box sandwich and fruit
TOTAL CARBOHYDRATE (G) 40

Snack
Fruit and Oat Bars
½ small glass of low-fat milk
TOTAL CARBOHYDRATE (G) 30

Dinner
Baked Pasta
served with green salad
TOTAL CARBOHYDRATE (G) 56

Dessert
Raspberry Whip with a scoop of low-fat ice cream
TOTAL CARBOHYDRATE (G) 10

ENERGY (CAL)	PROTEIN (G)	FAT (G)	SATURATED (G)	CARBOHYDRATE FAT (G)	FIBER (G)	SODIUM (MG)
1720	95	60	25	200	30	2000

Nutritional analysis of this daily menu

HIGH-FIBER CEREAL AND RAISINS

PREP TIME: 2 mins ■ COOKING TIME: none ■ SERVES: 1

1 cup high-fiber cereal flakes

⅔ cup low-fat, calcium-fortified milk

2 heaping tsp raisins

1. Place the cereal in a bowl. Top with milk and sprinkle over raisins.

PER SERVING
Energy (cal) 220 ■ Protein (g) 9 ■ Fat (g) 3 ■ Saturated fat (g) 2
Carbohydrate (g) 38 ■ Fiber (g) 6 ■ Sodium (mg) 140

LUNCH BOX

*S*andwich and fruit

PREP TIME: 10 mins ■ COOKING TIME: none ■ SERVES: 1

2 slices low-GI bread

2 tsp canola-based margarine

2 slices (1½ oz) chicken or turkey breast

1 small carrot, cut into sticks

1 stick celery, cut into sticks

2 whole-grain crackers

1 reduced-fat cheese stick

5–6 strawberries

1. Make up a sandwich with the bread, margarine and meat.

2. Put the celery and carrot in a small self-sealing plastic bag.

3. Wrap the crackers in plastic wrap with the cheese stick.

4. Wash and hull the strawberries and place in a small plastic container.

5. Pack all items together in a lunch box.

PER SERVING
Energy (cal) 500 ■ Protein (g) 26 ■ Fat (g) 19 ■ Saturated fat (g) 6
Carbohydrate (g) 54 ■ Fiber (g) 11 ■ Sodium (mg) 800

FRUIT AND OAT BARS

This one is easy enough for kids to make themselves!

PREP TIME: 10 mins ■ **COOKING TIME:** 40 mins ■ **MAKES:** 16 squares

---

1½ cups self-rising flour

1½ cups traditional rolled oats

½ cup dried coconut

½ cup brown sugar

⅓ cup raisins

⅓ cup currants

⅓ cup dates, chopped

½ cup canola oil

1 cup skim milk

1. Preheat the oven to 325°F. Grease and line a 9" × 9" square pan with parchment paper.
2. Combine the flour, oats, coconut, sugar and dried fruit in a bowl. Stir in the oil and milk, mixing with a wooden spoon until combined.
3. Press mixture evenly into the pan and bake for 40 minutes, or until golden and center is firm to touch.
4. Cool in the pan then turn out and cut into squares.

PER SERVING
Energy (cal) 210 ■ Protein (g) 3 ■ Fat (g) 10 ■ Saturated fat (g) 2 Carbohydrate (g) 27 ■
Fiber (g) 2 ■ Sodium (mg) 105

BAKED PASTA

PREP TIME: 30 minutes ■ **COOKING TIME:** 50 minutes ■ **SERVES:** 4

---

1 onion, halved and sliced into thin wedges

2½ cups (12 oz) peeled pumpkin or butternut squash, chopped into cubes about ½–1" square

1 tsp chopped fresh rosemary

1½ tbsp olive oil

3⅓ cups (9 oz) fusilli or spiral pasta

1 cup (3½ oz) cauliflower florets

1 cup (3 oz) broccoli florets

⅔ cup frozen peas

1 cup smooth ricotta

½ cup extra-light sour cream

2½ tbsp Dijon mustard

3½ oz diced ham

¼ cup chopped flat-leaf parsley

¾ cup pizza cheese

1. Preheat the oven to 390°F.
2. Place onions in one small bowl and pumpkin and rosemary in another. Toss each with 2 tsp oil. In a lined baking tray, roast pumpkin for 20 minutes, or until cooked. Add onions to tray after pumpkin has been cooking for 5 minutes. Toss once during cooking. Remove and turn oven temperature down to 350°F.
3. Meanwhile, in a large pot cook pasta according to directions on package. When pasta has 2 minutes left to cook add cauliflower and broccoli to pasta saucepan. Continue boiling for 2 more minutes. Drain pasta and vegetables and then pour them back into the saucepan. Stir in peas and pumpkin mix.
4. In a bowl, combine ricotta, sour cream and mustard. Stir this into pasta along with ham and parsley. Season with pepper.
5. Spread pasta mix into a 2.5-quart baking dish. Sprinkle top evenly with pizza cheese.
6. Bake for 25–30 minutes, or until top is golden.
7. Serve with a green salad.

PER SERVING
Energy (cal) 550 ■ Protein (g) 30 ■ Fat (g) 23 ■ Saturated fat (g) 10 Carbohydrate (g) 55 ■ Fiber (g) 6 ■ Sodium (mg) 695

RASPBERRY WHIP

PREP TIME: 5 mins ■ CHILLING TIME: 4 hours ■ SERVES: 4

1 package raspberry-flavored gelatin powder

¾ cup hot water

2 cups low-fat plain (unflavored) yogurt

1 cup (8 oz) cottage cheese

1 x container fresh strawberries or raspberries, to serve (about 2 cups)

1. Add the gelatin to the hot water and stir to dissolve. Add the yogurt and cottage cheese and blend with a food processor or electric mixer.

2. Pour into 4 × ¾–cup ramekins and refrigerate until set.

3. Serve garnished with fresh strawberries or raspberries, if desired.

PER SERVING
Energy (cal) 120 ■ Protein (g) 19 ■ Fat (g) 1 ■ Saturated fat (g) <1
Carbohydrate (g) 7 ■ Fiber (g) 0 ■ Sodium (mg) 160

Type 1 Diabetes and Teenagers

(Plus Daily Food Guide and Recipes)

The teenage years tend to be a time when you want to challenge the world. That's normal. It's all part of growing up, fitting in with your friends and what they are doing, experimenting, testing limits, and seeking independence from your family.

If you have diabetes, it's also a time when you have to start taking full responsibility for managing your own health—and when you'll discover firsthand the close relationship between what you do (or don't do) and your blood glucose levels (if you test). Progressing from depending on your parents for your diabetes management to doing it yourself can put strain on the family—but it's all part of letting go and trusting. On both sides. The evidence shows that the young people who manage self-care best are those who feel supported by their family and friends, their doctor and their diabetes team.

What with school and possibly extra coaching for exams, a part-time job, social life, sports and all the other things you like to do, your eating patterns may change, too. You'll find you are missing meals, grabbing snacks instead of sitting down to main meals or "grazing," and maybe eating more takeout and fast foods away from home.

Experimenting with alcohol and other recreational drugs can affect your appetite, too. Don't worry, all is not lost. Adolescents have higher total energy requirements than young adults (on average about 250 calories a day more) so there is room to enjoy some foods with higher energy density, such as takeout and other so-called junk foods.

It's in Your Mind

- If you think you can do it, you are more likely to do it, no matter what the barriers.
- If you believe that you are responsible for your own destiny, you are more likely to look after yourself.
- If you see lots of barriers to looking after yourself (cost, physical abilities, emotions), you need to tackle them first. Talk to someone about the problems.
- If you can't see any benefit (either short or long term) in looking after yourself, you're not very likely to do it.
- If you're worried about hypos, you are more likely to manage your diabetes in a way that avoids them, but often at the cost of running high blood glucose levels.

On top of this, with the emotional stress from making and breaking relationships, it's not surprising that your insulin requirements usually increase during these years. In fact, teenage boys sometimes need six times as much insulin as adults because their hormones are fluctuating so much. When you are ready for it, have a talk with your doctor or diabetes educator about switching to the more flexible daily multiple injection regimen.

■

If you are fudging test results or missing blood tests, you are not alone. It's what teenagers do to look as if they're managing their diabetes better than they actually are.

■

Teens and Food

IN ONE STUDY of 144 type 1 teens 11–19 years of age, 81 percent admitted to eating inappropriate food in the previous 10 days. It was the most frequently reported form of "mismanagement."

- 56 percent reported missing meals and snacks, and
- 34 percent reported taking extra insulin to cover what they considered inappropriate food.

YOUR GOOD FOOD AND MOVES GUIDE

▶ Have breakfast—it fills your tank after a night without food and it helps you do better in school. Great breakfasts include cereal and milk; whole-grain toast and peanut butter; yogurt and fruit.

▶ Snack smart—if your snacks are healthy you're halfway there. Grab an apple or banana, a glass of low-fat milk or container of yogurt, or a handful of dried fruit and nuts.

▶ Don't overdo any one food—you know it's okay to eat chocolate and French fries occasionally, but keep your food choices varied and team the ice cream with some fruit.

▶ Concentrate on eating more fruit, grains and vegetables—eat breakfast cereals, whole-grain toast, oat/granola bars, strawberries, bananas, or melon chunks.

▶ Don't think of foods as good or bad—if you want to eat pizza tonight with your friends, eat lighter during the day.

▶ Keep active—do at least 30 minutes of exercise a day: walking or riding to school or to see friends; training for sports; walking a dog . . . and don't forget to join in physical activity at school.

▶ Be active with family and friends—find someone to exercise with. Plan group activities such as dancing, cycling, skiing, roller-blading, skating . . . the possibilities are endless.

HANDLING HYPOS

Hypos can happen at any age, even if you take every known precaution to prevent them. Here are some foods suitable for managing a hypo (your friends need to know about these foods and when you might need them).

Start with easily absorbed carbohydrates, to raise your blood glucose levels quickly:

- ½–1 cup ordinary soft drink, fruit juice or punch
- 4 large jelly beans, or 7 small jelly beans
- 2–3 teaspoons of sugar, or
- glucose tablets or gels (10–20 grams).

Follow that, within 15–20 minutes, with carbohydrate foods that will maintain your blood glucose levels:

- 1 slice of low-GI bread
- 1 banana or apple
- 8 ounces plain yogurt or 4 ounces flavored yogurt, or
- 1 glass of milk.

Why Worry about Your HbA1c?

THERE IS NO HbA1c level below which the risk of complications is eliminated. But any improvement in HbA1c reduces your risk. In order to have an HbA1c less than 7.5 percent, you need to meet the following everyday blood glucose targets:

- A before-meal blood glucose level (BGL) of 65–110 mg/dL, and
- An after-meal blood glucose level (BGL) of less than 180 mg/dL.

EATING DISORDERS AND TYPE 1 DIABETES

Due to the necessary focus on the types and amounts of foods eaten each day, and the tendency of insulin to promote weight gain, it is perhaps not surprising to learn that eating disorders such as anorexia and bulimia are more common in young people with diabetes than in those without. Another related issue—omission of insulin to promote weight loss—is also not uncommon.

Of course such behaviors have predictable effects on blood glucose levels, and in the long term they increase the risk of developing diabetic complications substantially. Treating people with diabetes and an eating disorder is multifaceted—it typically includes a combination of psychotherapy and nutritional and pharmacological strategies.

YOUR DAILY FOOD GUIDE AND RECIPES

- 12 servings breads, cereals and other starchy foods
- 4 servings fruit
- 2 servings of milk products
- 2–3 servings meat and alternatives
- 4 servings fat-rich foods
- 5 or more servings vegetables

This food guide is based on the nutrition requirements of active 14–18 year olds. The energy content ranges from 1,790 to 2,500 calories with 50 percent of energy from carbohydrates.

Meal plan for a teenager with type 1 diabetes	Daily food servings	Example
Breakfast	4 servings bread, cereal or other starchy foods plus 1 serving fat rich food	4 slices of grain toast, topped with peanut butter and banana
	1 serving fruit	
	1 serving milk product	1 cup low-fat milk and Quik
Snack	2 servings bread, cereal or other starchy foods + 1 serving vegetables	a "salad" sandwich
Lunch	2 servings bread, cereal or other starchy foods and 1 fat serving	a seeded roll spread with mayonnaise or mustard
	1 serving vegetables	1 cup shredded lettuce
	1 serving meat or alternative	1 slice ham and 1 slice cheese
Lunch	1 serving fruit	an apple

Meal plan for a teenager with type 1 diabetes	Daily food servings	Example
Snack	1 serving fruit	
Dinner	4 servings bread, cereal or other starchy foods	1 cup mashed potato and 1 full corn cob
	4 servings vegetables	2 cups cooked mixed veggies
	2 servings meat or alternative	7-ounce piece of steak
	1 serving fat-rich food	2 teaspoons margarine in mashed potato
Snack	1 serving milk product + 1 serving fruit	4 scoops low-fat ice cream and ½ cup canned fruit

A MENU AND RECIPES FOR THE DAY

Breakfast
Breakfast on the Go
TOTAL CARBOHYDRATE (G) 60

Snack
2 Super Muesli Bars
TOTAL CARBOHYDRATE (G) 30

Lunch
Chicken Satay Wrap
1 banana
TOTAL CARBOHYDRATE (G) 45

Snack
Peanut butter sandwich
TOTAL CARBOHYDRATE (G) 30

Dinner
Stir-Fried Pork and Vegetables
TOTAL CARBOHYDRATE (G) 60

Dessert
2 servings Orange and Pineapple Whip
TOTAL CARBOHYDRATE (G) 20

Nutritional analysis of this daily menu

ENERGY (CAL)	PROTEIN (G)	FAT (G)	SATURATED FAT (G)	CARBOHYDRATE (G)	FIBER (G)	SODIUM (MG)
1790	95	45	10	245	25	1500

BREAKFAST ON THE GO

*I*t's quick, sustaining and delicious. What more could you want?

PREP TIME: 5 mins ■ **COOKING TIME: none** ■ **SERVES: 1**

---

1 cup low-fat milk or soy milk

½ cup low-fat vanilla yogurt

¼ small container strawberries
(about ½ cup)

1 ripe banana

1. Combine all ingredients in a food processor. Blend.
2. Pour into a glass. Drink and go.

PER SERVING
Energy (cal) 340 ■ Protein (g) 22 ■ Fat (g) 1 ■ Saturated fat (g) <1
Carbohydrate (g) 60 ■ Fiber (g) 4 ■ Sodium (mg) 235

SUPER MUESLI BAR

*T*his recipe is based on "Dad's Super Muesli Bar," which came from one of our readers, Piers Hartley.

PREP TIME: 25 mins ■ COOKING TIME: 25 mins ■ MAKES: 16 bars

---

1 cup rolled oats

½ cup roasted hazelnuts, chopped*

¼ cup sunflower seeds

2½ tbsp sesame seeds

¼ cup whole wheat self-rising flour

1 tsp cinnamon

½ cup dates, chopped

½ cup dried apricots, chopped

3½ tbsp margarine

2½ tbsp honey

1½ tbsp brown sugar

1 tsp vanilla extract

1 egg

1 egg white

1. Preheat the oven to 350°F and grease a 8" × 12" rectangular pan. Line the base and 2 long sides with parchment paper and extend the paper an inch or so above the edge of the pan to facilitate removing the cake later.

2. In a large bowl, combine oats, nuts, seeds, flour and cinnamon. Mix in dried fruit.

3. In a small saucepan, melt margarine, honey and sugar on a low heat, stirring until ingredients are melted and combined. Remove from heat and add vanilla extract.

4. In a small bowl, beat egg and egg white together.

5. Add margarine mixture and eggs to the oat mixture and mix until well combined.

6. Spoon into prepared pan and press down so it is an even level. Bake for 25 minutes, or until lightly golden. Cool in pan before cutting into bars.

*You can buy roasted hazelnuts from the supermarket, or roast them yourself, in a 325°F oven for 10–15 minutes, or until they begin to turn golden and the skins begin to flake off to the touch.

PER SERVING
Energy (cal) 140 ■ Protein (g) 3 ■ Fat (g) 8 ■ Saturated fat (g) 1
Carbohydrate (g) 15 ■ Fiber (g) 2 ■ Sodium (mg) 46

CHICKEN SATAY WRAP

*M*ost lavash bread provides about 1 exchange of carbohydrates, leaving plenty of space for additional carbohydrates from a low-fat flavored milk or fruit juice.

PREP TIME: 10 mins ■ COOKING TIME: none ■ SERVES: 1

---

1 whole wheat lavash or flat bread

1 lettuce leaf, shredded

1 small tomato, sliced and laid on paper towel

1½ oz chopped cooked chicken, skin removed (leftover BBQ chicken, for example)

1½ tbsp satay sauce

1. Lay the flat bread on a board. Lay the shredded lettuce over the top, leaving a margin of about 1½ inches along one long side. Top with the tomato slices and chicken, finishing with the sauce. Make a fold in the bread along the margin (to hold the filling at the bottom of the wrap), then roll from one of the short sides to enclose the filling.

2. Wrap firmly in paper then plastic wrap.

PER SERVING
Energy (cal) 285 ■ Protein (g) 20 ■ Fat (g) 10 ■ Saturated fat (g) 3
Carbohydrate (g) 25 ■ Fiber (g) 5 ■ Sodium (mg) 360

STIR-FRIED PORK AND VEGETABLES

PREP TIME: 25 mins ■ **COOKING TIME:** 15 mins ■ **SERVES:** 4

1½ cups basmati rice, rinsed

1 bunch baby bok choy

1½ tbsp sesame oil

9 oz stir-fry pork

1 small red onion, halved and
   thinly sliced

1 red pepper, cut into thin strips

1 cup mushrooms, sliced

2 garlic cloves, crushed

2 tsp ginger, grated

1 tsp red chili, chopped

1½ tbsp reduced-sodium soy
   sauce

1. Bring 2½ cups water to a boil in a large saucepan with a tight-fitting lid. Stir in the rice and quickly replace the lid. Reduce the heat to as low as possible and cook for 10 minutes. Remove from the heat and leave to stand, still covered, for 5 minutes.

2. Meanwhile, cut the bok choy in half to separate the leaves from the stems. Cut the leaves into wide shreds, and finely slice the stems.

3. Heat 2 tsp oil in a large wok over high heat. Stir-fry pork in two batches until well browned, about 3–4 minutes. Remove pork from wok.

4. Heat the remaining oil in the wok and add the onion. Stir-fry over a moderately high heat for 2 minutes, until just tender. Add the pepper and bok choy stems and stir-fry for 2 minutes.

5. Add the mushrooms, garlic, ginger and chili, and stir-fry for 3 minutes, or until the mushrooms are just soft.

6. Return the pork to the wok and add the bok choy leaves and soy sauce. Toss until heated through and bok choy has just started to wilt. Serve immediately with rice.

PER SERVING
Energy (cal) 405 ■ Protein (g) 22 ■ Fat (g) 7 ■ Saturated fat (g) 2
Carbohydrate (g) 62 ■ Fiber (g) 3 ■ Sodium (mg) 240

ORANGE AND PINEAPPLE WHIP

PREP TIME: 10 minutes ■ COOKING/SETTING TIME: few hours ■ SERVES: 4

½ x 12-oz can of light evaporated milk (chilled)

1 8-oz can of crushed pineapple (unsweetened)

½ cup pineapple juice

1 package orange-flavored gelatin powdered (sugar-free)

¼ tsp coconut extract (available at specialty foods stores)

1. Chill the evaporated milk overnight.
2. Drain the pineapple, saving ¼ cup of the juice.
3. Heat the saved juice in the microwave until near boiling.
4. Dissolve the gelatin in the juice, then leave to one side.
5. In a large bowl, beat the chilled milk with the coconut extract (using an electric beater) until thick.
6. Combine the gelatin juice with the drained pineapple, add to the whipped milk, and stir until combined.
7. Refrigerate until set.

PER SERVING
Energy (cal) 70 ■ Protein (g) 5 ■ Fat (g) 1 ■ Saturated fat (g) 0.5 Carbohydrate (g) 11 ■ Fiber (g) 1 Sodium (mg) 60

▪34▪

Type 1 Diabetes
and Adults
(Plus Daily Food Guide and Recipes)

*B*y now you will have settled down into some kind of a routine, and you'll know what to do to manage most aspects of your diabetes by yourself. With the exception of pregnancy, which we discussed in chapter 28, the main focus as an adult is preventing the complications that are part and parcel of diabetes.

Time for some good news. There is compelling evidence from the Diabetes Control and Complications Trial (DCCT), that "intensive management" dramatically reduces your risk of developing complications: by up to 50 percent for kidney disease and up to 76 percent for eye disease.

So, what's intensive management?

▶ Multiple daily insulin injections or insulin pump therapy
▶ Having a food and physical activity plan
▶ Testing your blood glucose levels four or more times a day, and
▶ Adjusting your insulin doses according to your food intake
  and physical activity.

Regular carbohydrate meals and snacks (depending on your insulin regimen) and having at least one low-GI food at each meal is enough to maintain optimal blood glucose levels in most adults with type 1 diabetes.

But because of the greater risk of developing heart disease, there's a greater focus on weight management, eating the right types and amounts of fats, and minimizing salt intake as you age.

The meal ideas in this chapter have been designed to help you achieve optimal management of your blood glucose levels, as well as your blood fats and blood pressure, without sacrificing variety and taste.

KEEPING UP WITH THE LATEST IN DIABETES MANAGEMENT

If you have had diabetes for many years, you may think that you do not need to see your diabetes team any more. But diabetes management is changing all the time—there are new insulins, new blood pressure medications, new monitors, and new dietary tools (such as the GI). So it's important to continue to see your "team" regularly, even if your diabetes management is working well—if you don't, you may miss out on developments that could improve the quality of your life.

HANDLING HYPO UNAWARENESS AND HYPOS

You can still get hypos, no matter how much you know or how careful you are in managing your blood glucose. Under most circumstances you can identify the symptoms and treat the hypo immediately, without any further problems. Here are the foods you need to keep on hand for treating hypos.

Start with easily absorbed carbohydrates to raise your blood glucose levels quickly:

- ½–1 cup ordinary soft drink, fruit juice or punch
- 4 large jelly beans, or 7 small jelly beans

▶ 2–3 teaspoons sugar, or
▶ glucose tablets or gels (10–20 grams).

Follow that, within 15–20 minutes, with carbohydrate foods that will maintain your blood glucose levels:

▶ 1 slice low-GI bread
▶ 1 banana or apple
▶ 8 ounces unsweetened yogurt or 4 ounces sweetened yogurt, or
▶ 1 glass of milk.

WHAT ABOUT HYPO UNAWARENESS?

Years of intensive diabetes management can sometimes create what has been termed hypo unawareness. Typical symptoms of a hypo can be completely absent, or even reversed. If you think this may be happening to you, don't despair: there are now a number of different therapies available to reverse hypo unawareness, from as simple as changes to your insulin regimen to complete cognitive-behavioral programs, depending on the underlying cause of the problem. New technologies such as the Gluco Watch (glucowatch.com) may also help. Have a talk with your diabetes management team if you think you are unaware of hypos and need help.

YOUR DAILY FOOD GUIDE AND RECIPES

▶ 8–10 servings bread, cereals and other starchy foods
▶ 2–3 servings fruit
▶ 2 servings of milk products
▶ 1–2 servings meat and alternatives
▶ 2–3 servings fat-rich foods
▶ 5–6 or more servings vegetables

The daily food guide provides between 1,500 and 2,000 calories, with 50–55 percent of energy coming from carbohydrates.

Meal plan for an adult with type 1 diabetes	Daily food servings	Example	Other ideas
Breakfast	2 servings bread, cereal or other starchy foods + 1 serving milk product	1½ cup cooked oatmeal with 1 cup milk	1 cup low-GI cornflakes with milk
	1 serving fruit	1 small diced banana	1 diced pear
	1 diced pear		
Lunch	3 servings bread, cereal or other starchy foods + 2 servings vegetables	1 Lebanese flatbread filled with tabbouleh, lettuce and tomato	2 slices grain bread with lettuce, tomato and 2 oatmeal cookies
	1 serving meat or alternative	1 ounces grated cheese	3½ oz canned salmon
	1 serving fat-rich food	2 tbsp hummus on a kebab	1 tbsp mayonnaise
	1 serving fruit	an orange	½ cup apple juice
Dinner	3 servings bread, cereal or other starchy foods	1 cup cooked rice	¾ cup roasted sweet potato plus 2 medium plain roasted potatoes
	3 servings vegetables + 1 serving fat-rich food	1½ cups stir-fried vegetables or more	½ cup peas ½ cup roasted pumpkin ½ cup broccoli
	1 serving meat or alternative	5 oz mixed seafood stir-fry	2–3 slices (3 ounces) roast lamb
	1 serving fruit	¼ small fresh pineapple, grilled with a sprinkle of brown sugar	A fruit pop
Snack	1 serving milk product	8 oz low-fat yogurt	1 cup skim milk with Quik

A MENU AND RECIPES FOR A DAY

The nutritional analysis of this day allows for ½ cup of skim milk for tea or coffee during the day.

Breakfast
Homemade Muesli with a diced peach
TOTAL CARBOHYDRATE (G) 60

Snack
1 serving seasonal fruit
TOTAL CARBOHYDRATE (G) 13

Lunch
Whole-Grain Salad Sandwiches
TOTAL CARBOHYDRATE (G) 60

Dinner
BBQ Lamb and Lentil Salad with Lemony Yogurt Dressing
TOTAL CARBOHYDRATE (G) 50

Dessert
Chocolate Mousse served with a handful of berries
TOTAL CARBOHYDRATE (G) 30

Nutritional analysis of this daily menu						
ENERGY (CAL)	PROTEIN (G)	FAT (G)	SATURATED FAT (G)	CARBOHYDRATE (G)	FIBER (G)	SODIUM (MG)
2080	120	70	20	220	35	2400

HOMEMADE MUESLI

PREP TIME: 5 minutes ■ **COOKING TIME:** none ■ **SERVES:** 2

---

1 cup rolled oats

1½ tbsp raisins

1½ tbsp dried apricots

1½ tbsp dried apple slices

2½ tbsp slivered almonds

1 cup low-fat calcium-enriched
   milk

1. Chop the dried apricots into slivers and combine with rest of the dry ingredients.
2. Pour into a breakfast bowl and add milk.

PER SERVING
Energy (cal) 35 ■ Protein (g) 13 ■ Fat (g) 10 ■ Saturated fat (g) 1 Carbohydrate (g) 48 ■
Fiber (g) 5 ■ Sodium (mg) 80

WHOLE-GRAIN SALAD SANDWICHES

PREP TIME: 5 minutes ■ COOKING TIME: none ■ SERVES: 1

4 slices whole-grain bread

2 tsp reduced-sodium canola margarine

2 slices (1½ oz) reduced-fat cheddar cheese

2 slices beet

4 slices tomato

½ cup mixed lettuce

¼ red onion

1 tsp extra-virgin olive oil

black pepper

1. Lightly spread the canola margarine on all the slices of bread.
2. Place the cheese on 2 slices of bread.
3. Add a slice of beet and tomato to each of those 2 slices of bread.
4. Chop the mixed lettuce and add half to each of those 2 slices of bread.
5. Dice the red onion and add half to each of those 2 slices of bread.
6. Drizzle olive oil over each salad, and grind over pepper to taste.
7. Add the second slice of bread.

PER SERVING
Energy (cal) 640 ■ Protein (g) 28 ■ Fat (g) 28 ■ Saturated fat (g) 9
Carbohydrate (g) 60 ■ Fiber (g) 8 ■ Sodium (mg) 810

BBQ LAMB AND LENTIL SALAD WITH LEMONY YOGURT DRESSING

*T*his recipe consists of simple steps and makes a superbly healthy meal.

PREP TIME: 20 mins ■ COOKING TIME: 10 mins ■ SERVES: 2

10–14 oz lamb tenderloin

2 tsp olive oil

1 clove garlic, crushed, or 1 tsp minced garlic

few sprigs of fresh oregano, roughly torn

finely grated rind of 1 lemon

Salad

1½ tbsp olive oil

1 x 15-oz can brown lentils, drained

2 medium tomatoes, diced

1 small bunch spinach, leaves

a squeeze of lemon juice

Dressing

juice of 1 lemon

½ cup low-fat natural yogurt

salt and pepper

1. Place the oil, crushed garlic, oregano and lemon rind in a glass or ceramic dish. Add the whole lamb fillets and turn to coat. Set aside for 20 minutes to marinate or cover and refrigerate overnight.

2. Heat a frying pan or grill over medium-high heat and cook the lamb for 3–4 minutes each side, turning once. Remove from the pan, cover and set aside while you prepare the salad.

3. For the salad, heat the olive oil in a frying pan and add the drained lentils, stirring over medium heat to warm through. Add the tomatoes, shredded spinach and the lemon juice and stir to combine. Remove from heat.

4. For the dressing, combine the lemon juice with the natural yogurt in a small jar. Season with salt and pepper. Put on the lid and shake to combine.

5. Slice the rested lamb, across the grain (about ½" thick).

6. Spoon the lentils and vegetables onto plates. Top with the sliced meat and pour over the dressing.

PER SERVING
Energy (cal) 515 ■ Protein (g) 55 ■ Fat (g) 22 ■ Saturated fat (g) 5
Carbohydrate (g) 17 ■ Fiber (g) 8 ■ Sodium (mg) 580

CHOCOLATE MOUSSE

PREP TIME: 10 mins ■ **COOKING TIME:** 5 mins ■
CHILLING TIME: 2–3 hours ■ **SERVES:** 6

⅓ cup cocoa powder

2 tsp gelatin powder

1 cup + 1 tbsp sugar

1½ cups skim evaporated milk

½ cup reduced-fat cream

⅔ cup strawberries or raspberries,
   to serve

1. Sift the cocoa into a saucepan, then stir in the gelatin and sugar. Stir in about ¼ cup of the milk, stirring to form a smooth paste. Put the saucepan over medium heat and stir for about 3 minutes to dissolve the sugar and gelatin, then gradually stir in the remaining milk. Heat until the liquid is hot but not boiling, stirring occasionally.

2. Remove from the heat, stir in the cream, then divide the mixture among 6 × ½-cup glasses or ramekins. Chill until set.

3. Serve with the fresh berries.

PER SERVING
Energy (cal) 190 ■ Protein (g) 8 ■ Fat (g) 5 ■ Saturated fat (g) 4
Carbohydrate (g) 28 ■ Fiber (g) 1 ■ Sodium (mg) 90

▪35▪

Managing Diabetes
When Eating Out

$\mathcal{E}$ ating out can really test your resolve as far as healthy eating goes. But, like most things, the more often you do it, the more important it is to get it right. If you only eat out once a month, there's no need to be too fussy with what you eat. But if it's three or four times a week, whether for business or pleasure, making good choices is critical to your nutritional well-being.

When we eat out we tend to eat more than we would at home. And in most places, we're likely to get a lot more salt, refined carbohydrates and fat than we would from home-cooked food. This chapter tells you the best menu choices for a wide range of cuisines, and gives you tips for eating out at the movies, lunch bars, cafés, bars, on a flight, and for fast food and takeout, including McDonald's and KFC.

But first, here are our tips on avoiding the traps when eating out.

Trap 1. Going out on an empty stomach

Don't starve yourself through the day in preparation for a big night out. All that does is reduce your metabolic rate.

What to do? Eat a light breakfast and lunch, and before you go, have a quick snack such as a slice of whole-grain bread, a sliced apple, or a glass of tomato/vegetable juice. This will take the edge off your appetite, and you'll be less likely to overeat.

Trap 2. Taking your diabetes medication

Don't take your diabetes medication before you go. If you're supposed to have it with meals, take it with you. You may not end up eating at the time you think you will, and before you know it you're having a hypo before dinner.

What to do? Take your medication with you and have it just before you eat.

Trap 3. Starting with bread

Bypass breads at the start of a meal unless you are in need of some carbs right away or are planning a low-carb appetizer. It is likely to be saturated with butter, and if you eat a couple of thick slices, you've probably eaten over half your usual carb intake for the meal. And its probable high GI could end up increasing your appetite rather than satisfying it.

What to do? Take the edge off your appetite with a garden salad or vegetable soup. The high water and fiber content of these will fill up your stomach, leaving less space for the more calorie-dense entrée or main course.

Trap 4. Giving in to fries

Whenever you can, hold the fries. French fries, potato chips or wedges, whatever you call them, often come with the meal whether you order them or not. Their high energy density, high-GI carbohydrate and high saturated fat content make them a major diabetes enemy.

What to do? If you feel you need the carbs, try a fruit juice instead.

Trap 5. Forgetting your 1 (carb), 2 (protein), 3 (veggies) model

No, we're not talking about three-course meals. We mean the three basic components of a healthy balanced meal: 1—carbs, preferably low GI; 2—protein, which might be meat, seafood, poultry or a vegetarian alternative such as legumes or tofu; and 3—vegetables or salad.

What to do? Make sure that what you pick from the menu gives you all three components.

Trap 6. Not being discerning with drinks

Sugary drinks tend to bypass your body's fullness-sensing mechanisms, and alcohol contains almost twice as many calories as carbohydrates.

What to do? Make water your first choice. Ask for some every time you go out to eat, whether you feel like it or not. Chances are you'll drink it if it's in front of you. It doesn't have to be tap water; ask for mineral water if you enjoy the bubbles. Mineral water with a dash of freshly squeezed lime juice is almost as good as an aperitif! And remember, no more than 1–2 glasses of alcohol.

Trap 7. Finishing everything on your plate

Portions are getting bigger these days. And in some restaurants, you have to order the sides separately. This generally means you end up with far more food than anyone would need.

What to do? You can't control how much you are served, but you can control how much you eat. You don't have to clean your plate. Try to notice when you feel full and put down your knife and fork. Encourage the waiters to clear your table quickly so you're not tempted to nibble away at what you originally left. Take your leftovers home if you don't want to waste them.

Trap 8. Eating in a hurry

If you gobble your food, you don't give the receptors in your stomach time to send an "I am full" signal to your brain, which makes it very easy to overeat.

What to do? If you usually eat quickly, eating out is a good opportunity to practice eating slowly. Look around, talk to your companions and pace yourself. Taking time over your meals can help you eat less.

Trap 9. Ordering too much

Most people's eyes are bigger than their stomach when it comes to a menu. It all looks so tempting and it is a special occasion . . .

What to do? Try not to order all your courses at the one time: order just one course, and see how you feel before you order more. Another option is to order an appetizer for your main course, or an appetizer size for your main course. In Asian restaurants, where sharing meals is part of the fun, you'll probably find that four people can share three meals plus rice very comfortably.

Trap 10. Overlooking the simple fare

Fusion food and fashion food abound these days, and many menu items seem to be laden with amazing combinations of ingredients and flavors, always including the latest "must have" ingredients.

What to do? Often simple fare is the healthiest—and the tastiest. You know where you stand with a crisp fresh salad with a simple dressing, a vegetable soup, oysters, shrimp or scallops simply prepared, steak, grilled fish and a fresh fruit plate. When these foods are beautifully prepared with quality ingredients, they are just as delicious as anything else.

THE HEALTH GUIDE TO WHAT'S ON THE MENU

Asian meals

Asian meals, including Chinese, Thai, Vietnamese, Indian and Japanese, offer a great variety of foods which you can put together to create a healthy meal.

Keeping in mind the three steps to a balanced meal, seek out a low-GI carb such as low-GI rice, dhal, sushi or noodles. Chinese and Thai traditionally use jasmine rice, and although it is high GI, a small serving of steamed rice is better for you than fried rice or fried noodles.

Adding some protein gives staying power—try marinated tofu, stir-fried seafood, tandoori chicken, sashimi tuna, fish tikka or lean beef. Be cautious with pork and duck—fattier cuts are often used—and avoid Thai curries and dishes made with coconut milk, because it's high in saturated fat.

Remember, the third dish to order is steamed or stir-fried vegetables! Go easy on extras, especially the deep-fried ones—spring rolls, dim sums, pakoras and tempura. These are often served as an appetizer, so they get you when your appetite is greatest. Don't order them if you can help it.

And remember, while someone's picking up the tandoori or teriyaki takeout you can be stir-frying the vegetables at home. In a frying pan or wok, heat a teaspoon of sesame oil and stir-fry 2 teaspoons crushed garlic, 1½ tablespoon crushed ginger and 3 finely chopped shallots for 30 seconds. Add 2 cups chopped broccoli with the stalks trimmed (plus other Asian greens if you have them on hand) and ½ cup chicken stock. Cover and steam. Serve with soy sauce.

Good menu options include all of the following:

Chinese

- Steamed dim sums or dumplings
- Clear soups containing noodles/wontons and vegetables
- Vegetable-based dishes such as chop suey
- Braised skinless chicken or beef dishes in chili, oyster, soy or garlic sauces
- Seafood dishes such as curried shrimp, scallops with ginger and shallots, steamed whole fish
- Stir-fried or steamed vegetables
- Noodles or smaller servings of steamed or boiled rice.

Thai

- Fresh spring rolls
- Hot and sour soup—it's a good low-calorie stomach filler
- Any Thai salad
- Noodles in soups rather than fried in pad thai
- Seafood braised in a sauce with vegetables
- Wok-tossed tofu (bean curd), seafood, chicken, beef, lamb or pork fillet with nuts, vegetables and sauce
- Smaller servings of steamed jasmine rice
- Stir-fried mixed vegetables with garlic and oyster sauce or Thai herbs.

Indian

- Unleavened bread such as chapatis, plain naan or roti
- Beef, chicken, seafood or vegetable curry
- Tikka (dry roasted) or tandoori (marinated in spices and yogurt) chicken, shrimp or fish
- Basmati rice—a great lower-GI accompaniment, but watch the quantity!
- Dhal—an even better accompaniment, being very low GI
- Vegetable dishes such as stir-fried vegetables, vegetable curry, channa (a delicious chickpea curry), spicy spinach (saag), fresh salad and side orders such as pickles, cucumber raita, tomato and onion.

Japanese

▶ Miso soup or the more substantial udon soup
▶ Sushi, with seafood, chicken or vegetable
▶ Teriyaki (grilled meat or seafood with a special sauce)
▶ Teppan yaki (grilled steak, seafood and veggies)
▶ Yakitori (skewered chicken and onions in teriyaki sauce)
▶ Sashimi (thinly sliced raw beef, salmon or tuna—a great way to stock up on omega-3 fats)
▶ Shabu-shabu (thin slices of beef quickly cooked with mushrooms, cabbage and other vegetables)
▶ Side orders like seaweed salad, edamame (young green soybeans), wasabi (horseradish), shoyu (soy sauce) and oshinko (pickled ginger).

Mexican and Spanish

Mexican restaurants are ideal for low-GI choices because they make such great use of beans. Many of the dishes are very high in carbohydrates, though, because they include rice and corn as well. Probably the biggest nutritional hazards are cheese—they use lots of it—and sour cream. You can ask for these to be served separately. They do some salads as accompaniments. Good menu options include:

▶ Bean and salsa dips
▶ Gazpacho or black bean soup
▶ Salads with grilled chicken or lamb
▶ Seafood
▶ Shellfish paella (spicy rice with seafood, tomato and saffron)
▶ Enchiladas (corn tortillas filled with meat or cheese with chili sauce)
▶ Burritos (filled flour tortillas) and fajitas.

Italian

You'll find lots of low-GI pasta in an Italian restaurant, but it might be best to order an appetizer-sized serving—it will be plenty big enough.

Many pasta dishes also use a lot of cheese, so balance your meal by having a fresh salad with it. Steer clear of breaded and deep-fried seafood and watch out for creamy sauces. Good menu options include:

▶ Minestrone, stracciatella (soups)
▶ Prosciutto (paper-thin slices of cured ham) wrapped around melon
▶ Barbecued marinated seafood dishes
▶ Appetizer-sized pasta with tomato (napolitana), bean (fagoli) or seafood (marinara) sauce (without cream)
▶ Cannelloni with ricotta and spinach
▶ Grilled fish
▶ Roast or grilled fillet of beef, lamb loin or poultry
▶ Green garden salad with olive oil and balsamic vinegar
▶ Tomato salads with basil, olive oil and lemon juice
▶ Vegetarian pizza
▶ Gelato or sorbet or a fresh fruit platter.

Greek and Middle Eastern

Mediterranean cuisine uses a lot of olive oil, lemon, garlic, onions and other vegetables. Many dishes are grilled—specialties such as barbecued octopus or grilled sardines are excellent choices. You'll find regular bread and potatoes replaced with flat bread and Turkish bread, and whole grains such as bulgur (cracked wheat) in tabbouleh and couscous (semolina pasta) in stuffed eggplant and pepper. Good menu options include:

▶ Meze platter with pita bread. Among the small appetizing dishes here you could pick and choose what you like. There are healthy dips to enjoy in small quantities, such as hummus, baba ghanoush, tzatziki and taramasalata with tasty extras of olives and dolmades
▶ Souvlaki—grilled skewers of meat or chicken with vegetables
▶ Kofta or kibbi balls of minced lamb with bulgur (cracked wheat)
▶ Stifatho—a lamb, potato and onion casserole

▶ Greek salad of fresh lettuce, tomato, olives, feta cheese, peppers, with balsamic dressing or oil and lemon (you could ask for the dressing on the side) or tabbouleh salad
▶ Cabbage rolls, stuffed tomatoes
▶ Fresh fruit platter.

HOW TO HURDLE NUTRITIONAL HAZARDS WITH FAST FOOD AND TAKEOUT

You're out and about, on the go and there it is, that grumbling grouch in your belly—hunger pangs have hit! You need to eat and you need to eat *now*! So how good are you at finding something decent to eat in the big wide world of fast food?

Did you think you were bypassing the fat with a new-fashioned warm salad or freshly made roll? The truth is you might do just as well with a burger, but remember, a decent burger with all the extras and cheese has about 30 grams of fat and over 1,100 milligrams of sodium. It probably shouldn't be your first choice if you're trying to lose weight and improve your ability to utilize insulin.

How do you decide what's good to eat when there's so much to choose from? If that angel inside you has been losing the argument in the "eat it"–"don't eat it" battle lately, you probably owe it the courtesy of taking a look at this . . .

CAFÉ AND BAR FOOD

NUTRITIONAL HAZARDS	BETTER OPTIONS
Beverages	**Beverages**
• Super-sized gourmet coffee and hot chocolate • Oversized juices • Regular soft drinks	• Coffee with skim milk • Water, mineral water or regular-sized freshly squeezed fruit and vegetable juices • Diet soft drinks
Light meals	**Light meals**
• Buttery herb or garlic bread • Spring rolls and other deep-fried morsels • Ham and cheese croissants • Club sandwich	• Bruschetta (with tomato, basil, olive oil) • Soups (watch out for cream or coconut milk) • Salads BLTs (go easy on the mayo) • Smoked salmon on a bagel (go easy on the cream cheese)
Entreés	**Entreés**
• Chicken cutlet • Beef and onion burger • Pasta carbonara • Large pasta with pesto and parmesan • Fried seafood basket • Nachos with corn chips, cheese and sour cream	• Grilled steak or skinless chicken breast • Vegetable-topped pizza (thin crust) • Appetizer-sized pasta dishes with tomato-based sauce (such as bolognese, marinara, napolitana, arrabiata) • Seafood such as marinated calamari, grilled with chili and lemon or steamed mussels with a tomato sauce
Sides	**Sides**
• French fries, mashed potato	• Steamed vegetables or side salads
Breakfasts	**Breakfasts**
• Sausage, bacon • Croissants • Hash browns • Pastries	• Smoked salmon • Poached eggs • Raisin toast • Sourdough or whole-grain bread
Sweets	**Sweets**
• Baked cheesecake, caramel slice, brownies, sticky date pudding	• A single little biscuit or slice or a fat-free chocolate milk

AT THE MOVIES

NUTRITIONAL HAZARDS	BETTER OPTIONS
• Anything beyond a small popcorn	• Small popcorn
• Anything beyond a 1-oz bag of chips	• 1-oz (30g) bag of chips (baked, Terra)
• Ice cream bars	• Soft-serve frozen yogurt, fruit pop
• Big chocolate bars	• Go for something smaller

LUNCH BARS

NUTRITIONAL HAZARDS	BETTER OPTIONS
• White bread	• Mixed-grain or sourdough bread
• Big bread like Turkish and focaccia (unless you want lots of carbs)	• Avocado or hummus instead of margarine or butter
• Salami, sausage	• Veggie fillings for sandwiches or as a side order instead of fries
• Cheese every day (a generous serving can add as much fat as fries)	• Container of fresh rice, bean, garden or Greek salad
• Fries, chips	• Pasta dishes with a mixture of vegetables and meat
• Milkshakes	• Lebanese kebabs with tabbouleh and hummus
• Anything deep-fried, including chicken cutlet, fish cocktails, spring rolls, scallops	• Grilled fish rather than fried fish
• A burger with "the works"	• Vegetarian pizza
	• Gourmet wraps
	• Containers of fruit salad
	• Burritos with beans, lettuce, tomato and a little cheese (skip the sour cream!)
	• Frozen yogurt or low-fat yogurt mixed with fresh fruits
	• A low-fat smoothie

IN-FLIGHT

NUTRITIONAL HAZARDS	BETTER OPTIONS
• White bread, cheese, pepperoni or salami, cookies and pastries (in airport lounges) • Packaged cakes or muffins, cheese and crackers, chocolate-coated ice cream or chocolate bar (offered as a snack in flight) • Too much alcohol	• Fresh fruit, soup and salad • Dried fruit, nut bars, bananas or apples that you have brought yourself • Plenty of water

FAST-FOOD WORLDS

Fast-food outlets do offer the advantage of having the nutritional composition of their menu available so we took a closer look to see what we could recommend. Some of the options stood out as being either

▶ too high in fat, or
▶ too high in carbohydrates for most people.

We've highlighted this with:

★ = more than 20 grams of fat per serving
❖ = more than 60 grams of carbohydrates per serving.

Boston Market

NUTRITIONAL HAZARDS	BETTER OPTIONS
Meals	**Meals**
• 3 Piece Dark chicken (with skin) ★ • Pastry Top Chicken Pot Pie ★❖ • Boston Meatloaf Carver ★❖	• ¼ White Rotisserie Chicken • Salad with rotisserie chicken and lite ranch dressing • Boston Turkey Carver
Extras	**Extras**
• Creamed Spinach★, Squash Casserole ★, Caesar Side Salad ★ • Desserts★ (Chocolate Cake ★, Chocolate Chip Fudge Brownie ★)	• Garlic Dill New Potatoes, Mashed Potatoes, Sweet Corn, Green Beans • Salads such as Coleslaw or Side Salad with lite dressing—eat first to fill your stomach • Fresh Fruit Salad

McDonald's

NUTRITIONAL HAZARDS	BETTER OPTIONS
Breakfast items	Breakfast items
• Hotcakes ❖	• English Muffin
• Hash Browns	• Egg McMuffin
• Big Breakfast ★	• Fruit 'n Yogurt Parfait
	• Biscuit with strawberry preserves
Meal items	Meal items
• Crispy Chicken Classic Sandwich ★	• Salad menu items with grilled chicken
• Asian Salad with Crispy Chicken	
• Quarter Pounder ★, Big Mac ★, Big N' Tasty ★	• Grilled snack wraps with ranch or honey mustard
	• 4 or 6 piece Chicken McNuggets
Extras	Extras
• McFlurry® ★❖	• Side salad
• French Fries	• Soft-serve ice cream cone
	• Apple dippers with caramel dip
Drinks	Drinks
• Soft drinks	• Water, Diet Coke, iced tea

Burger King

NUTRITIONAL HAZARDS	BETTER OPTIONS
Meal items	Meal items
• Whopper ★	• Whopper Jr. ★
• Bacon Cheeseburger ★	• Tendergrill Chicken Sandwich
• Tendercrisp Chicken Sandwich ★❖	• Tendergrill Chicken Garden Salad
Extras	Extras
• French Fries, Onion Rings	• Salads
Drinks	Drinks
• Milk shakes ❖ and soft drinks	• Diet sodas and water

KFC

NUTRITIONAL HAZARDS	BETTER OPTIONS
Meal items	Meal items
• Crispy Twister★ ❖	• KFC Snackers
• Original Recipe Chicken pieces, Popcorn Chicken ★	• Roasted BLT Salad with Light or Fat-Free Dressing
• BBQ, Buffalo, and Sweet & Sour Wings ★	
Extras	Sides
• Potato Wedges	• Chewy Granola Bar
• Pecan Pie Slice★, Lil' Buckets	• Green Beans, Corn on the Cob, Mashed Potatoes with Gravy
	• Coleslaw

ON THE ROAD

Traveling away from home means stepping out of your routine—it can be harder to eat well, and much, much easier to miss meals. Here are a few tips about what to take:

- Tuna and salmon in foil pouches (remember a plastic fork)
- Reduced-sodium instant soups (all you need is boiling water and a mug)
- Rice cakes
- Dried apricots, apples, etc.
- Dried fruit bars
- Portion-controlled packs of unsalted nuts or dried fruit.

▪ 36 ▪

How Do You Deal with Special Occasions . . . and What About Chocolate?

Christmas, **Thanksgiving, birthdays,** entertaining, celebrations, parties—all these events have one thing in common: food! The circumstances might present some challenges:

▶ The foods served may be new to you, so you won't be sure how to fit them into your diet
▶ The time of meals may be different from your usual schedule
▶ The amount of food may be more or less than you usually eat, and
▶ Special occasions are also occasions for treat foods—chocolate features in a big way at Halloween, Christmas, Easter and Hanukkah.

So what do you do? Kick back and let your hair down? Or hide away and avoid life? There is a middle path—you don't want to knock yourself around, but you want to have a good time, too. If you want to feel good after your next special occasion, try taking a positive approach to doing things a little differently.

When You Are the Host

WHEN YOU ARE entertaining, whether it's a special family event, a religious festival or simply a get-together with friends, you have to put yourself first. Here are some tips:

- Buy and prepare only as much food as you need
- Let your guests know that there's no need to bring any food: if it is a tradition that everyone contributes something, specify exactly what you would like them to bring, and
- Freeze leftovers as soon as possible—this means you're less likely to pick at them while you are cleaning up. Better still, give leftovers to guests when they leave or donate them to a charity that feeds underprivileged or homeless people.

10 TIPS TO SUCCESSFUL SOCIALIZING

- Don't arrive hungry: if you have a small healthy snack before you leave home, you'll reduce the chance that you'll overeat when you get to the party.
- Don't stockpile your plate with treats you don't need: if it's a buffet, take one or two items and only come back for more if you genuinely need to.
- Smaller portions can help you stay in control: try eating a small amount of several foods. This way you can eat what you like.
- Adopt a pastry-free policy: if you avoid these calorie-laden party foods, you'll be ahead.
- Talk more, eat less, and move away from the food table.
- Take to the dance floor to burn up some or all the excess energy.
- Alternate alcoholic and nonalcoholic drinks.

- Use small wine glasses: a standard glass of wine is ½ cup, not the 1½ cups the largest glasses can hold (incidentally, they aren't meant to be filled to the brim).
- Fill your glass yourself, and only when it's empty: it's very easy to lose count of top-offs from others.
- If you eat dessert as part of your meal, eat fewer carbohydrates (starch, fruit, milk) in the rest of the meal, or learn to adjust your short- or fast-acting insulin for larger portions.

CHRISTMAS

Christmas is one day of the year. Try to keep your celebratory eating separate from your regular meals instead of letting the whole Christmas period become a time of gorging and indulgence. At the same time, however, don't expect to lose weight; that would just be setting yourself up for failure.

The main course: The traditional meal—whether it's roast turkey or lamb barbecued steaks—should be okay, but you may need to keep an eye on the timing of the meal.

Dessert options: Prepare or buy lots of fruit salad. There's nothing more refreshing. A wonderful light alternative to traditional Christmas pudding is a Summer pudding—made in a mold lined with fresh bread and filled with a combination of fresh berries in syrup (which could be artificially sweetened).

Fruitcake: Take care with fruitcake too, even if your great-aunt makes one with no added sugar. Fruitcake is a very concentrated source of carbohydrates and (depending on the recipe) saturated fat, so one thick finger-sized piece would be enough at one sitting.

Because you're likely to be on vacation over the Christmas period, you may have time to fit in more activity. An aftermeal walk or backyard game will help you digest your food and counteract the calories. Try these ideas:

- A day out at the park, zoo, or indoor game center
- An adventure vacation (instead of the usual few lazy days poolside), and
- Asking for an active present, such as a gym membership, rock-climbing course, exercise machine or weekend at a health spa.

■

**Let people know if you don't want food—
especially chocolate and cookies and other
sweets—as gifts.**

■

EASTER

Again, because it comes but once a year, Easter is another time when a little indulgence is okay and shouldn't upset your diabetes management too much (depending on how much you like chocolate).

Obviously you need to try to keep to regular meals, but that is usually more difficult when you're socializing or traveling, so consider taking supplies with you. Some fresh fruit, a sandwich—something simple that may not be easily available when you're out.

It will also help to keep your carbohydrate intake under control if you know how to substitute Easter foods for your usual carbohydrates. If the information isn't available on a food label, here's a guide:

- Hot cross buns—count on their being about 50 percent carbohydrate, so an average bun of 80 grams will give you around 40 grams of carbohydrates.
- Chocolate Easter eggs—look for the serving size and assume a serving of chocolate containing 60 grams (4 exchanges) of carbohydrates.
- Chocolate—the carbohydrate content varies depending on the quality of the chocolate. Most chocolate is around 50–60 percent carbohydrate. The healthiest choice is the very dark (85 percent cocoa) variety because it's richest in antioxidants and is a low 20 percent carbohydrate.

Chocolate Easter eggs, being hollow, look like more chocolate than they actually are, so they aren't bad value for a child with diabetes. Easter-themed gifts could be a welcome addition to a big single chocolate egg for a child; an adult may prefer a bunch of flowers, a basket of fruit or a bottle of wine.

Don't bother with diabetic chocolate or eggs. They cost more and are still high in saturated fat and calories. They may be sugar free, but that isn't really the issue with chocolate.

The Real Deal on Chocolate

IF EATEN IN moderation, an occasional chocolate can be enjoyed by most people with diabetes or prediabetes—there is increasing scientific evidence that a little bit of chocolate each day may do you good.

CHOCOLATE AND YOUR BLOOD GLUCOSE

Although most chocolates have a relatively high sugar content, they don't have a big impact on your blood glucose levels. In fact, the average GI is around 45, because their high fat content slows the rate at which the sugars from the stomach are released into the intestine and absorbed into the blood. So people with diabetes don't need to eat low- or reduced-sugar chocolates to avoid high blood glucose levels. However, alternatively sweetened chocolates usually do have fewer calories—a big advantage if you are trying to lose weight.

CHOCOLATE AND YOUR WEIGHT

Most chocolates are what we call energy dense—you get a lot of calories in a little piece. This is good if you are trying to gain weight, travel long distances with limited storage space, or participate in an endurance sport where it is an advantage to be able to carry around a concentrated and highly palatable source of carbohydrates and energy. But it is obviously not good if you are trying to lose weight.

If you are overweight, buy only your favorite, high-quality chocolate, and be careful not to eat too much. Keep it for a treat.

Chocolate Checkout

PRODUCT NAME	ENERGY (CAL)	FAT (G)	SATURATED FAT (G)	CARBO-HYDRATE (G)	SUGARS (G)	FIBER (G)
Chocolate, with nuts	158	11.1	3.9	10.3	9.6	1.0
Chocolate, milk	149	8.5	5.0	15.8	15.1	0.2
Chocolate, dark	147	8.0	4.8	17.6	14.6	0.7
Chocolate, milk, with fruit and nuts	146	8.3	4.0	14.8	12.5	1.4
Chocolate, carbohydrate-modified, filled, with fructose	131	7.0	4.2	16.9	16.4	0.0
Chocolate, caramel filled	125	5.8	3.4	16.5	15.9	0.5
Bar, coconut cream-centered, milk chocolate-coated	121	6.3	4.8	14.6	12.4	2.1
Bar, cherry and coconut/fruit, chocolate-coated	119	6.2	4.8	14.7	13.6	1.3
Bar, peppermint crackle, milk chocolate-coated	119	4.5	4.1	19.6	18.0	0.1
Chocolate, dark, creme-filled	116	4.5	3.2	19.1	18.8	0.6
Chocolate, liqueur-filled	112	4.4	4.0	16.7	16.4	0.7
Chocolate, carbohydrate-modified, plain, artificially sweetened	108	7.8	4.7	17.3	1.5	0.2

CHOCOLATE AND YOUR BLOOD FATS

Chocolate is high in total and saturated fats. In high-quality chocolates, cocoa butter is the main source of fat. This is important, because cocoa butter is high in a particular kind of saturated fat called stearic acid. Stearic acid raises the bad LDL cholesterol less than all other saturated fats do, and it raises the good HDL cholesterol more, so the net effect on your total blood cholesterol levels is not bad at all.

However, the amount of cocoa butter—and therefore the amount of stearic acid as well—used in chocolate varies, and this information is usually not provided in any simple form on the wrapper. As a rough guide, the better-quality (and therefore more expensive) varieties generally have more cocoa butter, so they are usually a better choice.

CHOCOLATE AND ANTIOXIDANTS

Chocolate is one of nature's richest sources of a powerful group of antioxidants known as flavonoids—others are green and black tea, red wine, certain fruits (berries, red grapes, plums, apples) and vegetables (artichokes, asparagus, cabbage, russet and sweet potatoes). It's believed that these antioxidants may benefit people with diabetes or prediabetes by helping to keep cholesterol from sticking to the walls of blood vessels, relaxing major blood vessels and thereby decreasing blood pressure, and maybe even reducing the ability of the blood to form too many clots. A 1-ounce piece of dark chocolate (about one row of a bar) provides about the same amount of these antioxidants as half a cup of black tea or a glass of red wine.

Milk chocolate has only a third of the antioxidant dark chocolate has, and white chocolate has none at all.

RAMADAN

Generally, if you have type 1 diabetes, especially if it's poorly managed, you are strongly advised not to fast during Ramadan because of the risk of hypoglycemia and hyperglycemia. Dehydration and thrombosis are also possible risks.

If you do fast, make sure you check your blood glucose level (BGL) several times a day, and get some specific advice about the timing, type and dose of your insulin.

With type 2 diabetes, there is obviously less risk of hypoglycemia, but if you overindulge at sunset and before dawn, you run a real risk of hyperglycemia. It would be better to distribute your food over three smaller meals to prevent this. It's best to make your decision about fasting after talking with your doctor/diabetes team.

If you are considering fasting, see if you can have a checkup with your doctor/diabetes team 1–2 months before Ramadan. Make sure you're clear about dosing and timing of medications, how often to monitor, meal planning and what to do about physical activity.

The predawn meal: During Ramadan, the predawn meal would ideally be based on low-GI carbohydrates to help sustain you throughout the day.

The evening meal: The meal at sunset can be higher GI, but it's not a good idea to follow the common practice of eating large amounts of high-carbohydrate, high-fat foods at this time.

Make a deliberate effort to increase your fluid intake during non-fasting times.

You will have to end the fast immediately if your blood glucose level (BGL):

▶ Drops below 60 mg/dL (3.3 mmol/L)
▶ Is less than 70 mg/dL (3.9 mmol/L) in the first few hours after starting the fast (especially if you've taken insulin or sulphonylureas before dawn).

▪ 37 ▪

What to Do When You Get Sick or Go to the Hospital

*M*anaging your diabetes when you're sick is more demanding than when you're well, even though the basics don't change. You can apply the general principles we outline in this chapter to help you get through, but visit your doctor if the problem persists for more than a couple of days.

First, it's important to know that some illnesses will cause your blood glucose levels to go low, and others will cause them to go high.

Infections that usually cause low blood glucose levels are generally associated with nausea, vomiting and/or diarrhea, but with no accompanying fever, and there is no increase in insulin resistance or insulin requirements. Rather, the problem seems to be mainly with your inability to absorb or retain food. Common causes are viruses associated with mild gastritis (nausea and vomiting only) or a mild gastroenteritis (vomiting and diarrhea). Food poisoning may present a similar picture.

Infections that usually cause high blood glucose levels are more common, and they are generally associated with a fever. They tend to raise blood glucose levels because they involve higher levels of stress hormones and other factors, which increase gluconeogenesis and insulin resistance. In addition, ketones may appear in the urine. Illnesses that cause raised blood glucose levels are usually those associated with feelings of lethargy, weakness, irritability, muscle aches, headache, fever and obvious signs of an infection. And remember, many of these kinds of infections have a silent phase—you may have unexplained high blood glucose levels for several days before the illness itself becomes apparent.

The essential principles in sick-day management are:

- **Treat the underlying illness.** You may need to see your doctor for antibiotics or other prescription medications
- **Symptomatic relief.** If you have a fever, headache or aches and pains, take regular Tylenol (acetaminophen) or other similar medications in recommended doses
- **Rest.** Get plenty of bed rest, and whenever possible, stay at home
- **Lower-carbohydrate medications.** For young children, many syrups are available in sugar-free forms (antibiotics, acetaminophen, ibuprofen), and those that aren't sugar free are usually okay because the amount of carbohydrate in each dose is not large enough to cause a problem. For older children, adolescents and adults, most medications are available in pill or capsule form, and these are sugar free, and
- **Drink plenty of fluids.** People with diabetes and a fever lose fluid due to the increased body temperature; they may also be losing large volumes of fluid because of high blood glucose levels, which increase urination. If blood glucose levels are greater than 270 mg/dL, drink some water or low-calorie drinks to avoid raising blood glucose higher.

WHAT SHOULD BE IN YOUR SICK-DAY KIT?

Everyone with diabetes should have a sick-day kit prepared and ready to use when required. It should have in it:

- Local doctor's and hospital's phone number
- Diary, for recording and dating symptoms and blood glucose levels
- Thermometer
- Tylenol or alternative
- Low-calorie (diet) drinks or water
- Fruit juice/lemonade or other soft drinks (caffeine is not recommended)
- Rapid- or short-acting insulin and ketone test strips (if you use insulin)
- Glucagon (people with type 1).

WHAT YOU SHOULD EAT OR DRINK WHEN YOU AREN'T FEELING WELL

The following drinks and foods will give you about 15 grams of carbohydrates, and are usually well tolerated.

BEVERAGE/FOOD	AMOUNT/VOLUME
Milk	1 cup (8 oz)
Milk + flavoring	¾ cup milk + 1 tbsp Quik
Fruit juice	½–¾ cup
Tea or coffee, hot water with lemon juice	Add 1 tbsp sugar or honey
Sports (electrolyte) drink	1 cup
Pedialyte	4 packets
Ordinary soda or fruit punch (not low calorie or diet)	¾ cup
Canned soup	1 cup (8 oz) reconstituted
Breakfast cereals	⅔ cup Honey Nut Cheerios, ½ cup oatmeal
Dry toast	1 slice
Crackers or crisp bread	2 Ryvita, etc.
Plain sweet cookies	Vanilla wafers
Mashed potato	½ cup
Rice	⅓ cup
Ordinary Jell-O or pudding	½ cup
Low-fat ice cream	1–1½ scoops
Fruit pop	1 average

IN THE HOSPITAL

Generally, hospital admission is disruptive to glycemic management and to your diet—as much because it is different from your usual regimen as because of anything else. Lying in bed, invasive procedures, stress and pain and changes to medications can all increase your blood glucose levels. But good blood glucose levels are necessary for a speedy recovery, so it's important to do all you can to help keep your blood glucose in a healthy range.

■

A stay in the hospital is not a time to forget about your diet.

■

Hospital meals are very unlikely to be the same as what you eat at home. Although the food service differs from hospital to hospital, most have standard menus for people with diabetes—for meals and snacks. These days, you usually get to choose from the menu, but sometimes it can be a while before it finds you, so your first few meals are likely to have been chosen for you.

You may automatically receive a diabetic menu or you may be able to choose from the full menu. In either case, you may find limits applied to control the amount of carbohydrates you receive and to keep the meal low in saturated fat and sodium.

Sometimes you'll find you've been on the full menu by mistake, so don't assume that everything you're being offered is okay for you. If you think what you're being offered is not appropriate, say something to the nursing or food service staff.

Keep in mind that the hospital food service is trying to please the majority. This is why hospital food tends to be bland, soft and easy to chew. So if you need something different, ask for it. If you're finding it difficult to eat anything, for example, a restricted menu won't suit you and you'll need to ask for something else. If you usually have a snack in the evening before you go to bed and you're not receiving one, ask for it. If you are away from the ward during mealtime and no food is offered to you when you return, speak up.

The general rule is talk to the dietitian, diet technician aid, nurse or doctor if things are not working.

■

**Never assume that the nurses know you have
missed your meal or that you need something.**

■

Fluids only

You might be put on fluids only after surgery or as part of the preparation for a test. There are basically only two menus—free fluids or clear fluids. A clear-fluid diet consists of water, Jell-O, lemonade, fruit pops, clear soup (stock), black tea and coffee; a free-fluid diet includes milk, creamy soups, mousses and ice cream. Some of the fluids will be sugar sweetened and will act as an alternative source of carbohydrates while you're not eating.

Nothing by mouth

There may be times during a hospital stay when you will be put on "nothing by mouth." This is to keep your stomach empty—before surgery, for example. Even water isn't allowed. At these times your blood glucose levels should be closely monitored, and adjustments may have to be made to your diabetes medication or insulin to control them.

▪ 38 ▪

What if You Also Have Celiac Disease?

*C*eliac disease is a condition in which the body cannot tolerate gluten, a protein found in some cereal grains. The only treatment is a gluten-free diet.

Developing celiac disease on top of diabetes can be very upsetting. It brings another layer of dietary restriction on top of what you may have experienced upon developing diabetes. This additional and unwanted burden can be overwhelming, so the whole cycle of grief (see chapter 4) can recur.

For reasons that we don't yet completely understand, people with type 1 diabetes have a much greater risk of developing celiac disease than people who don't have diabetes. Celiac disease and type 1 diabetes are both autoimmune diseases, and they are "triggered" in genetically susceptible people by an as yet unknown factor in the environment.

What if you have type 2 diabetes or prediabetes? It seems that you have about the same level of risk as the rest of the population. You may develop celiac disease, of course, but you aren't at as big a risk as someone with type 1.

WHAT IS CELIAC DISEASE
AND HOW IS IT DIAGNOSED?

Celiac disease is a condition in which the lining of your small intestine becomes damaged due to an immune reaction from your body to a small protein known as gluten. Gluten is found in certain grain foods (wheat, rye, triticale and barley), and in much smaller amounts in oats (as a contaminant). Of course, many processed foods contain these grains as ingredients, and that's where things can get tricky—more about that later.

The first step in finding out whether or not you have celiac disease is to go to your doctor to discuss your symptoms, and you and your family's history. Your doctor will arrange a blood test if you:

▶ Have some of the symptoms of celiac disease
▶ Have a family history of celiac disease, and/or
▶ Are at higher risk because of having type 1 diabetes.

The test looks for raised levels of antigliadin, antiendomysial and/or transglutaminase antibodies in your blood. The blood test itself does not diagnose celiac disease—it merely suggests that further testing, in the form of a small-bowel biopsy, is required.

Celiac disease can only be diagnosed correctly when a small-bowel biopsy shows that the villi in your small intestine have been damaged. The villi are very small and dense "finger-like" projections that line the small intestine. You must be eating gluten-containing foods for a few months before the biopsy or you may not get true results.

In a person with celiac disease, the villi become "flattened" and reduced in number when exposed to gluten. These damaged villi can no longer completely absorb the nutrients from food, and this usually results in a broad range of nutritional deficiencies. These nutritional deficiencies are responsible for many of the common symptoms of celiac disease.

WHAT ARE YOUR CHANCES OF DEVELOPING CELIAC DISEASE?

Recent studies in the United States and Canada indicate that about 1 in 250 people have celiac disease at present—but only 1 out of 4,7000 people is diagnosed. People of Northern European descent seem to be more susceptible than other ethnic groups. There is also some evidence that the number of people with celiac disease is rising throughout the world, though some believe the increase may simply be due to more effective diagnostic techniques.

Somewhere between 30 and 80 out of 1,000 children with type 1 diabetes also have celiac disease. Because it is so much more common in this group, the American Diabetes Association recommends regular screening of all children with type 1.

WHAT ARE THE SYMPTOMS?

The symptoms of celiac disease are not always obvious—in fact celiac disease has been described as the "great imitator." Although you should never try to diagnose yourself, the following list of typical symptoms for children and adults may help you decide whether or not you should discuss celiac disease with your doctor.

Symptoms that are common in children

- Diarrhea or constipation
- Abdominal distension, pain and flatulence
- Large, bulky, foul stools
- Nausea and vomiting
- Poor weight gain and retarded growth in younger children
- Weight loss in older children
- Chronic anemia
- Irritability
- Difficulty in managing blood glucose levels, which may lead to hypoglycemia or hyperglycemia.

Symptoms do not occur until gluten has been introduced into an infant's diet.

Symptoms that are common in adults

- Diarrhea—this may begin at any age and often persists for many years. It may first appear after other illnesses, such as bacterial or viral gastroenteritis, or an abdominal operation
- Constipation—some people experience this more often than diarrhea
- Flatulence, abdominal distension/bloating and cramping
- Nausea and vomiting
- Unexplained weight loss
- Anemia—iron or folate/folic acid deficiency are the most common cause. The anemia will either not respond to appropriate treatment or will recur after treatment
- Fatigue and lethargy
- Difficulty in managing blood glucose levels, which may lead to hypoglycemia or hyperglycemia.

Symptoms that are less common in adults

- Vitamin B$_{12}$, A, D, E and/or K deficiency
- Low blood calcium levels, with muscle spasms
- Easy bruising of the skin—due to vitamin deficiencies
- Unusual skin rashes such as dermatitis herpetiformis
- Ulcerations and/or swelling of the mouth and tongue
- Bone and joint pains
- Miscarriages and infertility in women.

Sometimes, however, there are no recognizable symptoms at all—and this is particularly common in people with type 1 diabetes.

IF YOU DON'T HAVE ANY SYMPTOMS, WHY SHOULD YOU WORRY ABOUT IT?

If you have celiac disease and you don't treat it, your chances of developing other health problems increase significantly. First, if you are eating gluten, damage to the small intestinal villi can still occur, even if you are not experiencing symptoms. Severe villi damage can lead to a general malabsorption of vitamins, minerals and other nutrients from your food. This can result in anemia due to malabsorption of iron, or osteoporosis due to malabsorption of calcium, for example. Perhaps more seriously, there is a much greater risk of developing mouth, throat and intestinal cancers if you continue to eat gluten when you have celiac disease.

IF YOU GO ON A GLUTEN-FREE DIET, WILL ALL YOUR HEALTH PROBLEMS GO AWAY?

The good news is that most people experience a rapid decrease in their symptoms soon after they remove gluten from their diet, and your risk of developing cancers will go back to being about the same as the rest of the population's risk. However, just because you don't have symptoms, it doesn't mean that your celiac disease has been "cured" and you can start eating food containing gluten again. Some people can eat small amounts of food containing gluten without experiencing symptoms, or without their symptoms recurring, but it is strongly recommended that you do not do this—if you do, you will increase your risk of developing these health problems again. The gluten-free diet is for life.

HOW DO YOU MANAGE CELIAC DISEASE?

At the moment, the only treatment for celiac disease is a lifelong gluten-free diet. That means no gluten-containing grains—wheat, rye, triticale and barley—and no products that contain ingredients made from these grains.

This means that most breads, some breakfast cereals, most cookies, cakes, scones and pizza, as well as many other processed foods have to go.

Don't despair; there are lots of gluten-free alternatives. The following foods are gluten free:

- Corn, rice, sago, tapioca, buckwheat, potato flour, soy flour and arrowroot, and products that are made from these foods
- Fruits and vegetables

▶ Meat (except most processed meats), chicken, fish and eggs, and
▶ Milk and most other dairy foods.

Many processed foods contain gluten. One way of finding out which ones to avoid is to check the ingredient list. Ingredients such as wheaten cornstarch or wheat starch and malt or malt extract contain small amounts of gluten and should be avoided.

Others, such as maltodextrin and certain food starches, may also be derived from wheat starch and so may have very small amounts of gluten. However, they might also be derived from corn, tapioca, rice or potato and so may not contain gluten.

To help you figure it out, all ingredients derived from wheat, rye, oats and barley must be declared on the food label. For example, flour derived from wheat would appear on the label as "enriched flour (wheat, malted barley)."

What does "gluten free" mean on food labels?

In January 2007, the Food and Drug Administration (FDA) began regulating the "gluten-free" label on foods in the United States. As currently defined by the FDA, foods are gluten free "if they don't contain wheat, barley, rye or their hybrids, or if they contain fewer than 20 parts per million gluten." Foods that have gluten-free claims on their labels can be safely consumed by people with diabetes and celiac disease.

Low-GI gluten-free foods

Many gluten-free foods, such as dairy foods, legumes and most fruits, have a low GI. Unfortunately, many of the gluten-free breads and cereals in supermarkets have not had their GI measured yet. Foods that have been tested and found to have a lower GI are listed in the following table. In the tables at the end of the book, there is a section on commercial gluten-free products.

Lower-GI Foods that Are Gluten Free

FOOD GROUP	FOOD NAME
Grains	Buckwheat
	Corn tortilla*
	Basmati rice
	Rice vermicelli
Fruit	Most fresh, frozen, dried, glacé or canned* fruits, apples, apricots, grapefruit, grapes, oranges, peaches, pears, plums, raisins
	Most fruit juices
Vegetables	Sweet corn
	Yam
Dairy and soy	Low-fat ice cream*
	Low-fat and reduced-fat milk
	Low-fat and reduced-fat soy milk*
	Low-fat pudding*, pudding mix*
	Yogurt*
Legumes, seeds and nuts	All dried and canned beans, peas, lentils, chickpeas
Breakfast cereals	Rice bran
Snack food	Plain popcorn
	Nuts*
	Dried fruit and nut mixes*
	Sunflower and pumpkin seeds*

*May contain gluten but gluten-free brands can be found

In addition to these low-GI carbohydrates, comprehensive lists of gluten-free foods are available from the Celiac Disease Foundation.

For more information on celiac disease

The Celiac Disease Foundation (CDF) has a comprehensive list of books about living with celiac disease at their Web site, www.celiac.org (click on "Books & More"), where you can also order their guidelines for living gluten-free. *Gluten-Free Diet* by Shelley Case provides a comprehensive resource, covering 2,600 gluten-fee foods available in the United States and Canada.

Gluten-Free Foods for Hypos

THE GLUTEN-FREE foods in the following list are suitable for treating a hypo:

Easily absorbed carbohydrates to begin with, to raise blood glucose levels quickly. For example, one of the following:

- 2–3 teaspoons sugar or honey
- 4 cubes sugar
- 10–15 grams glucose tablets (check sizes, as some contain 1½ grams glucose and others 5 grams)
- ½–¾ cup (4–6 oz) fruit juice
- ⅓ cup (2½ oz) Lucozade*, or
- soft sugar candies (about 6)*.

Followed within 15–20 minutes by carbohydrate foods that will maintain blood glucose levels. For example, one of the following:

- 1 cup milk
- 1 container gluten-free yogurt, or
- 1 piece of fruit, such as an apple, banana or pear.

Note: *May contain glucose syrup, glucose and/or maltodextrin derived from wheat starch, so may contain traces of gluten. Check ingredient list, which must say if this is the case.

·39·

Do You Need to Take a Supplement?

*I*f you're generally healthy and eat a wide variety of foods as part of a well-balanced diet, including fruits, vegetables, dairy, whole grains, legumes and lean meats and fish, it's very unlikely that you need to take a supplement. There are some times, however, when your doctor or dietitian may recommend you take one.

If you're pregnant or planning to have a baby, a folate supplement is recommended. It helps protect your baby against neural tube birth defects such as spina bifida. As we said in chapter 28, it's important to start taking this before you become pregnant.

Men and women over 50 may need a calcium and vitamin D supplement. This helps keep your bones strong and decrease bone loss after menopause if you don't get enough calcium and vitamin D from your diet.

Some vegetarians and vegans may need supplements. Although it is possible to meet your nutrient requirements from nonmeat sources, if your diet isn't optimal, or you're going through a time of increased requirements, you may not get enough. Vitamin B_{12} is the one that can cause problems, especially for vegans, as it isn't naturally found in plant foods. So if you don't eat meat, dairy foods or eggs, your only reliable source of B_{12} will be fortified vegetarian foods or a dietary supplement.

When you are first diagnosed with diabetes, your blood glucose levels may have been high for some time, which means you may be deficient in a number of vitamins and minerals, because many are either lost in the urine, or because the amount you need is higher because of the diabetes itself. The most common problems are the vitamins E, B_6, folate, B_{12}, and the minerals calcium, zinc, magnesium and possibly chromium. Sometimes people taking the medication metformin develop a B_{12} deficiency, so a B_{12} supplement may be necessary.

After a few months, when your blood glucose levels have returned to normal (or close to it) through healthy eating, regular physical activity and appropriate medication, your vitamin and mineral requirements will return to normal too.

Whatever your situation is, it's best to discuss which vitamin and mineral supplements you need, if any, with your dietitian or doctor. Most of the rest of us don't need to worry about supplementation—it's just not necessary.

HOW COMMON ARE VITAMIN AND MINERAL DEFICIENCIES?

True vitamin and mineral deficiencies can result in poor wound healing, bruising, anemia, increased risk of infections, cognitive (mental) impairment, neurological disorders, stroke and some cancers. Luckily, these levels of deficiency are rare. They are usually only seen in cases of extreme poverty, or if you:

▶ Have a very poor diet
▶ Are on a very restricted weight loss diet (less than 1,200 calories [5,040 kJ] a day)
▶ Have a medical condition such as undiagnosed celiac disease that affects how your body absorbs, uses or excretes nutrients

- Smoke—tobacco decreases the absorption of many vitamins and minerals, including vitamin C, folate, magnesium and calcium, and/or
- Drink excessively—long-term excessive alcohol consumption can impair the digestion and absorption of several vitamins and minerals, including vitamin B_1, iron, zinc, magnesium and folate.

True vitamin or mineral deficiency is rare in people with diabetes. However, high blood glucose levels can lead to increased urination, which means you can lose some B vitamins, vitamin C, and certain minerals in your urine.

On the other hand, some minerals—copper and iron, for instance—seem to be more easily stored in the bodies of people with diabetes, so taking supplements of these can be dangerous.

WHAT'S THE BEST WAY TO MAKE SURE YOU ARE GETTING ENOUGH VITAMINS AND MINERALS?

The best way to ensure that you are getting the right amount of all vitamins and minerals is to eat a well-balanced diet. As a rule, vitamins and minerals are absorbed more effectively from foods than they are from supplements. Also, they are usually cheaper that way—and definitely much tastier!

It can be dangerous to self-treat a vitamin or mineral deficiency without knowing the underlying cause. For example, what looks like a simple iron deficiency can be caused by internal bleeding due to a cancer somewhere in the digestive tract—this happens much too often with American adults. Make sure you check out any suspected deficiency with your doctor.

SHOULD YOU TAKE A SUPPLEMENT "JUST IN CASE"?

If you eat a healthy diet and your diabetes is well managed, but you still want some "just in case" nutrition insurance, what should you do?

Ask yourself these two questions:

▶ Are your blood glucose levels kept within the recommended range most of the time? If they're not, talk to your dietitian and/or diabetes educator about how you can improve your blood glucose, and

▶ Do you think you have clear symptoms of deficiency? If you do, see your doctor, because he or she knows your medical history best.

If you do have a vitamin or mineral deficiency, talk to your dietitian about how you can change your diet so that you get all the nutrients you need from food. Don't head straight for the pharmacy or vitamin store for pills to pop.

DOES IT REALLY MATTER IF YOU TAKE A SUPPLEMENT EVEN IF YOUR DIET ISN'T DEFICIENT?

Yes, it does. Some vitamins and minerals can be toxic if you take them in amounts that are much more than the recommended daily allowance.

On top of this, too much of one can actually cause a deficiency of another. For example, large doses of vitamin C can decrease your body's ability to absorb vitamin B_{12}, and large doses of zinc can interfere with the absorption of copper. So remember, no megadoses.

THE CHROMIUM QUESTION

Chromium is an essential mineral. Originally, scientists thought it formed a part of a glucose tolerance factor, in combination with some B vitamins and amino acids. However, glucose tolerance factor has never been isolated in humans or animals, or synthesized in a laboratory. No one has yet proved that it actually exists!

New research suggests that rather than being a part of the glucose tolerance factor, chromium is at the center of a very small protein molecule that helps activate insulin receptors in your body's cells. If this is true, it means that chromium may help insulin work more effectively in the cells of your body. This in turn helps your body manage blood glucose levels more effectively.

How much chromium do you need?

A minute amount. It has been estimated that 25 micrograms a day for women and 35 micrograms a day for men is all you need. This amount is easy to get from the food you eat. Good sources are:

- bran-based breakfast cereals and whole-grain breads and cereals
- egg yolk
- brewers' yeast and yeast extract
- cheese
- fruits such as apples, oranges and pineapples
- vegetables such as broccoli, mushrooms, potatoes with their skin on, tomatoes
- liver, kidney and lean meat
- peanuts
- oysters
- some spices (pepper, chili)

What happens if you don't get enough chromium?

In the past, hospitalized patients living on intravenous nutrient solutions that lacked chromium were seen to develop high blood glucose levels. When chromium was added to the intravenous solutions, the symptoms were reversed. This sparked speculation that poor chromium intake could contribute to the development of type 2 diabetes.

Many scientists believe that people with a poor or inadequate chromium intake may be more responsive to supplementation than those who are well nourished. In other words, if your diet is low in chromium, a supplement may improve glucose control.

How do you know if you are low in chromium?

A person's chromium status seems to be hard to measure. Blood, urine, nail and even hair samples have been used, but none of these seems to be ideal. Despite years of research, there is still no universally accepted way of determining whether or not a person is deficient in chromium.

Should you take a chromium supplement "just in case"?

Probably not. There are risks in taking large amounts of chromium as it accumulates in the body. What's more, there is no evidence of widespread chromium deficiency in the United States and Canada. What we do know is that eating a varied, balanced diet will give you all the chromium you need—remember, it's a minute amount.

Chromium Studies

A NUMBER OF studies have been done to see whether or not people with diabetes benefit from a chromium supplement. One study in China showed a significant improvement in blood glucose levels after taking either 200 or 1,000 micrograms of chromium (picolinate) each day for 4 months. Other studies have shown no benefit from supplementation.

•40•

What About Herbal Therapies?

*I*f **you check** out an herbal remedies encyclopedia, you'll find hundreds of plants that have a reputation for lowering blood glucose and were once "used for treating diabetes." However, most have not been scientifically evaluated and many are consumed regularly as part of a normal healthy diet, for example:

HERBS AND SPICES	VEGETABLES	FRUIT
Agrimony	Cabbage	Apples
Burdock	Celery	Blackberries
Chili pepper	Garlic	Elderberries
Coriander	Navy beans	Guavas
Dandelion	Leeks	Hops
Ginger	Lettuce	Lemons
Juniper	Mushrooms	Limes
Liquorice	Onions	Lychees
Nettles	Peas	Papayas
Sage	Potatoes	Raspberries
Tarragon	Sweet corn	
Thyme	Turnips	

HOW DO THEY WORK?

For most of these plants, very little is known about how they might work to lower blood glucose. Some of the active components that have been analyzed include:

- *Alkaloids*, which are found in mulberry, fenugreek and black bean. They also may work by slowing the rate of digestion and absorption of carbohydrates, and possibly by reducing glucose production from the liver
- *Flavonoids*, which are found in grapes and wine, tea, cocoa and soybeans, and the herb false teak. They may help stimulate insulin release from the pancreas
- *Glucosides*, which are found in bilberry, blackberry and raspberry. They may improve insulin action in the muscles and some organs, making the insulin you produce or inject work more effectively, and
- *Propionic acid*, which is found in unripe fruits, and more specifically, the Jamaican ackee apple. It may reduce glucose stores in the liver and glucose production by the liver.

SHOULD YOU USE HERBAL REMEDIES?

There is some evidence that some plants can decrease glucose absorption, decrease glucose production, increase insulin secretion, or improve insulin action. However, there is no evidence that plants can be a substitute for insulin, so herbal remedies are unlikely to be of any use if you have type 1 diabetes.

However, they may be useful for people with type 2 diabetes, or those trying to prevent it, but there are issues with toxicity, potency, and quality control. Why?

A couple of reasons. First, as well as the active ingredients that may help lower blood glucose levels, herbs may contain other substances that are poisonous.

Second, the amount of the active ingredient may vary considerably from batch to batch, depending on the season, where the plant was grown and how it was processed and stored. This variation could contribute to major swings in your blood glucose levels, which may be life-threatening.

What's the solution? Herbs are probably best used as a basis for research into new medicines. When the active ingredient has been identified, it can be produced in large quantities in a purified form so that there are no accompanying toxins, the dose is always the same and the quality is strictly controlled—basically, so you know you'll get what you are paying for. For example, guanidine, from the plant goat's rue (*Galega officinalis*), provided the design template for metformin (diabex, diaformin, glucophage, etc.).

What about Cinnamon?

A RECENT STUDY found that by taking 1–6 grams of cinnamon each day for 40 days, people with type 2 diabetes experienced significant improvements in blood glucose levels, LDL cholesterol and triglycerides.

However, the researchers did not state whether or not the people in the study made any changes to their diets or physical activity levels, and as we know, eating a healthy diet and increasing physical activity levels can also improve blood glucose, cholesterol and triglyceride levels. Therefore, more research is needed to work out whether or not cinnamon itself can really help people with diabetes.

BUYER BEWARE!

Stevia rebaudiana

Stevia is a South American herb, first discovered by scientists in the late 1800s. Its extract, stevioside, is 250–300 times sweeter than sucrose, but unlike sugars, it does not have any calories. Advertising material claims that stevia:

- "Is better . . . than pharmaceutical sweeteners"
- "May actually lower blood sugar levels," and
- "Stimulates mental alertness, counters fatigue, facilitates

digestion, regulates metabolism, and has a therapeutic effect on the liver, pancreas and spleen."

Despite all the claims, there has been very little scientific research done on the therapeutic properties of stevia, and what has been done suggests that it is little more than a nonnutritive alternative sweetener (see chapter 16).

Tahitian noni juice

Noni (*Morinda citrifolia*) is a shrub or small tree that is native to Southeast Asia but has spread extensively throughout India, and into the Pacific Islands as far as Tahiti. The fruit has a pungent odor when ripening and is therefore also known as cheese fruit or even vomit fruit. Tahitian noni juice is extracted from the fruit and mixed with large quantities of "natural fruit juices" (such as blackcurrant), then sold as a tonic—noni juice. It is supposed to contain the active ingredient "xeronine," which is claimed to:

- Lower blood pressure
- Regulate sleep, temperature and moods
- Increase body energy
- Alleviate pain
- Have antibacterial properties
- Inhibit growth of cancer tumors, and autoimmune diseases.

Unfortunately, there is no evidence so far that Tahitian noni juice has any therapeutic benefits for humans, so it seems to be little more than a very expensive fruit juice!

Glossary

A1c (also called HbA1c, hemoglobin A1c or glycosylated or glycated hemoglobin) is a blood test that measures your average blood glucose level (BGL) over the previous 2–3 months. It indicates the percentage of hemoglobin (the part of the red blood cell that carries oxygen to the cells and sometimes joins with glucose in the bloodstream) that is "glycated." Glycated means it has a glucose molecule riding on its back. This is proportional to the amount of glucose in the blood. The higher the level of HbA1c, the greater the risk of developing diabetic complications. If you have diabetes, you should have the A1c test 2–4 times a year, depending on your type, and you should aim to keep it under 7 percent.

Acanthosis nigricans is sandpaper-like dark skin in the armpits or neck—or, in severe cases, over joints. It is the result of severe **insulin resistance**. It is often one of the first physical signs that you have diabetes or prediabetes.

Alternative sweeteners are substances used to sweeten foods instead of sugar. The term includes nutritive sweeteners (which add calories to the diet) and nonnutritive sweeteners (no calories).

Acarbose is a blood glucose-lowering medication that works by slowing the rate of digestion of carbohydrates in the small intestine.

Arteries are blood vessels carrying oxygenated blood from the lungs and heart to the rest of the body.

Atherosclerosis or hardening of the arteries is a slowly developing condition that produces problems such as angina, stroke or a heart attack. Most heart disease is caused by atherosclerosis—clogging on the inside wall of the arteries through the slow buildup of fatty deposits (called plaques) which narrow the arteries and reduce the blood flow. If the plaques rupture, clots form, causing a more acute, total blockage. If the blood vessel is providing blood to the heart, the result would be a heart attack. Atherosclerosis can affect the arteries to the heart, and those in the brain, kidneys, arms and legs.

Autoimmune diseases are diseases in which the immune system mistakenly attacks and destroys body tissue or organs which it believes to be foreign. Type 1 diabetes, celiac disease and rheumatoid arthritis are autoimmune diseases.

Basal insulin is like background insulin. The term can be used to refer to the insulin produced by your pancreas, or long-acting injected insulin, or insulin trickled in by your pump, which helps manage your blood glucose levels in the fasting state—between meals and overnight.

Beta cells produce the hormone insulin. They are found grouped together in the islets of Langerhans in the pancreas.

Biguanides are a commonly used type of medication that lower blood glucose levels by increasing insulin sensitivity and decreasing glucose production by the liver. Metformin is the most widely used form.

Blood glucose, also known as blood sugar, is the most common kind of sugar found in the blood. It is the main source of energy for most of the body's organs and tissues and the only source of fuel for the brain.

Blood glucose level (BGL) is the concentration of glucose in the bloodstream. If you haven't eaten in the past few hours (and you don't have diabetes), your blood glucose level will normally fall within the range of 65–110 mg/dL (3.5–6 mmol/L). If you eat, this will rise, but rarely above 180 mg/dL (10 mmol/L). It is measured in milligrams per deciliter (mg/dL) in the United States and millimoles per liter (mmol/L) in journals and the rest of the world (including Canada).

Blood pressure is the pressure of the blood on the inside walls of arteries caused by the beating of the heart. It is expressed as a ratio, such as 120/80. The first number is the systolic pressure, or the pressure when the heart pushes the blood out into the arteries. The second number is the diastolic pressure, or the pressure when the heart rests between beats. High blood pressure (hypertension)— above 140/90—is the most common cardiovascular disease risk factor. High blood pressure is more common in people with diabetes and increases the risk of stroke, heart attack, and kidney and eye diseases. Your blood pressure should be measured when you visit your doctor for a checkup, or at least twice a year. Your blood pressure goals will vary depending on your age and other factors.

Body Mass Index (BMI) is a measure of body weight relative to height. It is calculated by multiplying weight in pounds by 705, divided by height in inches squared (in^2). It has limitations, because it does not take account of body composition. It can overestimate body fat in athletes and others who have a muscular build (such as bodybuilders), and in pregnant women, and underestimate body fat in older people or people with a disability who have lost muscle mass. For an easy online calculator visit: www.nhlbisupport.com/bmi.

BMI categories:

Less than 18.5	Underweight
18.5–24.9	Healthy weight range
25–29.9	Overweight
Over 30	Obese

Bolus insulin (also known as insulin bolus) refers to the burst of insulin that is delivered by your pancreas, or to short-acting insulin given by injection or by an insulin pump to "cover" a meal or snack or to correct for a high blood glucose level (BGL).

Calorie (or kilocalorie, to be technically correct) is the unit that measures the energy we get from food. Carbohydrates, protein, fat and alcohol all provide the body with energy. Carbs and protein provide 4 calories per gram, fat gives 9 calories per gram, and alcohol gives 7 calories per gram. A kilocalorie is the amount of energy (or heat) needed to increase the temperature of 1 kilogram of water by 1°C. The equivalent metric unit is the **kilojoule** (kJ). You can convert calories to kilojoules by multiplying by 4.2.

Carbohydrate is one of the three main nutrients in food—protein and fat are the other two. Carbohydrate is the starchy part of foods such as rice, bread, legumes, potatoes and pasta, and the sugars in foods such as fruit, milk and honey, and certain types of fiber. Some foods contain a large amount of carbohydrates (cereals, potatoes, sweet potatoes, yams and legumes); other foods, such as carrots, broccoli and salad vegetables, are very diluted sources.

See also **fiber, starch** and **sugars.**

Carbohydrate counting is a method of meal planning for people with diabetes based on counting the grams of carbohydrates in food.

Carbohydrate exchange is an amount of food typically containing an average of 15 grams (12–17 grams) of carbohydrates. It is one of several approaches to meal planning for people with diabetes. Lists set out the serving sizes of different carb foods and assign a certain number of exchanges to each meal over the course of the day. The system is intended to promote consistency in the amount of carbohydrates eaten every day. It was developed long before research on the glycemic index (GI) was published, so it focuses purely on carbohydrate quantity, not on carbohydrate quality.

Cardiovascular disease (CVD) refers to the diseases that involve the heart and/or blood vessels (arteries and veins), particularly those related to **atherosclerosis.**

Cardiovascular system is the heart and blood vessels. It is the means by which blood is pumped from the heart and circulated through the body. As it circulates, the blood carries nourishment and oxygen to all the body tissues. It also removes waste products.

Central obesity (your waist measurement) is often a better predictor of your health risks than Body Mass Index (BMI). Abdominal fat increases your risk of heart disease, high blood pressure and diabetes.

Cholesterol is a soft waxy substance found in the blood and in all the body's cells. It is an important part of a healthy body because it is part of the walls around all the body's cells and is a major component of many of the hormones the body produces. Most of the cholesterol the body needs is manufactured by the liver. It is also found in some animal foods (eggs, milk, cheese, liver, meat and poultry). High levels of cholesterol in the blood can lead to blocked arteries, heart attack and stroke. Cholesterol and other fats can't dissolve in the blood—they have to be transported to and from the cells by special carriers called lipoproteins. The most common ones are low-density lipoprotein (LDL) cholesterol and high-density lipoprotein (HDL) cholesterol.

HDL cholesterol is known as "good" cholesterol because higher levels of HDL seem to protect against heart attack and stroke; HDL tends to sweep excess cholesterol from the blood back to the liver.

LDL cholesterol is the main form of cholesterol in the blood and does most of the damage to blood vessels—high levels are a red flag for cardiovascular disease. If there is too much LDL cholesterol in the blood, it can slowly build up in the walls of the blood vessels that feed the heart, brain and other important organs, causing a heart attack or stroke.

Recommended ranges for people with diabetes

Total cholesterol	< 200 mg/dL (< 5.1 mmol/L)
Triglycerides	< 150 mg/dL (< 1.7 mmol/L)
HDL cholesterol	
men	> 40 mg/dL (> 1.0 mmol/L)
women	> 50 mg/dL (> 1.3 mmol/L)
LDL cholesterol	< 100 mg/dL (< 2.5 mmol/L)
Total cholesterol/HDL ratio	men: <5.0; women: < 4.0

Celiac disease is a condition in which the lining of the small intestine is damaged due to an immune reaction from the body to gluten, a protein found in certain grain foods, such as wheat, rye, triticale and barley, and in much smaller amounts in oats. The only treatment for celiac disease at the moment is a gluten-free diet.

Complications are the harmful effects of diabetes including damage to the blood vessels, heart, nervous system, eyes, feet, and kidneys, teeth and gums. Studies show that keeping blood glucose, blood pressure and cholesterol levels within the recommended ranges can help prevent or delay these problems.

Chromium is an essential mineral that the body needs in very small amounts. It helps insulin work more effectively. People with a chromium deficiency develop symptoms characteristic of diabetes.

However, chromium deficiency is thought to be very rare, and is not likely to be the cause of diabetes or prediabetes in most people. Likewise, taking chromium supplements is not likely to cause a dramatic improvement in blood glucose levels in most people.

Dawn phenomenon is the rise in blood glucose levels that occurs in the early morning hours before waking. It is due to the body's release of hormones.

Diabetes

Type 1 diabetes is characterized by high blood glucose levels due to the body's complete inability to produce insulin. It occurs when the body's immune system attacks the insulin-producing beta cells in the pancreas and destroys them. The pancreas then produces very little or no insulin. Type 1 diabetes occurs most often in young people but can develop in adults.

Type 2 diabetes is characterized by high blood glucose levels caused by an insufficiency of insulin and the body's inability to use insulin efficiently. It is thought to occur when the body becomes **insulin resistant**. The pancreas compensates initially by producing more insulin but eventually becomes exhausted and doesn't produce enough insulin. Type 2 diabetes occurs most often in middle-aged and older people but is being seen increasingly in younger people—even adolescents.

See also **gestational diabetes**.

Diabetic ketoacidosis (also called ketoacidosis or DKA) is the result of a severe lack of insulin leading to high blood glucose levels and an accumulation of **ketones** in the blood and urine. It is an emergency condition, and can lead to coma and death if it is not treated. The symptoms are nausea, stomach pain, vomiting, fruity breath odor, chest pain, rapid shallow breathing and difficulty staying awake.

Dyslipidemia refers to abnormal levels of cholesterol and triglycerides in the blood.

Energy (fuel for the body) is provided by the foods we eat. How much energy a food provides depends on the amount of carbohydrates, protein and fat it contains. This energy is measured in calories or kilojoules: these words allow us to talk about how much energy a food contains and how much energy is burned up during exercise.

Fasting blood glucose is a blood test in which a sample of your blood is drawn after an overnight fast (8–12 hours) to measure the amount of glucose in your blood. The test is used to diagnose diabetes and prediabetes and to monitor people who already have type 2 diabetes.

Fat is one of the three main nutrients in food and provides 9 calories per gram. The idea is to focus on the good fats (monounsaturated and polyunsaturated fats) and avoid the bad fats (trans fats and saturated fats). You don't actually need to eat any saturated fat, since your body can make all it needs, but it is fairly difficult not to eat some, since all fats are actually mixtures of saturated and unsaturated fats.

Saturated fats are solid or semisolid at room temperature. These are the fats on meat, and in chicken skin, butter, cheese, palm oil and coconut oil. Saturated fats raise blood cholesterol levels by increasing the amount of cholesterol produced by the liver, causing it to build up in the bloodstream and become part of the plaque that forms on the walls of the blood vessels.

Unsaturated fat is liquid at room temperature and comes primarily from plant foods and fish. Monounsaturated and polyunsaturated fats provide the essential fatty acids that form your cell membranes, help you absorb the fat-soluble vitamins A, D, E and K, form part of your body's hormones, provide insulation, and help you absorb some antioxidants from fruit and vegetables. Polyunsaturated and monounsaturated fats help lower blood cholesterol levels and may help raise HDL cholesterol levels.

Trans fats occur naturally in small amounts in the fat of dairy products and meat. They are also formed by hydrogenation—a chemical process that changes a liquid oil into a solid fat. Foods high in trans fats include fried fast foods, some margarines, crackers, cookies and snack foods—the United States and Canada require manufacturers to list the amount of trans fat in nutrition information panels. Trans fats can raise cholesterol levels and are linked to an increased risk of cardiovascular disease.

Fatty liver is the buildup of excessive amounts of **triglycerides** and other fats inside liver cells. It may progress to the medical condition known as NASH (nonalcoholic steatohepatitis), which is more common in type 2 diabetes.

Fiber, in terms of food or dietary fiber, is mainly carbohydrate molecules made up of many different sorts of monosaccharides. They are different from starches and sugars in that they are not broken down by human digestive enzymes and they reach the large intestine mostly unchanged. Once there, bacteria begin to ferment and break down the fibers. Dietary fiber comes mainly from the outer bran layers of grains (corn, oats, wheat and rice, and foods containing these grains), fruit and vegetables and nuts and legumes (dried beans, peas and lentils). There are two main types of fiber—soluble and insoluble.

Soluble fiber can be dissolved in water—it is things such as the gel, gum and often jellylike components of apples, oats and legumes. Some soluble fibers are very viscous when in solution. By slowing down the time it takes for food to pass through the stomach and small intestine, soluble fiber can lower the glycemic response to a food. Good sources include oatmeal, oat bran, nuts and seeds, legumes (beans, peas and lentils), apples, pears, strawberries and blueberries.

Insoluble fiber, such as cellulose, is not soluble in water and does not directly affect the speed of digestion. It is dry and branlike and commonly called roughage. All cereal grains and products that retain the outer coat of the grain they are made from are sources of insoluble fiber—whole-wheat bread and All-Bran, for example— but not all foods containing insoluble fiber are low GI. Insoluble fiber will only lower the GI of a food when it exists in its original, intact form, such as in whole grains of wheat. In this form it acts as a physical barrier, delaying the access of digestive enzymes and water to the starch within the cereal grain. Good sources include whole rains, whole wheat breads, barley, couscous, brown rice, bulgur, wheat bran, seeds, and most vegetables.

See also **resistant starch**.

Fructose *see* **sugars**.

Fuel hierarchy is the order in which the body burns different types of fuel. The body runs on fuel, just like a car runs on gasoline. These fuels are derived from the protein, fat, carbohydrates and alcohol you consume. Alcohol is burned first because the body has no place to store unused alcohol and it is potentially toxic to many of the body's organs and tissues. Protein comes second, then carbohydrates, then fat—the last in line. In practice, the fuel mix is usually a combination of carbohydrates and fat in varying proportions—after meals the mix is mainly carbohydrate; before meals it is mainly fat.

Gestational diabetes is diabetes that develops during pregnancy. It usually goes away after the baby is born. Hormones released by the placenta during pregnancy reduce the effectiveness of the mother's insulin and will unmask any predisposition she has to diabetes. It is managed with diet, exercise and sometimes insulin.

Glucagon is a hormone produced by the alpha cells in the pancreas. Between meals, blood glucose levels start to fall. As this happens, the pancreas releases glucagon into the blood, causing blood glucose levels to rise by promoting the conversion of glycogen (glucose stores) in the liver to glucose. An injectable form of glucagon can be used to treat severe **hypoglycemia**.

Glucose is a simple form of sugar (a monosaccharide) that is created when the body's digestive processes break down the carbohydrate foods you eat (such as bread, cereals and fruit). It is this glucose that is absorbed from the intestine and becomes the fuel that circulates in the bloodstream.

Glucose tolerance test (GTT) is a test used in the diagnosis of diabetes and prediabetes. Glucose in the blood is measured at regular intervals for a couple of hours before and after a person has drunk either 50 or 75 grams of pure glucose after an overnight fast.

Glycemia is the concentration of glucose in the blood (adjective, **glycemic**).

Glycemic index (GI) relates to the fact that different carbohydrate foods behave differently in the body. Some break down quickly during digestion and release glucose rapidly into the bloodstream; others break down gradually and slowly trickle glucose into the bloodstream. The glycemic index, or GI, is a numerical ranking on a scale of 0 to 100 that describes this difference. It is a measure of carbohydrate quality. After testing hundreds of carbohydrate foods around the world, scientists have found that foods with a low GI will have less effect on your blood glucose than foods with a high GI. High-GI foods tend to cause spikes in your glucose levels, whereas low-GI foods tend to cause gentle rises. All foods are compared with a reference food and tested following an internationally standardized method. For more information, visit the official glycemic index Web site: www.glycemicindex.com.

Glycemic Index Symbol Program (GISP) is a program that encourages manufacturers to have their carbohydrate foods GI tested at an accredited laboratory, and to list the results on the labels of their foods. Foods that are part of the GISP must meet strict nutrition criteria to ensure that they are healthy foods. They are easily identified by the program's logo. For more information, visit the official glycemic index symbol program's Web site: www.gisymbol.com.

Glycemic load (GL) is how high your blood glucose actually rises and how long it remains high when you eat a meal containing carbohydrates. The levels depend on both the quality of the carbohydrate (its GI) and the quantity of carbohydrate in the meal. Researchers at Harvard University came up with the term "glycemic load" to describe this. It is calculated by multiplying the GI of a food by the available carbohydrate content (carbohydrate minus fiber) in the serving (expressed in grams), divided by 100 (GL = GI × 100 available carbs per serving).

Glycemic potential or **glycemic potency** refers to a food or meal's predicted blood glucose-raising effect.

Glycemic response (also known as **glycemic impact**) refers to the change or pattern of change in blood glucose after consuming a food or meal. Glucose responses can be fast or slow, short or prolonged. It is primarily determined by the food's carbohydrate content. Other factors include how much food you eat, how processed the food is and even how the food is prepared (for example, pasta that is cooked al dente has a slower glycemic response than pasta that is overcooked).

Glycogen is the name given to the glucose stored in the body. It can be readily broken down into glucose to maintain normal blood glucose levels. In men, approximately two-thirds of the body's glycogen is in the muscles and one-third is in the liver. The total amount of glycogen in the body is relatively small, though—it will be exhausted in about 24 hours during fasting or starvation.

Glycosylated hemoglobin *see* **A1c**.

Gram is a unit of weight in the metric system: 1 ounce equals 28 grams (often rounded up to 30 grams). A typical sandwich-thickness slice of bread weighs 30 grams.

Hba1c *see* **A1c**.

HDL cholesterol *see* **cholesterol**.

High blood glucose *see* **hyperglycemia**.

Honeymoon phase is a temporary remission of hyperglycemia that occurs in some people when they are newly diagnosed with type 1 diabetes—some insulin secretion resumes for a short time, usually a few months, but then it stops again.

Hormones are "chemical messengers" made in one part of the body and released into the bloodstream to trigger or regulate particular functions of another part of the body. For example, insulin is a hormone made in the pancreas that lets glucose into cells throughout the body so that they can produce energy.

Hyperglycemia is a condition that occurs when there are excessively high levels of glucose in the blood. The symptoms usually occur when blood glucose levels go above 270 mg/dL (15 mmol/L). They include extreme thirst, large volumes and frequent urination, weakness, and weight loss. If hyperglycemia is not treated, it can lead to the production of ketones, deep breathing, abdominal pain, drowsiness and eventually unconsciousness, coma and death.

Hyperinsulinemia is a condition when the level of insulin in the blood is higher than normal. It is caused by overproduction of insulin by the body and is related to insulin resistance.

Hypoglycemia (also called an insulin reaction) occurs when a person's blood glucose falls below normal levels—usually less than 65 mg/dL (3.5 mmol/L). You can treat it by consuming a carb-rich food such as a glucose tablet or juice. It can also be treated with an injection of glucagon if the person is unconscious or unable to swallow. *See also* **reactive hypoglycemia**.

Hypertension *see* **blood pressure**.

Immune system is the body's defense system protecting itself from viruses, bacteria and any "foreign" substances.

Impaired fasting glucose is a condition in which the fasting blood glucose level (BGL) is raised (100–125 mg/dL [6.0–6.9 mmol/L]) after an overnight fast but is not high enough to be classified as diabetes. It is sometimes called **prediabetes**.

Impaired glucose tolerance is a condition in which the blood sugar level is raised (140–199 mg/dL [7.8–11 mmol/L]) after a 2-hour oral glucose tolerance test, but is not high enough to be classified as diabetes. It is sometimes called **prediabetes**. People with impaired glucose tolerance are at increased risk of developing diabetes, heart disease and stroke.

Insulin is a hormone produced by the pancreas that helps glucose pass into the cells, where it is used to create energy for the body. The pancreas should automatically produce the right amount of insulin to move glucose into the cells. When the body cannot make enough insulin, it has to be taken by injection or through use of an insulin pump. It can't be taken by mouth because it will be broken down by the body's digestive juices. As well as being involved in regulating blood glucose levels, insulin also plays a key part in determining whether we burn fat or carbohydrates to meet our energy needs—it switches muscle cells from fat burning to carb burning. This is why lowering your insulin levels is one of the secrets to lifelong health.

Insulin bolus *see* **bolus insulin**.

Insulinemia means the presence of insulin in the blood; **hyperinsulinemia** means excessive amounts of insulin in the blood.

Insulin resistance is when your muscle and liver cells are not good at taking up glucose unless there's a lot of insulin around. If you have this condition, chances are you'll have very high insulin levels even long after a meal as your body tries to metabolize the carbohydrates in the meal. When insulin levels in the body are chronically raised, the cells that usually respond to insulin become resistant to its signals. The body then responds by secreting more and more insulin, a never-ending vicious cycle that spells trouble on many fronts. Insulin resistance is at the root of prediabetes and type 2 diabetes, many forms of heart disease, and polycystic ovarian syndrome (PCOS).

Insulin resistance syndrome *see* **metabolic syndrome**.

Insulin sensitivity occurs when your muscle and liver cells take up glucose rapidly, without the need for a lot of insulin. Exercise keeps you insulin sensitive; so does a moderately high carbohydrate intake.

Islets of Langerhans are small clusters or islands of cells within the pancreas. They are made up of alpha and beta cells—the beta cells produce insulin and the alpha cells produce glucagon.

Ketones are the breakdown products of fat which some of the body's cells can use for fuel. They occur in higher concentrations when the body is unable to use glucose as a fuel because there is insufficient insulin. Ketones are strong acids, and when they are produced in large quantities they can upset the body's delicate acid-base balance. They are normally released into the urine, but if levels are very high or if the person is dehydrated, they may begin to build up in the blood. High blood levels of ketones may cause fruity-smelling breath, loss of appetite, nausea or vomiting, fast, deep breathing (to blow off the acid in the form of carbon dioxide) and excessive urination (to eliminate the extra acid). In severe cases, it may lead to coma and death. In a pregnant woman, even a moderate amount of ketones in the blood may harm the baby and impair brain development. Excessive formation of ketones in the blood is called ketosis. Large amounts of ketones in the urine may signal **diabetic ketoacidosis**, a dangerous condition that is caused by very high blood glucose levels.

Ketosis is the metabolic state in which the body is burning fat for fuel—normally carbohydrates are the main source of fuel for your brain, nervous system, kidneys and many other organs.

Kilojoules (kJ) are the metric equivalent of calories—a measure of the amount of energy a food provides when burned for fuel in the body. They are also used to describe the amount of fuel needed by the body. To convert kilojoules into calories, divide by 4.2.

LDL cholesterol *see* **cholesterol**.

Lipid profile is a series of blood tests measuring total cholesterol, triglycerides and HDL cholesterol. LDL cholesterol is then usually calculated from those results, but it can sometimes be measured separately. Your lipid profile is one measure of your risk of cardiovascular disease.

Lipids is a term for fats in the body.

Metabolic syndrome is a cluster of serious heart disease risk factors. A person with metabolic syndrome will have central or abdominal obesity plus two of the following risk factors: high triglycerides, low HDL cholesterol, raised blood pressure, raised blood glucose. Tests on patients with the metabolic syndrome show that insulin resistance is very common.

Metabolism refers to how the cells of your body chemically change the food you consume and make the protein, fats and carbohydrates into forms of energy, or use them for growth and repair.

mg/dL stands for milligrams per deciliter—a unit of measurement that shows the concentration of a substance in a specific amount of fluid. In the United States, blood glucose test results are reported as mg/dL. Medical journals and other countries, including Canada, use millimoles per liter (**mmol/L**). To convert blood glucose levels from mmol/L to mg/dL, multiply mmol/L by 18: 10 mmol/L × 18 = 180 mg/dL.

mmol/L stands for millimoles per liter—a unit of measurement that shows the concentration of a substance in a specific amount of fluid. In most of the world, blood glucose test results are reported as mmol/L. In the United States, milligrams per deciliter (mg/dL) is used. To convert blood glucose results from mg/dL to mmol/L, divide mg/dL by 18: 180 mg/dL ÷ 18 = 10 mmol/L.

Monounsaturated fat *see* **fats**.

Nephropathy is another name for kidney damage. Higher than normal blood glucose and blood pressure levels cause damage to the kidneys, making them leaky, so that protein (albumin) appears in the urine. If blood glucose and blood pressure levels are not treated promptly, the damage can progress to complete kidney failure.

Neuropathy is another name for damage to the nerves, and is usually caused by high blood glucose levels. Occasionally it is caused by excessive alcohol consumption. It most commonly affects the sexual organs (as impotence, for instance), the stomach (delayed emptying of the stomach into the small intestine) and the lower legs and feet (numbness, coldness or tingling).

Obesity is when a person's **Body Mass Index** is greater than 30 kg/m². The risk of developing prediabetes, type 2 diabetes, heart disease, stroke and arthritis is very high when a person is obese.

Overweight is when a person's **Body Mass Index** is 25–29.9 (the healthy weight range is 18.5–24.9). The risk of developing prediabetes, type 2 diabetes, heart disease and stroke starts to increase when a person is overweight.

Pancreas is a vital organ near the stomach that secretes the digestive juices that help break down food during digestion, and produces the hormones insulin and glucagon.

PCOS (polycystic ovarian syndrome) can have a number of different causes. Elements of PCOS are thought to affect one in four women in developed countries. At the root of PCOS is **insulin resistance**. The signs of PCOS range from subtle symptoms such as faint facial hair to a "full house" syndrome—lack of periods, infertility, heavy body-hair growth, acne or skin pigmentation, obstinate body fat, diabetes and cardiovascular disease.

Postprandial glycemia describes the rise in blood glucose that occurs immediately after a meal that contains appreciable (greater than 10 grams per serving) amounts of carbohydrates.

Prediabetes is a condition in which blood glucose levels are higher than normal, but not high enough for a diagnosis of diabetes. People with prediabetes may have **impaired fasting glucose** or **impaired glucose tolerance**. Some people have both. Studies show that most people with prediabetes will develop type 2 diabetes within 10 years if they don't make lifestyle changes such as losing weight, eating a healthy diet and exercising more. They are also at increased risk of having a heart attack or stroke.

Preeclampsia is a serious complication of late pregnancy characterized by a sudden increase in blood pressure, excessive weight gain, swelling and protein in the urine. It requires immediate medical attention.

Protein is one of the three main nutrients we get from food (the other two are fat and carbohydrates). The body uses protein to build and repair body tissue—muscles, bones, skin, hair and virtually every other body part are made of protein. The best sources are meat, eggs, fish, seafood, poultry and dairy foods. Other sources are plant proteins—legumes (beans, chickpeas and lentils), tofu, cereal grains (especially whole grains), and nuts and seeds. Because the body can't stockpile amino acids (the building blocks of protein) from one day to the next, the way it does with fat and carbohydrates, we need a daily supply. Women (on average) need about 45 grams of protein a day (more if they are pregnant or breastfeeding) and men about 55 grams. Active people, and growing children and teenagers, may need more.

Polyunsaturated fats *see* **fats**.

Resistant starch is the starch that completely resists digestion in the small intestine. It cannot contribute to the glycemic effect because it is not absorbed; it passes through to the large intestine, where it acts just like dietary fiber to improve bowel health. Sources of resistant starch are unprocessed cereals and whole grains, firm (unripe) bananas, legumes, potatoes and starchy foods that have been cooked, then cooled (such as cold potatoes or rice, sushi or pasta salads). Resistant starch is added to some refined cereal products, including breads and breakfast cereals, to increase their fiber content.

Retinopathy is damage to the retina of the eye caused by high blood glucose and blood pressure. It was once a major cause of blindness in people with diabetes, but modern laser therapy can now successfully treat many people with this condition.

Risk factor is anything that increases your chances of developing a disease.

Saturated fats *see* **fats**.

Starches are long chains of sugar molecules. They are called polysaccharides (poly meaning many). They are not sweet-tasting. There are two sorts—amylose and amylopectin.

Amylose is a straight-chain molecule, like a string of beads. These tend to line up in rows and form tight compact clumps that are harder to gelatinize and therefore digest.

Amylopectin is a string of glucose molecules with lots of branching points, such as you see in some types of seaweed. Amylopectin molecules are larger and more open and the starch is easier to gelatinize and digest. *See also* **resistant starch**.

Starch gelatinization is what happens when starch granules have swollen and burst during cooking—the starch is said to be fully gelatinized. The starch in raw food is stored in hard, compact granules that make it difficult to digest. This is why most starchy foods need to be cooked. During cooking, water and heat expand the starch granules to different degrees; some granules actually burst and free the individual starch molecules. The swollen granules and free starch molecules are very easy to digest because the starch-digesting enzymes in the small intestine have a greater surface area to attack. A food containing starch that is fully gelatinized will therefore have a very high GI value.

Sugars are one type of carbohydrates. The simplest is a single sugar molecule called a monosaccharide (mono meaning one, saccharide meaning sweet). Glucose is a monosaccharide that occurs in food (as glucose itself, and as the building block of starch). If two monosaccharides are joined, the result is a disaccharide (di meaning two). Sucrose, or common table sugar, is a disaccharide, as is lactose, the sugar in milk. As the number of monosaccharides in the chain in-creases, the carbohydrate becomes less sweet. Maltodextrins are oligosaccharides (oligo meaning a few) that are 5 or 6 glucose residues long; they are often used as food ingredients. They taste only faintly sweet.

Sugars found in food:

Monosaccharides	**Disaccharides**
(single-sugar molecules)	(two single-sugar molecules)
Glucose	Maltose = glucose + glucose
Fructose	Sucrose = glucose + fructose
Galactose	Lactose = glucose + galactose

Sulphonylureas are a group of diabetes medications that are used to lower blood glucose levels in people with type 2 diabetes. They work by increasing the amount of insulin produced by the pancreas, and because of this they are capable of causing hypoglycemia.

Syndrome X *see* **metabolic syndrome**.

Trans fats *see* **fats**.

Triglycerides (also known as **triacylglycerols** or **blood fats**) are another type of fat linked with increased risk of heart disease. Having high levels of triglycerides often goes hand in hand with having too little HDL cholesterol—this can be inherited, but it's most often associated with being overweight or obese. Normal ranges for triglycerides are 90–205 mg/dL (1.0–2.3 mmol/L). People with diabetes should aim to keep their triglyceride levels under 150 mg/dL (1.7 mmol/L), because they are already at greater risk of cardiovascular disease.

Unsaturated fat is fat containing double bonds, giving it a flexible structure that makes it liquid at room temperature. Plant oils contain large proportions of unsaturated fat.

Veins are blood vessels that transport carbon dioxide—they carry blood from tissues to the lungs, to be resupplied with oxygen.

Nutritional Tables

Introduction to the
Nutritional Tables

*H*ealthy **eating for** preventing or managing your diabetes involves choosing a variety of foods from all of the food groups. To help make things as easy as possible, we have grouped foods into two broad categories: 1) those that are sources of carbohydrates, and as a consequence have had their GI values measured; and 2) those that provide very little carbohydrate, so they will essentially have no effect on your blood glucose levels.

1. Carbohydrate-containing foods

Because it is important that you try to spread the amount of carbohydrates you eat evenly throughout the day, we have listed all of the carbohydrate-containing foods in amounts that provide approximately 15 grams of carbohydrates per serving. This amount is equivalent to a "carbohydrate exchange" and you can use them with the meal plans we have provided or develop your own meal plan, perhaps in conjunction with your dietitian. However, we also tried our hardest to list all foods in amounts that are commonly used, and easily estimated without resorting to the kitchen scale! Therefore, the actual amounts of carbohydrates in each serving can vary from around 12 to 19 grams. Don't worry that they are not exact—exchanges are just approximations, and you should not be thinking that any of the values are absolutely correct—foods are grown, not produced in a pharmaceutical laboratory, and as such they vary naturally anyway. Just use the guides we have given you along with the GI value. Research has proved that together the amount and GI of the food account for about 90 percent of the variability in blood glucose levels after a meal—a very powerful combination!

In addition to the carbohydrate and GI values, we have listed the amounts of calories, total and saturated fat, dietary fiber and sodium, as these factors are all important components to consider when choosing a healthy diet.

2. Low- or carbohydrate-free foods

As we have done for the carbohydrate-containing foods, we have listed all of the other foods in amounts that constitute typical servings. Because they contain little or no carbohydrates they do not have GI values, but of course this does not necessarily mean that you can or should eat them freely. In our current "obesogenic" environment we all need to make sure that we eat enough of a broad range of foods to provide all the essential nutrients we need for optimal health, but not so much that we gain too much weight. We have listed the caloric content of all of these foods to help prevent unwanted weight gain. In addition, we have provided a range of other nutrients that are relevant to each particular food group to help you make the best choice for your personal needs. Use the information we have provided to choose the foods that are best for your health, but don't forget to make sure that you enjoy them, too!

Finally, don't forget to use the label-reading tips in chapter 15 so that you can include more than those foods that we have listed here. Each year new foods come in to your local supermarket and others disappear—so knowing how to find suitable alternatives is all part of your diabetes and prediabetes management plan.

CARBOHYDRATE-RICH FOODS

Food	Serve Size	Household Measure	Calories	Fat (g)	Saturated Fat (g)	Carbo-hydrate (g)	Fiber (g)	Sodium (mg)	GI	LOW MED HIGH
BEANS, PEAS & LEGUMES										
Baked beans, canned in tomato sauce	5 oz	½ cup (or ⅓ can)	106	0.7	0.1	15.3	6.6	548	49	low
Baked beans, canned in tomato sauce, Heinz®	5 oz	½ cup (or ⅓ can)	114	0.5	0.1	17.9	5.5	411	55	low
Beans, canned refried, Casa Fiesta	4 oz	½ cup (or ⅓ can)	117	1.4	0.4	16.6	6.7	538	38	low
Black beans, boiled	2¼ oz	⅓ cup	86	0.4	0.1	15.4	5.7	1	30	low
Black-eyed beans, soaked, boiled	4¼ oz	⅔ cup	125	0.6	0.1	17.2	7.8	5	42	low
Borlotti beans, canned, drained	2¼ oz	⅓ cup	92	0.4	0.1	17.1	2.3	1	41	low
Broad beans, boiled	6 oz	1 cup	151	1.2	0.2	14.6	9.5	7	79	high
Butter beans, canned, drained	6 oz	1 cup	118	0.3	0	16.7	7.8	711	36	low
Butter beans, dried, boiled	5¼ oz	⅔ cup	120	0.5	0	17	8	11	31	low
Butter beans, soaked overnight, boiled 50 minutes	5¼ oz	⅔ cup	120	0.5	0	17	8	11	26	low
Cannellini beans, dried, boiled	4 oz	⅔ cup	118	0.5	0.1	16.2	8	3	31	low
Chickpeas, canned in brine	4 oz	⅔ cup	123	2.4	0.3	15.8	5.4	288	40	low
Chickpeas, dried, boiled	3 oz	½ cup	115	2.2	0.3	13.6	4.8	9	28	LOW
Four bean mix, canned, drained	3½ oz	½ cup	97	0.4	0.1	14.3	6.2	310	37	low
Haricot beans, cooked, canned	2¼ oz	⅓ cup	74	0.3	0.1	13.3	3.3	291	38	low
Haricot beans, dried, boiled	4 oz	⅔ cup	126	0.8	0.1	15.2	10.1	9	33	low
Kidney beans, dark red, canned, drained	3½ oz	½ cup	98	0.6	0.1	13.7	6.2	304	43	low
Kidney beans, red, dried, boiled	3 oz	½ cup	119	0.3	0	13.3	9	2	28	low
Kidney beans, red, soaked overnight, boiled 60 mins	3 oz	½ cup	119	0.3	0	13.3	9	2	51	low
Lentils, green, canned	4¾ oz	⅔ cup	87	0.4	0	13.4	4.1	419	48	low
Lentils, green, dried, boiled	4½ oz	⅔ cup	96	0.5	0.1	12.2	4.6	10	30	low
Lentils, red, dried, boiled	4½ oz	⅔ cup	96	0.5	0.1	12.2	4.6	10	26	low
Lentils, red, split, boiled 25 mins	4½ oz	⅔ cup	96	0.5	0.1	12.2	4.6	10	21	low
Lima beans, baby, frozen, reheated	4 oz	⅔ cup	126	0.8	0.1	15.2	10.1	9	32	low
Mung beans, boiled	5 oz	⅔ cup	152	3	0.9	16.4	10.7	17	39	low
Peas, dried, boiled	6¼ oz	1 cup	118	0.7	0	13.1	7	16	22	low
Peas, green, frozen, boiled	5½ oz	1 cup	113	0.6	0	12.6	9.3	5	48	low
President's Choice® Blue Menu™ low fat 4-bean salad	3 oz	⅓ cup	70	0	0	9	5	320	13	low
Soy beans, canned, drained	15 oz	2½ cups	432	23.7	3.4	12.5	20.6	1590	14	low

Ⓖ program participant

Food	Serve Size	Household Measure	Calories	Fat (g)	Saturated Fat (g)	Carbo-hydrate (g)	Fiber (g)	Sodium (mg)	GI	LOW MED HIGH
Soy beans, dried, boiled	18¼ oz	3 cups	736	39.7	5.7	12.4	37.2	46	18	low
Split peas, yellow, boiled 20 mins	6¼ oz	1 cup	118	0.7	0	13.1	7	16	32	low
Split peas, yellow, dried, soaked overnight, boiled 55 mins	6¼ oz	1 cup	118	0.7	0	13.1	7	16	25	low

BEVERAGES

Food	Serve Size	Household Measure	Calories	Fat (g)	Saturated Fat (g)	Carbo-hydrate (g)	Fiber (g)	Sodium (mg)	GI	LOW MED HIGH
AllSport Body Quencher	8 fl oz	1 cup	60	0	0	16	0	55	53	low
Apple and Cherry juice, pure	4 fl oz	½ cup	69	0	0	16.5	0.3	5	43	low
Apple and Mango juice, pure	4 fl oz	½ cup	63	0.1	0	15	1.7	1	47	low
Apple juice, filtered, pure	4 fl oz	½ cup	65	0.3	0	15		4	44	low
Apple juice, Granny Smith, unsweetened	4 fl oz	½ cup	50	0	0	12.7	0	11	44	low
Apple juice, no added sugar	4 fl oz	½ cup	50	0	0	12.7	0	11	40	low
Apple juice with fiber	4 fl oz	½ cup	60	0.3	0	14	0.3	4	37	low
Apple, pineapple	4 fl oz	½ cup	63	0.1	0	15	0.3	4	48	low
Beer (4.6% alcohol)	25 fl oz	2 cans	279	0	0	15.1	0	53	66	med
Blackcurrant fruit syrup (reconstituted)	5 fl oz	⅔ cup	82	0.7	0	14	0	11	52	low
Campbell's V8 Splash, tropical blend fruit drink	8 fl oz	1 cup	110	0	0	27	0	50	47	low
Campbell's, tomato juice	12 fl oz	1 bottle	75	0	0	11	3	1125	33	low
Campbell's, 100% vegetable juice	6 fl oz	1 can	38	0	0	6	2	465	43	low
Carrot juice, freshly made	8 fl oz	1 cup	71	0.3	0	13.9	2.4	118	43	low
Chocolate-flavored milk	5 fl oz	⅔ cup	139	6.3	4.2	15.6	0	100	37	low
Coca-Cola®	4 fl oz	½ cup	57	0	0	14.8	0	16	53	low
Cocoa with water	8 fl oz	1 cup	6	0.4	0.2	0.4		13		
Coffee, black	8 fl oz	1 cup	3	0	0	0.2		9		
Coffee, cappuccino	8 fl oz	1 cup	55	2.9	1.8	4.4		42		
Coffee, white	8 fl oz	1 cup	29	1.3	0.9	2.4		26		
Cola, artificially sweetened	8 fl oz	1 cup	2	0	0	0		32		
Cordial, orange, reconstituted	1 fl oz	⅛ cup	54	0	0	13.7	0	15	66	med
Cordial with water, artificially sweetened	8 fl oz	1 cup	4	0	0	0.9		9		
Cranberry Juice Cocktail	4 fl oz	½ cup	67	0.1	0	17.1	0	3	52	low
Diet Coke®	8 fl oz	1 cup	1	0	0	0.2		30		
Diet dry ginger ale	8 fl oz	1 cup	3	0	0	0		20		
Diet ginger beer	8 fl oz	1 cup	1	0	0	0.3		48		
Diet lemonade	8 fl oz	1 cup	2	1.8	1.8	1.8		14		

Ⓖ program participant

Food	Serve Size	Household Measure	Calories	Fat (g)	Saturated Fat (g)	Carbo-hydrate (g)	Fiber (g)	Sodium (mg)	GI	LOW MED HIGH
Diet orange fruit drink	12 fl oz	1 can	11	0	0	2.6		30		
Ensure®, vanilla drink	3 fl oz	⅓ cup	101	2.4	0.2	16	0.4	80	48	low
Fanta orange lite	8 fl oz	1 cup	6	1.8	0	1		26		
Fanta orange soft drink	4 fl oz	½ cup	64	0.6	0	15.4	0	6	68	med
Gatorade®	8 fl oz	1 cup	63	0	0	15	0	118	78	high
Grapefruit juice, unsweetened	8 fl oz	1 cup	84	0.3	0	17.9	0	13	48	low
Jevity®, fiber-enriched drink	3 fl oz	⅓ cup	101	2.4	0.2	16	0.4	80	48	low
Lemonade	4 fl oz	½ cup	52	0	0	13.5	0	21	54	low
Lemonade, artificially sweetened	8 fl oz	1 cup	4	0	0	0		41		
Lemon squash soft drink	4 fl oz	½ cup	64	0	0	15.5	0	14	58	med
Mango smoothie	4 fl oz	½ bottle	61	0.5	0.2	15.3	0.2	14	32	low
Malted powder in full fat milk	4 fl oz	½ cup	139	6.1	3.9	15	0.3	103	33	low
Malted powder in reduced fat milk	4 fl oz	½ cup	115	3	2.1	15.4	0.6	85	36	low
Malted powder in skim milk	4 fl oz	½ cup	97	1.4	1	14.7	0.6	95	39	low
Mineral water	8 fl oz	1 cup	0	0	0	0		23		
Nesquik® powder, Chocolate, in 1.5% fat milk	4 fl oz	½ cup	85	1.9	1.1	12.6	0	63	41	low
Nesquik® powder, Strawberry, in 1.5% fat milk	4 fl oz	½ cup	85	1.6	1	13.3	0	59	35	low
Orange juice, unsweetened, fresh	8 fl oz	1 cup	86	0.3	0	18.6	0.8	13	50	low
Orange juice, unsweetened, from concentrate	8 fl oz	1 cup	86	0.3	0	18.6	0.8	13	53	low
Pepsi Max	8 fl oz	1 cup	1	0	0	0.1		8		
Pineapple juice, unsweetened	4 fl oz	½ cup	52	0.1	0	12.3	0	1	46	low
President's Choice® Blue Menu™ Oh Mega j orange juice	8 fl oz	1 cup	130	0	0	30	0	25	48	low
President's Choice® Blue Menu™ Orange Delight Cocktail with pulp	8 fl oz	1 cup	70	0	0	16	0	5	44	low
President's Choice® Blue Menu™ tomato juice, low sodium	8 fl oz	1 cup	45	0	0	7	2	310	23	low
Prune juice	4 fl oz	½ cup	72	0	0	17.6	0.7	5	43	low
Blackcurrant fruit syrup (reconstituted)	5 fl oz	⅔ cup	82	0.7	0	14	0	11	52	low
Soda water	8 fl oz	1 cup	0	0	0	0		61		
Solo light	8 fl oz	1 cup	5	0	0	0.9		50		
Sprite Zero lemonade	8 fl oz	1 cup	2	0	0	0.2		30		
Strawberry-flavored milk	5 fl oz	⅔ cup	139	6.2	4.1	15.9	0	71	37	low
Sustagen® Drink, Dutch Chocolate	3 fl oz	⅓ cup	84	1.2	0.4	13.7	0	92	31	low
Tea, black	8 fl oz	1 cup	3	0.2	0	0		7		
Tea, white	8 fl oz	1 cup	16	0.9	0.5	1.1		16		
Tomato juice, no added sugar	12 fl oz	1½ cups	86	0	0	16.9	2	1130	38	low

Ⓖ program participant

Food	Serve Size	Household Measure	Calories	Fat (g)	Saturated Fat (g)	Carbo-hydrate (g)	Fiber (g)	Sodium (mg)	GI	LOW MED HIGH
Tomato juice, unsweetened	4 fl oz	½ cup	22	0	0	2.7		342		
Tonic water, artificially sweetened	8 fl oz	1 cup	0	0	0	0		0		

BREAD

Food	Serve Size	Household Measure	Calories	Fat (g)	Saturated Fat (g)	Carbo-hydrate (g)	Fiber (g)	Sodium (mg)	GI	LOW MED HIGH
9 Grain muffin	1 oz	2 muffins	79	1.5	0.3	11.2	1.8	86	43	low
9 Grain, multigrain bread	1¼ oz	1 slice	69	1.9	0.3	13	2.2	167	43	low
Bagel, white	1 oz	½ average	85	0.4	0.1	15.7	1	152	72	high
Black rye bread	1½ oz	1 slice	98	0.7	0.1	17.8	3.1	252	76	high
Bread Roll, white	1 oz	½ large (4 inch diameter)	97	1.3	0.2	17.4	1.2	188	71	high
Bread Roll, wholewheat	1¼ oz	½ large (4 inch diameter)	99	1.3	0.2	16.8	2.16	202	70	high
ⓖ Bürgen® Fruit and Muesli	1½ oz	1 slice	117	3.1	0.4	13.2	4.5	85	53	low
ⓖ Bürgen® Mixed Grain	1½ oz	1 slice	92	1.3	0.2	14.7	1.7	155	52	low
ⓖ Bürgen® Oat Bran and Honey bread	1½ oz	1 slice	94	2.2	0.3	13.4	3.8	153	45	low
ⓖ Bürgen® Rye bread	1½ oz	1 slice	89	1.5	0.2	12.8	2.1	150	51	low
ⓖ Bürgen® soy and flaxseed bread	1½ oz	1 slice	98	2.8	0.4	11.9	2.2	146	36	low
ⓖ Bürgen® Wholewheat and Grain	1½ oz	1 slice	90	1.3	0.2	13.6	2.2	151	43	low
Continental fruit loaf	¾ oz	1 slice	65	0.8	0.1	12.2	1	51	47	low
ⓖ Country Life Country Grain and Organic Rye	1¾ oz	1½ slices	123	2	0.5	15.3	5.9	125	48	low
Country Life gluten-free multigrain bread	1 oz	1 slice	81	1.6	0.7	13.6	0	74	79	high
ⓖ Country Life PerforMAX	2 oz	1½ slices	137	2.7	0.4	17.2	6	172	38	low
ⓖ Country Life Rye Hi-soy and flaxseed	1¾ oz	1½ slices	111	2	0.4	13.8	4.8	110	42	low
ⓖ Cripps 9 Grain loaf	1 oz	1 slice	85	1.8	0.3	11.9	2	153	43	low
Croissant, plain	1 oz	½ average	140	8.0	4.4	13.1	1	126	67	med
Crumpet	1¼ oz	1 round	78	0.3	0	15.9	1.1	389	69	med
ⓖ EnerGI white sandwich bread	1¼ oz	1 slice	93	1.1	0.3	16.6	1.5	162	54	low
Hamburger bun, white	1 oz	1 large (4 inch diameter)	97	1.3	0.2	17.5	1.2	188	61	med
Helga's™ Classic Seed Loaf	1¼ oz	1 slice	106	2.1	0.2	15.9	2.2	213	68	med
Helga's™ Traditional Wholewheat Bread	1¼ oz	1 slice	99	1.3	0.2	16.4	2.5	209	70	high
Hi Fibre, Lo GI white bread, Bakers Delight	1¼ oz	1 slice	86	0.6	0.2	15.3	4.2	218	52	low

ⓖ program participant

Food	Serve Size	Household Measure	Calories	Fat (g)	Saturated Fat (g)	Carbo- hydrate (g)	Fiber (g)	Sodium (mg)	GI	LOW MED HIGH
Homemade white bread	1¼ oz	1 thin slice	87	0.3	0	17.6	0.9	0.72	70	high
Italian bread	1¼ oz	1 slice	98	1	0.2	17.9	1.2	204	73	high
Kaiser rolls, white	1 oz	¼ roll	77	0.6	0.1	15.3	0.7	161	73	high
Lebanese bread, white	1 oz	½ medium (6 x 7 inch diameter)	98	0.7	0.1	18.9	1.1	158	75	high
Light rye bread	1 oz	¾ slice	82	0.9	0.2	14.4	1.9	176	68	med
Melba toast, plain	½ oz	1 slice	59	0.6	0.1	10.9	0.6	104	70	high
Multigrain sandwich bread	1 oz	1 slice	77	0.8	0.2	14.1	1.3	135	65	med
Organic stoneground wholewheat sourdough bread	1¼ oz	1 slice	95	0.6	0.1	17.2		218	59	med
Pita bread, white	1¼ oz	½ medium (6 x 7 inch diameter)	98	0.7	0.1	18.9	1.1	158	57	med
President's Choice® Blue Menu™ 100% Whole Wheat Gigantico Burger Buns	2¾ oz	1 bun	200	2.5	0.5	31	6	440	62	med
President's Choice® Blue Menu™ 100% Whole Wheat Gigantico Hot Dog Rolls	3¼ oz	1 roll	230	3	0.5	36	6	450	62	med
President's Choice® Blue Menu™ multi-grain flax loaf	3 oz	2 slices	220	3.5	1	32	6	260	51	low
President's Choice® Blue Menu™ tortillas, whole wheat	2 oz	1 tortilla	190	5	1	27	4	470	59	med
President's Choice® Blue Menu™ tortillas, flax	2 oz	1 tortilla	140	5	1	29	3	480	53	low
President's Choice® Blue Menu™ Whole Grain Baguette	1¾ oz	1 thick slice (2 inches wide)	130	1.5	0.3	21	3	260	73	high
President's Choice® Blue Menu™ whole wheat soy loaf	3 oz	2 slices	210	3	1	27	7	240	45	low
President's Choice® Blue Menu™ whole grain English muffins	2 oz	1 muffin	140	2.5	0.3	20	3	130	51	low
President's Choice® Blue Menu™ Whole Grain Multi-Grain English Muffins	2 oz	1 muffin	140	2.5	0.3	20	3	130	45	low
Pumpernickel bread	1 oz	⅔ slice	74	0.4	0.1	13.9	2.8	226	50	low
Raisin toast	1 oz	1 slice	90	0.8	0.2	17.4	1	74	63	med
Schinkenbrot, dark rye bread	1¼ oz	1 slice	102	0.9	0.1	18.1	2.8	217	86	high
Sourdough rye bread	1¼ oz	1 slice	96	0.6	0.1	18.2	1.7	211.	48	low
Sourdough wheat bread	1 oz	1 slice	62	0.6	0.1	11.2	1.1	134	54	low
Spelt multigrain bread	1¼ oz	1 slice	85	0.9	0.2	13.5	2.9	188	54	low
Stuffing, bread	2¾ oz	½ cup	152	6.6	2.1	17.1	1.9	410	74	high
Ⓖ Vogel's Original Mixed Grain	1½ oz	1 slice	105	1.4	0.2	16.2	2.6	176	54	low
Ⓖ Vogel's Rye with Sunflower	1½ oz	1 slice	108	2.1	0.2	14.6	3.3	172	47	low

Ⓖ program participant

Food	Serve Size	Household Measure	Calories	Fat (g)	Saturated Fat (g)	Carbo-hydrate (g)	Fiber (g)	Sodium (mg)	GI	LOW MED HIGH
Ⓖ Vogel's Seven Seed	1½ oz	1 slice	110	3.3	0.5	11.7	3.7	167	50	low
Ⓖ Vogel's Soy and flaxseed with Oats	1½ oz	1 slice	106	3	0.4	11.3	3.7	176	49	low
White bread, regular, sliced	1 oz	1 slice	69	0.7	0.1	12.5	0.8	143	71	high
Wholewheat sandwich bread	1 oz	1 slice	75	0.9	0.2	12	1.8	135	71	high
Wonder White®	1 oz	1 slice	69	0.8	0.2	11.9	1.3	128	80	high
Ⓖ Wonder White Low GI sandwich bread	1 oz	1 slice	81	0.9	0.1	13.3	2.6	151	54	low

BREAKFAST CEREALS

Food	Serve Size	Household Measure	Calories	Fat (g)	Saturated Fat (g)	Carbo-hydrate (g)	Fiber (g)	Sodium (mg)	GI	LOW MED HIGH
All-Bran® Fruit 'n' Oats, Kellogg's®	1 oz	⅓ cup	104	1.3	0.2	16.4	5.6	57	39	low
All-Bran®, Kellogg's®	1 oz	½ cup	101	0.9	0.2	14.2	8.3	114	34	low
Bran Flakes, Kellogg's®	¾ oz	½ cup	72	0.3	0.1	13.8	2.7	66	74	high
Ⓖ Bürgen® Fruit and Muesli	1 oz	¼ cup	86	1.5	0.4	15	2.3	43	51	low
Ⓖ Bürgen® Rye Muesli	1 oz	¼ cup	89	2.5	0.3	12.6	3.2	38	41	low
Ⓖ Bürgen® Soy-Flax Muesli	1 oz	¼ cup	92	2.7	0.4	12.5	2.5	37	51	low
Coco Pops®, Kellogg's®	½ oz	⅓ cup	59	0.3	0.2	13.2	0.1	101	77	high
Corn Flakes®, Kellogg's®	½ oz	½ cup	57	0.1	0	12.7	0.5	165	77	high
Crispix®, Kellogg's®	½ oz	½ cup	59	0	0	13.1	0.2	109	87	high
Crunchy Nut Corn Flakes, Kellogg's®	¾ oz	½ cup	76	0.8	0.2	15.3	1.1	158	72	high
Froot Loops®, Kellogg's®	¾ oz	½ cup	78	0.3	0.1	17.1	0.5	94	69	med
Frosted Flakes®, Kellogg's®	¾ oz	½ cup	75	0.1	0	17.4	0.5	141	55	low
Gluten-free Muesli	1½ oz	½ cup	183	10.9	4.9	13.3	7.3	12	39	low
Hi-Bran Weet-Bix®, regular	1 oz	1½ biscuits	107	1.5	1	16.8	5.5	122	61	med
Mini Wheats®, Blackcurrant, Kellogg's®	¾ oz	10 biscuits	76	0.4	0.1	14.8	2.1	3	72	high
Mini Wheats®, Wholewheat, Kellogg's®	¾ oz	13 biscuits	90	0.3	0	15.1	2.6	2	58	med
Muesli, gluten and wheat free with psyllium	1½ oz	½ cup	183	10.9	4.9	13.3	7.3	12	50	low
Muesli, Morning Sun Apricot and Almond cereal	1 oz	⅓ cup	107	1.9	0.5	17	3.7	8	49	low
Muesli, Natural	1 oz	¼ cup	106	2.6	0.4	16	2.5	4	40	low
Muesli, Swiss Formula	1 oz	⅓ cup	110	2	0.4	17.9	3.3	33	56	med
Muesli, toasted, Purina	1 oz	⅓ cup	131	4.8	1.3	17.6	2.5	50	43	low
Muesli, yeast and wheat free	1½ oz	½ cup	163	9.2	4.8	13.3	3.9	2	44	low
Nutri-Grain®, Kellogg's®	¾ oz	½ cup	77	0.1	0	13.9	0.5	120	66	med
Oat bran, raw, unprocessed	1 oz	⅓ cup	74	2.1	0.3	15.1	4.8	1	55	low

Ⓖ program participant

Food	Serve Size	Household Measure	Calories	Fat (g)	Saturated Fat (g)	Carbo-hydrate (g)	Fiber (g)	Sodium (mg)	GI	LOW MED HIGH
Oats, rolled, raw	1 oz	⅓ cup	114	2.3	0.5	17	3	3	59	med
Porridge, oatmeal, instant, made with water	6 oz	¾ cup	101	3	0	18	2.5	0	82	high
Porridge, oatmeal, made from steel-cut oats with water	6 oz	¾ cup	101	3	0	18	2.5	0	52	low
Porridge, multigrain, made with water	1 oz	⅓ cup	96	1.4	0.2	17.4	2.7	1	55	low
Porridge, oatmeal, regular, made from oats with water	6 oz	¾ cup	101	3	0	18	2.5	0	58	med
President's Choice® Blue Menu™ Bran Flakes	1 oz	¾ cup	110	0.5	0	19	5	190	65	med
President's Choice® Blue Menu™ Fiber-First, multi-bran cereal	1 oz	½ cup	110	1	0	10	13	270	56	med
President's Choice® Blue Menu™ Granola Clusters, original, low-fat	2 oz	⅔ cup	220	3	1	40	4	55	63	med
President's Choice® Blue Menu™ Granola Clusters, Raisin Almond, low-fat	2 oz	⅔ cup	220	3	1	40	3	50	70	high
President's Choice® Blue Menu™ Multi Grain Instant Oatmeal– Regular and Cinnamon & Spice	1½ oz	1 pouch	170	2.5	0.5	26	6	160	55	low
President's Choice® Blue Menu™ Soy Crunch Multi-Grain Cereal	2 oz	¾ cup	230	3	0.5	36	4	130	47	low
President's Choice® Blue Menu™ steel-cut oats	1½ oz	¼ cup	150	2	0.4	25	4	0	51	low
Puffed buckwheat	¾ oz	½ cup	67	0.5	0.1	14.5	0.9	0	65	med
Puffed wheat	¾ oz	⅔ cup	74	0.3	0.1	14.7	1.3	1	80	high
Quick Oats Porridge	1 oz	⅓ cup	115	2.6	0.5	18.5	2.1	1	50	low
Rice Bran, extruded, Ricegrowers	1 oz	⅓ cup	90	5.9	1.2	14.1	6	1	19	low
Rice Krispies®, Kellogg's®	¾ oz	½ cup	77	0.1	0	17.3	0.2	144	87	high
Semolina, cooked	8 oz	1 cup	86	0.2	0	17.3	0.7	0	55	low
Shredded wheat	1 oz	1 biscuit	84	0.3	0.1	16.4	3.1	2	75	high
Special K®, regular, Kellogg's®	¾ oz	½ cup	76	0.1	0	14.2	0.5	107	56	med
Raisin Bran®, Kellogg's®	1 oz	¾ cup	85	0.4	0.1	15.9	3.6	68	73	high
Weet-Bix®, regular	¾ oz	1½ biscuits	80	0.3	0.1	15.1	2.5	65	69	med

CAKES & MUFFINS

Food	Serve Size	Household Measure	Calories	Fat (g)	Saturated Fat (g)	Carbo-hydrate (g)	Fiber (g)	Sodium (mg)	GI	LOW MED HIGH
9 Grain muffin	1 oz	2 muffins	79	1.5	0.3	11.1	1.8	86	43	low
Angel food cake	1 oz	1 small piece (⅛ of a 10 inch cake)	77	0.7	0.3	15.3	0.3	137	67	med

Ⓖ program participant

Food	Serve Size	Household Measure	Calories	Fat (g)	Saturated Fat (g)	Carbo-hydrate (g)	Fiber (g)	Sodium (mg)	GI	LOW MED HIGH
Apple muffin, home-made	1½ oz	⅓ large	129	5.9	1.3	17	0	150	**46**	**low**
Banana cake, home-made	1½ oz	1 thin slice (⅛ of a 10 inch)	138	6.7	2.1	17.3	0.7	210	**51**	**low**
Blueberry muffin, commercially made	1½ oz	⅓ large	127	5.9	1.3	16.9	0	150	**59**	**med**
Bran muffin, commercially made	1½ oz	¾ average (2¾ inch diameter)	120	4.7	1.5	16.1	2.2	207	**60**	**med**
Carrot muffin, commercially made	1½ oz	⅓ large	127	5.9	1.3	16.9	0	150	**62**	**med**
Chocolate cake, made from packet mix with frosting, Betty Crocker	1 oz	1 small piece (1/12 of a 6 x 2½ x 2½ inch cake)	110	5.6	3.4	13.5	0.4	91	**38**	**low**
Chocolate Muffin	1½ oz	½ medium (2¾ inch diameter)	150	7.3	1.3	18.2	0.6	93	**53**	**low**
Croissant, plain	1 oz	½ average	140	8	4.4	13.1	1	126	**67**	**med**
Crumpet, white	1½ oz	1 round	86	0.3	0.1	17.5	1.2	425	**69**	**med**
Cupcake, strawberry-iced	1 oz	⅓ cupcake	84	2	1.2	14.7	0	91	**73**	**high**
Doughnut, cinnamon sugar	1½ oz	1 small	168	9.3	4.1	17.9	1	171	**76**	**high**
Egg custard	4 oz	1 small	117	4.2	2.4	15.4	0.4	109	**35**	**low**
NutriSystem, blueberry bran muffin	2 oz	1 container	100	1.5	0.5	11	8	130	**28**	**low**
Oatmeal muffin, made from	1½ oz packet mix	⅓ large	129	5.9	1.3	17	2	150	**69**	**med**
Pancakes, buckwheat, gluten-free, packet mix	¾ oz	1 small	67	0.2	0	15.2	0.8	95	**102**	**high**
Pancakes, prepared from mix (6 inch diameter)	2 oz	1 medium	143	6.5	2.6	17.7	0.5	111	**67**	**med**
President's Choice® Blue Menu™ Apple Berry Crumble	5¾ oz	1 dessert	210	2.5	1	34	9	65	**41**	**low**
President's Choice® Blue Menu™ Cranberry & Orange Soy Muffin	2½ oz	1 muffin	180	2	1	29	3	260	**48**	**low**
President's Choice® Blue Menu™ Raisin Bran Flax Muffin	2½ oz	1 muffin	200	3	1	33	5	210	**51**	**low**
President's Choice® Blue Menu™ Raspberry & Pomegranate Whole Grain Muffin	2½ oz	1 muffin	190	2	1	33	5	280	**58**	**med**
President's Choice® Blue Menu™ Raspberry Coffee Cake	1¾ oz	1 thin slice (1/12 of a cake)	160	6	1		222	160	**50**	**low**
President's Choice® Blue Menu™ Wild Blueberry 10-Grain Muffins	2½ oz	1 muffin	220	3	1	39	3	190	**57**	**med**
Scones, plain, made from packet mix	1 oz	1 small	110	3.0	1.1	17.1	0.9	182	**92**	**high**

Ⓖ program participant

Food	Serve Size	Household Measure	Calories	Fat (g)	Saturated Fat (g)	Carbo-hydrate (g)	Fiber (g)	Sodium (mg)	GI	LOW MED HIGH
Sponge cake, plain, unfilled	1 oz	1 cake (3 inch diameter)	72	1.1	0.31	13.9	0.3	60	46	low
Vanilla cake, made from packet mix with vanilla frosting, Betty Crocker	1½ oz	1 thin slice (¹⁄₂₄ of a 10 inch cake)	151	7.1	1.6	19		150	42	low
Waffles, plain	1¼ oz	1 square	141	6.9	2.9	15.6	0.8	335	76	high
Waffle, toasted	1¼ oz	1 square	141	6.9	2.9	15.6	0.8	335	76	high

CEREAL GRAINS

Food	Serve Size	Household Measure	Calories	Fat (g)	Saturated Fat (g)	Carbo-hydrate (g)	Fiber (g)	Sodium (mg)	GI	LOW MED HIGH
Barley, pearled, boiled	2 oz	⅓ cup	74	0.6	0.1	13.7	2.3	9.1	25	low
Buckwheat, boiled	3 oz	½ cup	89	0.5	0.1	17.2	0.8	3.6	54	low
Bulgur, cracked wheat	3 oz	⅓ cup	85	0.4	0.1	15.4	3.8	9	48	low
Couscous, boiled 5 mins	5½ oz	1 cup	73	0.2	0	14.6	0.2	1.5	65	med
Millet, boiled	2½ oz	½ cup	83	0.7	0.1	16.2	0.4	1.4	71	high
Polenta (cornmeal), boiled	6¾ oz	¾ cup	46	0.4	0	16.4	0.7	0	68	med
Quinoa, raw	1 oz	2 tbsp	84	1.5	0.3	15	2	1	51	low
Rye, whole kernels, raw	1 oz	2 ttbsp	67	0.5	0.1	14	2.9	1	34	low
Semolina, cooked	6 oz	¾ cup	65	0.2	0	13	0.6	0	55	low
Whole-wheat kernels, boiled	4 oz	½ cup	79	0.4	0.1	16.3	2	0	41	low

COOKIES

Food	Serve Size	Household Measure	Calories	Fat (g)	Saturated Fat (g)	Carbo-hydrate (g)	Fiber (g)	Sodium (mg)	GI	LOW MED HIGH
Apricot fruit cookies (97% fat free)	1 oz	1 cookie	84	0.7	0.1	15.9	3	73	47	low
Blueberry fruit cookies (97% fat free)	1 oz	1 cookie	84	0.7	0.1	15.9	3	73	47	low
Breton wheat crackers	1 oz	7 crackers	118	5.4	2.4	14	1	279	67	med
Corn Thins, puffed corn cakes, gluten-free	1 oz	4 slices	89	0.7	0.2	16.4	2.3	60	87	high
Digestives, plain	¾ oz	1½ cookies	110	4.8	2.2	14.9	0.6	154	59	med
Kavli Norwegian crispbread	¾ oz	4 crackers	68	0.3	1	14	2.5	70	71	high
Milk Arrowroot	¾ oz	2 cookies	77	1.9	0.9	13.1	0.5	47	69	med
Oatmeal cookies	¾ oz	2 cookies	103	4.7	2.7	13.9	0.6	141	54	low
President's Choice® Blue Menu™ Ancient Grains Snack Crackers	¾ oz	10 crackers	80	1.5	0.2	12	2	160	65	med
President's Choice® Blue Menu™ Cranberry Orange Cookies	¾ oz	2 cookies	110	4	1	16	1	55	60	med

Ⓖ program participant

Food	Serve Size	Household Measure	Calories	Fat (g)	Saturated Fat (g)	Carbo-hydrate (g)	Fiber (g)	Sodium (mg)	GI	LOW MED HIGH
President's Choice® Blue Menu™ Crunchy Oat Cookies	¾ oz	2 cookies	110	4	1	15	2	60	62	med
President's Choice® Blue Menu™ Fat-free Fruit Bar, Apple	1½ oz	2 cookies	130	0	0	30	1	115	90	high
President's Choice® Blue Menu™ Fat-free Fruit Bar, Raspberry	1½ oz	2 cookies	130	0	0	31	1	105	74	high
President's Choice® Blue Menu™ Fruit Bar, Fig	1½ oz	2 cookies	130	0	0	30	1	110	70	high
President's Choice® Blue Menu™ Ginger and Lemon Cookies	¾ oz	2 cookies	110	4	1	16	1	60	64	med
President's Choice® Blue Menu™ Wheat Snack Crackers	¾ oz	9 crackers	90	2	0.2	14	1	135	65	med
President's Choice® Blue Menu™ Wheat and Onion Snack Crackers	¾ oz	9 crackers	90	2	0.2	14	1	125	60	med
President's Choice® Blue Menu™ Wheat and Sesame Snack Crackers	¾ oz	9 crackers	80	2	0.2	14	1	135	56	med
President's Choice® Blue Menu™ Whole Wheat Fig Bar, 60%	1½ oz	2 cookies	130	0	0	29	2	110	72	high
Puffed crispbread	1 oz	3 crispbreads	95	1	0.4	17.9	0.7	137	81	high
Puffed Rice Cakes, white	¾ oz	2 rice cakes	75	0.7	0.1	14.8	0.8	1	82	high
Rich Tea biscuits®	¾ oz	3 cookies	111	3.6	1.6	17.6	0.5	116	55	low
Ryvita® Currant crispbread	¾ oz	1 ½ slices	82	0.6	0.1	15.6	2.7	5	66	med
Ryvita® Original Rye crispbread	¾ oz	2 slices	70	0.4	0.1	12.8	3.3	68	65	med
Ⓖ Ryvita® Pumpkin Seeds and Oats crispbread	1 oz	2 slices	98	2.5	0.5	13.9	3.6	100	48	low
Ryvita® Sesame Rye crispbread	¾ oz	2 slices	74	1.3	0.2	12.1	3.1	84	64	med
Ⓖ Ryvita® Sunflower Seeds and Oats crispbread	1 oz	2 slices	92	2.1	0.3	13.7	4	96	48	low
Shortbread biscuits, plain	1 oz	2 cookies	119	5.8	3.1	14.7	0.5	110	64	med
Shredded Wheat cookies	¾ oz	2 cookies	102	3.8	1.8	14.7	1.2	94	62	med
Snack Right® Fruit Roll, Spicy Apple and Raisin	¾ oz	1 cookie	66	1.2	0.3	12.4	0.9	40	45	low
Snack Right® Fruit Slice, Apricot	¾ oz	2 slices	72	0.5	0.1	15.4	1.1	32	52	low
Snack Right® Fruit Slice, Mango and Passionfruit	¾ oz	2 slices	75	0.6	0.1	15.8	1.1	30	49	low
Snack Right® Fruit Slice, Mixed Berry	¾ oz	2 slices	74	0.6	0.1	15.7	1	31	50	low
Snack Right® Fruit Slice, Raisin	1 oz	2 slices	82	0.7	0.2	17.2	1.1	35	48	low
Snack Right® Fruit Slice, Raisin and Chocolate	1 oz	2 slices	100	2.4	1.3	17.5	0.9	33	45	low
Spicy Apple fruit cookies (97% fat free)	1 oz	1 cookie	84	0.7	0.1	15.9	3	73	47	low

Ⓖ program participant

Food	Serve Size	Household Measure	Calories	Fat (g)	Saturated Fat (g)	Carbo-hydrate (g)	Fiber (g)	Sodium (mg)	GI	LOW MED HIGH
Sticky Date fruit cookies (97% fat free)	1 oz	1 cookie	84	0.7	0.1	15.9	3	73	47	low
Vanilla wafer cookies, plain	1 oz	2 cookies	132	7.4	7.1	15.5	0	17	77	high
Water crackers, plain	¾ oz	7 crackers	87	2	1	14.9	0.6	125	78	high
Zesty Ginger fruit cookies (97% fat free)	1 oz	1 cookies	84	0.7	0.1	15.9	3	73	47	low

DAIRY PRODUCTS: ICE-CREAM, CUSTARDS & DESSERTS

Food	Serve Size	Household Measure	Calories	Fat (g)	Saturated Fat (g)	Carbo-hydrate (g)	Fiber (g)	Sodium (mg)	GI	LOW MED HIGH
Chocolate Mousse, Nestlé®	3 oz	1½ container	98	2.2	1.7	14.5		45	37	low
Chocolate Mousse, Diet, Nestlé®	2¾ oz	⅓ cup	100	4.7	2.1	13.3	0.1	113	31	low
Chocolate pudding, instant, made from packet with full fat milk	4½ oz	⅙ packet	133	4.4	2.7	19.6		240	47	low
Crème Caramel, Diet, Nestlé®	4 oz	1 tub	76	1	0.8	12.5		85	33	low
Custard, home-made from milk, wheat starch and sugar	2 oz	¼ cup	83	2.1	1.3	14	0	29	43	low
Frutia, low fat frozen fruit dessert, Mango, Weiss	2 fl oz	¹⁄₁₀ tub	73	0	0	17.2		3	42	low
Ice-cream, light creamy low fat, chocolate	2½ fl oz	1½ scoops	104	1.4	0.9	16.3		35	27	low
Ice-cream, light creamy low fat, English toffee	2½ fl oz	1½ scoops	74	1	0.9	13.5	0.9	30	27	low
Ice-cream, light creamy low fat, mango	2½ fl oz	1½ scoops	72	1	0.9	13.2	0.9	25	30	low
Ice-cream, light creamy low fat, vanilla	2½ fl oz	1½ scoops	93	1.2	0.8	17	0.8	38	36	low
Ice-cream, regular, full fat, average of several types	2½ fl oz	1½ scoops	138	8	5.2	14.8	0	44	47	low
Ice-cream, Sara Lee®, full fat, French Vanilla	1¾ fl oz	1 scoop	202	12.9	8.6	18.1		41	38	low
Ice-cream, Sara Lee®, full fat, Ultra Chocolate	1¾ fl oz	1 scoop	196	12	8.1	18.8		53	37	low
Nestlé® Citrus Flavor Mousse dessert mix	1 oz	2 scoops	110	5	2.8	13.8		84	47	low
President's Choice® Blue Menu™ Frozen Yogurt, Mochaccino	4 fl oz	½ cup	120	2	1	21	0	65	51	low
President's Choice® Blue Menu™ Frozen Yogurt, Strawberry Banana	4 fl oz	½ cup	110	2	1	20	0	60	55	low
President's Choice® Blue Menu™ Frozen Yogurt, Vanilla	4 fl oz	½ cup	110	2	1	21	0	65	46	low

Ⓖ program participant

Food	Serve Size	Household Measure	Calories	Fat (g)	Saturated Fat (g)	Carbo-hydrate (g)	Fiber (g)	Sodium (mg)	GI	LOW MED HIGH
Tapioca pudding, boiled, with milk	4 oz	½ cup	125	4.2	2.1	17.5	0	57	81	high
Vanilla pudding, instant, made from packet mix with full fat milk	3 oz	⅛ packet prepared	103	3.2	2	15.3		190	40	low
Vanilla pudding, Sustagen®,	1 oz	½ scoop powdered mix	139	5.7		17.7		288	27	low
Wild Berry, non-dairy, frozen	1¾ fl oz	1 scoop fruit dessert	48	0.1	0	12		10	59	med
Yoplait Le Rice, dairy rice desserts, Apple Cinnamon	3 oz	½ container	104	1.8	1.2	18.9		52	52	low
Yoplait Le Rice, dairy rice desserts, Apricot and Almond Muesli	3 oz	½ container	105	1.9	1.2	18.6		64	45	low
Yoplait Le Rice, dairy rice desserts, Caramel	3 oz	½ container	105	1.8	1.2	19		53	41	low
Yoplait Le Rice, dairy rice desserts, Classic Vanilla	3 oz	½ container	105	2	1.3	18.5		59	36	low
Yoplait Le Rice, dairy rice desserts, Forest Berries	3 oz	½ container	99	1.8	1.2	17.4		64	45	low
Yoplait Le Rice, dairy rice desserts, Raspberry and Apple	3 oz	½ container	104	1.8	1.2	19.1		55	52	low
Yoplait Le Rice, dairy rice desserts, Strawberry	3 oz	½ container	104	1.7	1.2	19.1		53	54	low
Yoplait Le Rice, dairy rice desserts, Tropical Mango	3 oz	½ container	103	1.7	1.2	18.9		51	54	low

DAIRY PRODUCTS: MILK & ALTERNATIVES

Food	Serve Size	Household Measure	Calories	Fat (g)	Saturated Fat (g)	Carbo-hydrate (g)	Fiber (g)	Sodium (mg)	GI	LOW MED HIGH
Chocolate-flavored milk	5¼ fl oz	½ small carton	120	4.2	2.7	15.3		69	37	low
Strawberry-flavored milk	5¼ fl oz	½ small carton	116	4.2	2.7	14.7		65	37	low
Condensed milk, sweetened, full fat	1 oz	1 tablespoon	82	2.3	1.5	13.8	0	27	61	med
Lite White, reduced fat (1.4%) milk	8 fl oz	1 cup	127	3.5	2.3	13.7		128	30	low
Milk (3.6% fat)	8 fl oz	1 cup	168	9.8	6.5	12.1	0	106	27	low
Shape, calcium-enriched, low fat (0.1%) milk	8 fl oz	1 cup	121	0.3	0.3	16.8	0	173	34	low
Skim, low fat (0.1%) milk	8 fl oz	1 cup	89	0.3	0.3	12.2	0	128	32	low

Ⓖ program participant

Food	Serve Size	Household Measure	Calories	Fat (g)	Saturated Fat (g)	Carbo- hydrate (g)	Fiber (g)	Sodium (mg)	GI	LOW MED HIGH
ⒼSo Natural Calciforte, soy milk, calcium-enriched, full fat	8 fl oz	1 cup	171	7.25	0.8	18.7	1.3	233	**40**	low
So Natural Light, soy milk, reduced fat, calcium-fortified	8 fl oz	1 cup	105	1.23	0.3	14.2	1.2	98	**44**	low
So Natural Original, soy milk, full fat (3%)	8 fl oz	1 cup	150	7.3	0.7	18.5	1.3	225	**44**	low
Vitasoy® Light Original, soy milk	12 fl oz	1½ cups	106	2.6	0.4	15	0	161	**45**	low
Vitasoy® Premium Calci Plus® High Fiber, soy milk, 98.5% fat free	8 fl oz	1 cup	121	3.8	0.8	13.8	3.8	110	**16**	low
Vitasoy® Premium Calci Plus®, soy milk	8 fl oz	1 cup	160	7.5	1.5	15	1.3	120	**24**	low
Vitasoy®, rice milk, calcium-enriched	5 fl oz	⅔ cup	77	1.7	0.2	14.7	0.8	98	**79**	high

DAIRY PRODUCTS: YOGURT

Food	Serve Size	Household Measure	Calories	Fat (g)	Saturated Fat (g)	Carbo- hydrate (g)	Fiber (g)	Sodium (mg)	GI	LOW MED HIGH
Diet, low fat, no added sugar, vanilla	11 oz	1½ container	156	0.6	0.3	17	0	230	**20**	low
ⒼNestlé® All Natural 99% Fat Free Plain Natural	7 oz	1 container	136	2.1	1.5	16.8		134	**14**	low
ⒼNestlé® All Natural Apple & Cinnamon	7 oz	1 container	83	0.2	0.1	11.2		90	**30**	low
ⒼNestlé® All Natural Black Cherry	7 oz	1 container	83	0.3	0.2	11		87	**55**	low
ⒼNestlé® All Natural Light Apricot	7 oz	1 container	83	0.2	0.2	11		87	**49**	low
ⒼNestlé® All Natural Light Tropical Fruit Salad	7 oz	1 container	84	0.2	0.2	11.2		87	**38**	low
ⒼNestlé® All Natural Light Vanilla	7 oz	1 container	80	0.2	0.2	10.8		88	**37**	low
ⒼNestlé® All Natural Passionfruit	7 oz	1 container	82	0.3	0.2	10.6		90	**47**	low
ⒼNestlé® All Natural Peaches & Cream	7 oz	1 container	82	0.2	0.1	10.8		90	**28**	low
ⒼNestlé® All Natural Peach Mango	7 oz	1 container	85	0.2	0.2	11.6		88	**33**	low
ⒼNestlé® diet, low fat, all flavors	7 oz	1 container	82	0.2	0.2	10.8		88	**19–21**	low
Yoplait Lite Apricot yogurt	3½ oz	½ container	89	0.8	0.5	15.7	0	72	**27**	low
Yoplait Lite Berry Bliss yogurt	3½ oz	½ container	90	0.8	0.5	16	0	77	**25**	low
Yoplait Lite Blueberry Crème yogurt	3½ oz	½ container	95	0.8	0.5	17.2	0	78	**25**	low
Yoplait Lite Blueberry yogurt	3½ oz	½ container	94	0.8	0.5	16.9	0	75	**25**	low
Yoplait Lite Creamy Vanilla yogurt	3½ oz	½ container	94	0.8	0.5	17.2	0	76	**27**	low
Yoplait Lite Field Strawberries yogurt	3½ oz	½ container	94	0.8	0.5	17	0	85	**25**	low

Ⓖ program participant

Food	Serve Size	Household Measure	Calories	Fat (g)	Saturated Fat (g)	Carbo-hydrate (g)	Fiber (g)	Sodium (mg)	GI	LOW MED HIGH
Yoplait Lite French Cheesecake yogurt	3½ oz	½ container	100	0.8	0.5	18.4	0	76	27	low
Yoplait Lite Fruit Salad yogurt	3½ oz	½ container	92	0.8	0.5	16.5	0	78	32	low
Yoplait Lite Lemon Meringue yogurt	3½ oz	½ container	90	0.8	0.5	15.9	0	101	27	low
Yoplait Lite Mango Passion yogurt	3½ oz	½ container	93	0.8	0.5	16.6	0	77	37	low
Yoplait Lite Mango yogurt	3½ oz	½ container	94	0.8	0.5	17.2	0	76	37	low
Yoplait Lite Passionfruit yogurt	3½ oz	½ container	89	0.8	0.5	15.4	0	76	37	low
Yoplait Lite Peach Mango yogurt	3½ oz	½ container	92	0.8	0.5	16.5	0	78	37	low
Yoplait Lite Rhubarb Custard yogurt	3½ oz	½ container	95	0.8	0.5	17.1	0	87	27	low
Yoplait Lite Strawberry yogurt	3½ oz	½ container	90	0.8	0.5	16	0	81	25	low
Yoplait Lite Tropical Mango yogurt	3½ oz	½ container	94	0.8	0.5	17.2	0	76	32	low
Yoplait Lite Tropical yogurt	3½ oz	½ container	90	0.8	0.5	16	0	82	37	low
Yoplait Lite Vanilla Strawberry yogurt	3½ oz	½ container	93	0.8	0.5	16.8	0	79	25	low
Yoplait No Fat Apple Pie yogurt	7 oz	1 container	99	0.2	0.2	14.2	0	154	18	low
Yoplait No Fat Apricot yogurt	7 oz	1 container	100	0.2	0.2	14.4	0	162	20	low
Yoplait No Fat Banana Creamy Honey yogurt	7 oz	1 container	102	0.2	0.2	15	0	148	18	low
Yoplait No Fat Berry Brulée yogurt	7 oz	1 container	100	0.2	0.2	14.4	0	160	18	low
Yoplait No Fat Berry Crème yogurt	7 oz	1 container	98	0.2	0.2	13.8	0	158	16	low
Yoplait No Fat Black Cherry yogurt	7 oz	1 container	97	0.2	0.2	13.8	0	150	16	low
Yoplait No Fat Boysenberry yogurt	7 oz	1 container	96	0.2	0.2	13.2	0	168	16	low
Yoplait No Fat French Cheesecake yogurt	11 oz	1½ container	153	0.3	0.3	14.4	0	225	18	low
Yoplait No Fat French Vanilla yogurt	7 oz	1 container	92	0.2	0.2	13.6	0	150	20	low
Yoplait No Fat Mango yogurt	7 oz	1 container	85	0.2	0.2	13.8	0	160	20	low
Yoplait No Fat Passionfruit Crëme yogurt	7 oz	1 container	99	0.2	0.2	14	0	192	18	low
Yoplait No Fat Passionfruit yogurt	7 oz	1 container	99	0.2	0.2	13.8	0	192	20	low
Yoplait No Fat Peach Crëme yogurt	7 oz	1 container	98	0.2	0.2	14	0	154	18	low
Yoplait No Fat Peach Mango yogurt	7 oz	1 container	96	0.2	0.2	13.4	0	152	20	low
Yoplait No Fat Raspberry yogurt	7 oz	1 container	96	0.2	0.2	13.6	0	158	16	low
Yoplait No Fat Strawberry yogurt	7 oz	1 container	93	0.2	0.2	12.6	0	152	16	low
Yoplait No Fat Tropical yogurt	7 oz	1 container	97	0.2	0.2	13.6	0	178	20	low

FAST FOOD & CONVENIENCE MEALS

Food	Serve Size	Household Measure	Calories	Fat (g)	Saturated Fat (g)	Carbo-hydrate (g)	Fiber (g)	Sodium (mg)	GI	LOW MED HIGH
Chicken nuggets, frozen, reheated in microwave 5 mins	4 oz	6 nuggets	288	16.6	6.9	15.8	0.7	454	46	low
Fish fingers	2½ oz	3 fingers	156	7.8	2.1	13.2	0.7	220	38	low

Ⓖ program participant

Food	Serve Size	Household Measure	Calories	Fat (g)	Saturated Fat (g)	Carbo-hydrate (g)	Fiber (g)	Sodium (mg)	GI	LOW MED HIGH
French fries, frozen, reheated in microwave	5 oz	10 fries	120	3.4	0.4	18.7	1.9	25	75	high
ⓖ Lean Cuisine®, Burmese Vegetable Curry and Rice	3 ½ oz	⅓ meal	94	2.5	0.3	14	1.7	185	50	low
ⓖ Lean Cuisine®, Chicken Pomodoro	5 oz	½ meal	134	3.08	0.3	18.2	1.7	308	47	low
ⓖ Lean Cuisine®, Honey Soy Beef	5 oz	½ meal	133	2.5	0.4	19.6	1.4	511	47	low
Mashed potato, instant	4 oz	½ cup	74	0.1	0	14.1	2.2	4	85	high
NutriSystem, Beef Stroganoff with Noodles	9 oz	1 container	270	9	4.5	22	2	680	41	low
NutriSystem, Cheese Tortellini	8 oz	1 container	150	2	1	22	2	530	41	low
NutriSystem, Chicken Cacciatore Parmesan	8 oz	1 container	130	2	1	16	2	590	27	low
NutriSystem, Chicken Pasta	9 oz	1 container	180	3	1	23	3	610	41	low
NutriSystem, Hearty Beef Stew	8 oz	1 container	180	5	2	15	2	650	26	low
NutriSystem, Lasagna with Meat Sauce	8 oz	1 container	260	8	6	26	6	730	26	low
NutriSystem, Pot Roast	10 oz	1 container	270	7	2	16	2	780	31	low
NutriSystem, Rotini with Meatballs	9 oz	1 container	250	9	4	25	4	770	29	low
NutriSystem, Thin Crust Pizza with Cheese	3 oz	1 container	220	10	6	23	1	760	36	low
NutriSystem, Whipped Sweet Potatoes	2 oz	1 container	200	5	3	24	5	630	36	low
Party pies, beef, cooked	4 oz	2 small	231	12.1	5.7	14.2	0.8	256	45	low
President's Choice® Blue Menu™ Barley Risotto with Herbed Chicken	10 oz	1 container	290	6	1.5	37	5	800	38	low
President's Choice® Blue Menu™ Cauliflower Topped Shepherd's Pie	8 oz	¼ pie	220	9	5	13	1	590	21	low
President's Choice® Blue Menu™ Chicken Curry with Vegetables	10 oz	1 container	190	5	1	11	6	560	26	low
President's Choice® Blue Menu™ Deluxe Cheddar Macaroni & Cheese Dinner	2 oz	⅓ packet	230	3	1.5	39	3	450	34	low
President's Choice® Blue Menu™ Ginger Glazed Salmon	11 oz	1 container	300	4	0.5	45	5	570	40	low
President's Choice® Blue Menu™ Lentil and Bean Vegetarian Patty	4 oz	1 patty	170	2	0	27	4	490	55	low
President's Choice® Blue Menu™ Linguine with Shrimp Marinara	11 oz	1 container	240	4	1	28	8	750	40	low
President's Choice® Blue Menu™ Pasta Sauce, Tomato and Basil	4 oz	½ cup	70	2	0.4	8	2	480	33	low

ⓖ program participant

Food	Serve Size	Household Measure	Calories	Fat (g)	Saturated Fat (g)	Carbo-hydrate (g)	Fiber (g)	Sodium (mg)	GI	LOW MED HIGH
President's Choice® Blue Menu™ Penne with Roasted Vegetable Entrée	11 oz	1 container	320	6	2.5	43	9	750	39	low
President's Choice® Blue Menu™ Stone Baked Whole Wheat Pizza-Vegetable, Pesto and Feta Cheese	4¾ oz	½ pizza	240	7	2	28	5	650	54	low
Pizza, Super Supreme, pan, Pizza Hut	1¾ oz	1/16 slice of large pizza	127	5.1	2.4	13.5	1	241	36	low
Pizza, Super Supreme, thin and crispy, Pizza Hut	2½ oz	⅛ slice of large pizza	197	8.3	4.4	18.3	1.5	566	30	low
Pizza, Vegetarian Supreme, thin and crispy, Pizza Hut	1¾ oz	1/16 slice of large pizza	123	4.1	2.3	14.7	1.3	284	49	low
Shepherds pie	6¾ oz	¾ cup	204	8.8	3.5	15.2	1.5	720	66	med
Sushi, salmon	2¾ oz	3 pieces	102	1.4	0.4	17.5	1.3	291	48	low
Taco shells, cornmeal-based, baked	1 oz	2 regular size	120	5.9	0.9	14.1	2.1	95	68	med

FRUIT

Food	Serve Size	Household Measure	Calories	Fat (g)	Saturated Fat (g)	Carbo-hydrate (g)	Fiber (g)	Sodium (mg)	GI	LOW MED HIGH
Apple	4 oz	1 small	58	0.1	0	13.2	2.2	1	38	low
Apple, dried	1 oz	4 rings	69	0.1	0	16	2.4	1	29	low
Apricot, dried	1 oz	10 pieces	75	0.1	0	15.5	3.2	13	31	low
Apricots	6 oz	2 large	70	0.3	0	12.8	3.5	3.3	57	med
Apricots, canned, in light syrup	4½ oz	½ cup	72	0	0	15.8	2.3	3	64	med
Apricots, dried	1 oz	10 pieces	75	0.1	0	15.5	3.2	13	30	low
Banana	3 oz	1 small	73	0.1	0	16.1	1.8	1	52	low
Breadfruit	2 oz	¼ cup	57	0.1	0	14.9	2.7	1	68	med
Blueberries, wild	3½ oz	½ cup	45	0	0	8.8	4.2	0	53	low
Cantaloupe	12 oz	2 cups	80	0.3	0	15.9	3.4	34	65	med
Cherries, dried, tart	1½ oz	¼ cup	153	0.1	0	30	2.6	4	58	med
Cherries, frozen, tart	3½ oz	⅔ cup	50	0	0	6.4	0.6	18	54	low
Cherries, dark	4½ oz	1 cup	73	0.3	0	15.2	2.2	1	63	med
Cranberries, dried, sweetened	¾ oz	3 tbsp	62	0.3	0	16.5	1.1	1	64	med
Custard apple	3 oz	¼ large custard apple	64	0.5	0.2	12.9	2.1	3	54	low
Dates, Arabic, vacuum-packed	2 oz	3 medium	78	0.1	0	18	2.6	4	39	low
Dates, pitted	1 oz	5 average	72	0.1	0	16.8	2.4	4	45	low
Figs, dried, tenderized, Dessert Maid	1 oz	1½ figs	78	0.2	0	16.3	4.3	12	61	med
Fruit and nut mix	1¼ oz	¼ cup	158	8.3	2.2	17	2.7	19	15	low
Fruit cocktail, canned	5 oz	½ cup	68	0.1	0	15.8	1.5	5	55	low

Ⓖ program participant

Food	Serve Size	Household Measure	Calories	Fat (g)	Saturated Fat (g)	Carbo-hydrate (g)	Fiber (g)	Sodium (mg)	GI	LOW MED HIGH
Grapefruit	11 oz	1 large	86	0.6	0	14.9	1.9	12	25	low
Grapes	3½ oz	25 grapes (1 small bunch)	63	0.1	0	15	0.9	6	53	low
Kiwifruit	6¾ oz	2 small	108	0.4	0	18.6	7.6	11	53	low
Lychees, canned, in syrup, drained	3 oz	7 average	65	0.1	0	15.3	1.1	5	79	high
Mango	3½ oz	½ average	60	0.2	0	12.6	1.5	1	51	low
Mixed fruit, dried	1 oz	2 tbsp	78	0.3	0.1	18.2	1.6	22	60	med
Mixed nuts and raisins	1 oz	¼ cup	158	8.3	2.2	17	2.7	19	21	low
Nectarine, fresh	4 oz	1 average	50	0	0	10	2	0	43	low
Orange	7 oz	1 large	78	0.2	0	15.4	3.9	4	42	low
Papaya	7 oz	1 small	66	0.2	0	13.5	4.5	14	56	med
Peach	7 oz	2 small	69	0.2	0	12.8	2.8	4	42	low
Peaches, canned, in heavy syrup	5 oz	½ cup	66	0	0	14.4	1.8	7	58	med
Peaches, canned, in light syrup	4½ oz	½ cup	73	0	0	16.5	1.9	4	57	med
Peaches, canned, in natural juice	5½ oz	¾ cup	69	0	0	14.5	2.2	8	45	low
Peaches, dried	1 oz	3 halves	80	0.2	0	15.6	3.4	5	35	low
Pear	4 oz	1 small	68	0.1	0	15.7	2.9	2	38	low
Pear, canned, in natural juice	5 oz	¾ pear	65	0	0	14.8	2.4	7	44	low
Pear halves, canned, in reduced-sugar syrup, Lite	3½ oz	½ pear	62	0	0	14.5	1.8	2	25	low
Pears, dried	1 oz	1 ½ halves	68	0.1	0	16.3	2.6	3	43	low
Pineapple	6 oz	1 large slice	69	1.7	0	13.2	3.5	3	59	med
Plum	9 oz	2 large	103	0.3	0	18.7	5.5	5	39	low
Prunes, pitted, Sunsweet	1 oz	4 prunes	65	0.1	0	14	2.5	2	29	low
Raisins	¾ oz	6 tsp	60	0.2	0.1	14.2	1	12	64	med
Strawberries	17 oz	3 cups	115	0.5	0	13	10.6	29	40	low
Tropical fruit and nut mix	1 oz	3 tbsp	120	4.2	0.8	17.2	1.4	14	49	low
Watermelon	10 oz	1 large slice	69	0.6	0	14.2	1.7	6	76	high

GLUTEN-FREE PRODUCTS

Food	Serve Size	Household Measure	Calories	Fat (g)	Saturated Fat (g)	Carbo-hydrate (g)	Fiber (g)	Sodium (mg)	GI	LOW MED HIGH
Apricot and Apple Fruit Strips	¾ oz	1 strip	71	0	0	15.9	1.9	5	29	low
Apricot spread, no added sugar	1 oz	1 tbsp	56	0.1	0	13.3	0	3	29	low
Breakfast cereal, Vita-Pro®	1 oz	⅔ cup	104	0.5	0.2	14.4	5.9	88	52	low
Buckwheat pancakes, gluten-free, packet mix	¾ oz	1 small	67	0.2	0	15.2	0.8	95	102	high
Cookie, chocolate-coated, LEDA	1½ oz	2 cookies	183	10.8	6	18	2.6	52	35	low
Corn pasta	2 oz	½ cup	78	0.5	0.1	15	3.1	0	78	high

Ⓖ program participant

Food	Serve Size	Household Measure	Calories	Fat (g)	Saturated Fat (g)	Carbo-hydrate (g)	Fiber (g)	Sodium (mg)	GI	LOW MED HIGH
Corn Thins, puffed corn cakes, gluten-free	¾ oz	4 slices	89	0.7	0.2	16.4	2.3	60	87	high
Marmalade spread, no added sugar	1 oz	1 tbsp	61	0.2	0	14.4	0	3	27	low
Muesli (Gluten and Wheat free with Psyllium)	1½ oz	½ cup	183	10.9	4.9	13.3	7.3	12	50	low
Muesli Breakfast Bar, gluten-free	¾ oz	½ bar	97	3.7	1.5	13.1	1.9	6	50	low
Multigrain bread, Country life	1 oz	1 slice	91	1.8	0.8	15.3	1.7	83	79	high
Omega Bar (Gluten, Wheat and Dairy free)	1¼ oz	1 bar	174	4.2	1.5	14.7	2.7	4	21	low
Pasta, rice and maize, dry	1 oz	⅙ cup	79	0.1	0	18.7	0.6	2	76	high
Peach and Pear Fruit Strips	¾ oz	1 strip	71	0	0	15.4	2.8	14	29	low
Plum and Apple Fruit Strips	1 oz	1½ strip	77	0	0	16	4.2	10	29	low
Raspberry spread, no added sugar	1 oz	1 tbsp	60	0	0	14	0	17	26	low
Rice pasta, enriched (Gluten, Maize, Wheat and Soya free), Freedom Foods	¾ oz	⅙ cup	80	0.2	0	17.9	1.2	3	51	low
Spaghetti, Enriched (Gluten, Wheat and Soya free), Freedom Foods	¾ oz	⅙ cup	79	0.1	0	18.7	1.2	3	51	low
Spaghetti, rice and split pea, canned in tomato sauce, Orgran	4 oz	½ Can	69	0.3	0.1	13.6	0.9	440	68	med
Strawberry spread, no added sugar	1 oz	1 tbsp	60	0.2	0	14.2	0	3	29	low

NUTS & SEEDS

Food	Serve Size	Household Measure	Calories	Fat (g)	Saturated Fat (g)	Carbo-hydrate (g)	Fiber (g)	Sodium (mg)	GI	LOW MED HIGH
Almonds, raw	½ oz	1 tbsp	79	7.2	0.5	0.6	1.1	1		
Almonds, roasted	½ oz	1 tbsp	84	7.9	0.5	0.5	1.1	1		
Brazil nuts	½ oz	1 tbsp	90	8.9	1.9	0.3	1.1	0		
Cashew nuts, raw	½ oz	1 tbsp	76	6.4	1.1	2.2	0.8	1		
Cashew nuts, roasted and salted	½ oz	1 tbsp	83	6.7	1.1	3.4	0.6	38		
Coconut cream	4 fl oz	½ cup	263	26	22.8	4.7	2.2	27		
Coconut fresh	½ oz	1 tbsp	37	3.6	3.1	0.5	1	2		
Coconut milk, canned	4 fl oz	½ cup	261	25.8	22.6	4.7	2.2	27		
Coconut milk, fresh	4 fl oz	½ cup	302	30.2	26.8	4.2	2.8	19		
Hazelnuts	½ oz	1 tbsp	84	8	0.4	0.7	1.4	0		
Linseeds (flaxseeds)	½ oz	1 tbsp	46	3.4	0.3	2		7		
Macadamia nuts, raw	½ oz	1 tbsp	96	9.9	1.3	0.6	0.8	0		
Macadamia nuts, roasted	½ oz	1 tbsp	96	10	1.4	0.6	0.8	72		
Mixed nuts, fruit, seeds	½ oz	1 tbsp	62	4.1	0.8	4.1	1.1	5		
Mixed nuts, raw	½ oz	1 tbsp	79	7	0.9	1	1.1	0		
Mixed nuts, roasted, unsalted	½ oz	1 tbsp	81	7.2	0.9	1	1.1	0		

Ⓖ program participant

Food	Serve Size	Household Measure	Calories	Fat (g)	Saturated Fat (g)	Carbo-hydrate (g)	Fiber (g)	Sodium (mg)	GI	LOW MED HIGH
Nut & raisin mix	½ oz	1 tbsp	68	4.6	0.6	4.7	0.8	21		
Nut & seed mix	½ oz	1 tbsp	81	7	0.9	1.4	1.1	21		
Peanut butter	½ oz	3 tsp	104	8.4	1.4	1.7	1.8	51		
Peanut butter, no added sugar	½ oz	3 tsp	107	8.8	1.5	1.4	1.9	51		
Peanuts, raw	1 oz	1 tbsp	155	13.2	2	2.5	2.3	0		
Peanuts, roasted	½ oz	3 tsp	115	9.5	1.4	2.5	1.1	61		
Pecan pieces	1¾ oz	½ cup	349	36	2.3	2.5		2		
Pecans, natural	½ oz	1 tbsp	93	9.3	0.6	0.6	1.1	0		
Pine nuts	½ oz	1 tbsp	91	9.1	0.5	0.6	0.7	0		
Pistachio nuts, roasted	½ oz	1 tbsp	77	6.2	0.7	2.1	1.2	83		
Pistachio nuts, raw	½ oz	1 tbsp	79	6.6	0.8	2	1.2	1		
Poppy seeds	¼ oz	2 tsp	26	2.2	0.2	0.2	1	1		
Pumpkin seeds, raw	½ oz	1 tbsp	75	5.9	0.9	1.8	1.3	2		
Sesame seeds	½ oz	1 tbsp	79	7.2	0.9	0.1	1.3	3		
Sunflower seeds, raw	½ oz	1 tbsp	75	6.6	0.6	0.3	1.4	0		
Sunflower seeds, roasted	½ oz	1 tbsp	77	7	0.7	0.3	1.4	81		
Walnuts	½ oz	1 tbsp	90	9	0.6	0.4	0.8	0		

PASTA & NOODLES

Food	Serve Size	Household Measure	Calories	Fat (g)	Saturated Fat (g)	Carbo-hydrate (g)	Fiber (g)	Sodium (mg)	GI	LOW MED HIGH
Capellini pasta, white, boiled	2 oz	⅓ cup	74	0.18	0	14.7	1.08	34	45	low
Cheese tortellini, cooked	1¾ oz	⅓ cup	98	1.9	0.9	15.4		115	50	low
Corn pasta, gluten-free, boiled	1¾ oz	⅓ cup	59	0.3	0.1	13	2.2	0	78	high
Fettuccine, egg, boiled	2 oz	⅓ cup	75	0.3	0.1	14.3	1.01	38	40	low
Fuselli twists, tricolor, boiled	2½ oz	½ cup	90	0.2	0	18.8		35	51	low
Gnocchi, cooked	1¾ oz	¼ cup	74	0.5	0.2	14.5	1.15	30	68	med
Lasagna sheets, boiled	1¾ oz	1 small sheet	86	0.5	0.2	16		2	53	low
Linguine, thick, durum wheat, boiled	2 oz	⅓ cup	74	0.2	0	14.7	1.08	34	46	low
Linguine, thin, durum wheat, boiled	2 oz	⅓ cup	74	0.2	0	14.7	1.08	34	52	low
Macaroni and cheese, from packet mix, Kraft	2½ oz	⅛ packet	138	5.2	3.5	19	0.8	186	64	med
Macaroni, white, durum wheat, boiled	2 oz	⅓ cup	74	0.2	0	14.7	1.08	34	47	low
Ⓖ Maggi 2 Minute Noodles, Beef	4¼ oz	⅓ pack	89	0.4	0	17.5		388	52	low
Ⓖ Maggi 2 Minute Noodles, Chicken	4¼ oz	⅓ pack	125	5.3	0.8	16.2		331	52	low
Ⓖ Maggi 2 Minute Noodles, Curry	4¼ oz	⅓ pack	126	5.3	0.8	16.2		344	52	low
Ⓖ Maggi 2 Minute Noodles, Oriental	4¼ oz	⅓ pack	126	5.3	0.8	16.2		394	52	low

Ⓖ program participant

Food	Serve Size	Household Measure	Calories	Fat (g)	Saturated Fat (g)	Carbo-hydrate (g)	Fiber (g)	Sodium (mg)	GI	LOW MED HIGH
Ⓖ Maggi 2 Minute Noodles, Tomato	4¼ oz	⅓ pack	126	5.3	0.75	16.2		350	52	low
Mung bean (Lungkow bean thread) noodles, dried, boiled	1¾ oz	⅓ cup	53	0	0	12.7	0.8	2	33	low
Noodles, dried rice, boiled	2½ oz	⅓ cup	75	0.3	0	16	0.4	11	61	med
Noodles, fresh rice, boiled	2½ oz	⅓ cup	81	0.3	0	17.1	0.4	11	40	low
President's Choice® Blue Menu™ 100% Whole Wheat Spaghettini	3¼ oz	⅕ package	320	1	0	56	4	0	56	med
President's Choice® Blue Menu™ whole wheat rotini	3 oz	⅕ pack	330	2	0.5	56	9	85	45	low
President's Choice® Blue Menu™ whole wheat pasta	3 oz	⅕ pack	330	2	0.5	56	9	85	57	med
Ravioli, meat-filled, durum wheat flour, boiled	2 oz	⅓ cup	114	4.2	1.9	13.4		228	39	low
Rice and maize pasta, gluten-free	2½ oz	⅓ cup	99	0.1	0	16.3	0.3	46	76	high
Rice vermicelli noodles, dried, boiled, Chinese	2 oz	⅓ cup	75	0.2	0.1	16.3		4	58	med
Soba noodles, instant, served in soup	1¾ oz	⅓ cup	62	0.2	0	13.6		5	46	low
Spaghetti, gluten-free, canned in tomato sauce	4 oz	½ can	69	0.3	0.1	13.6	0.9	440	68	med
Spaghetti, protein-enriched, boiled	1¾ oz	⅓ cup	77	0.1	0	14.8	0.8	2	27	low
Spaghetti, white, durum wheat, boiled 10–15 mins	2 oz	⅓ cup	74	0.2	0	14.7	1.1	34	44	low
Spaghetti, wholewheat, boiled	2 oz	⅓ cup	74	0.2	0	14.7	1.1	34	42	low
Spirali, white, durum wheat, boiled	2 oz	⅓ cup	74	0.2	0	14.7	1.1	34	43	low
Udon noodles, plain, Fantastic, boiled	2 oz	⅓ cup	66	0.5	0	13.4	0	95	62	med
Vermicelli pasta, white, durum wheat, boiled	2 oz	⅓ cup	74	0.2	0	14.7	1.1	34	35	low

RICE

Food	Serve Size	Household Measure	Calories	Fat (g)	Saturated Fat (g)	Carbo-hydrate (g)	Fiber (g)	Sodium (mg)	GI	LOW MED HIGH
Arborio risotto rice, white, boiled, SunRice®	2 oz	⅓ cup	82	0.1	0	18.2	0.3	90	69	med
Basmati rice, white, boiled, Mahatma	2 oz	⅓ cup	82	0.1	0	18.2	0.3	90	58	med
Broken rice, Thai, white, cooked in rice cooker	2 oz	⅓ cup	82	0.1	0	18.2	0.3	90	86	high
Brown Pelde rice, boiled	2 oz	⅓ cup	92	0.6	0.1	19	0.9	66	76	high
Calrose rice, brown, medium-grain, boiled	2 oz	⅓ cup	92	0.6	0.1	19	0.9	66	87	high

Ⓖ program participant

Food	Serve Size	Household Measure	Calories	Fat (g)	Saturated Fat (g)	Carbo-hydrate (g)	Fiber (g)	Sodium (mg)	GI	LOW MED HIGH
Calrose rice, white, medium-grain, boiled	2 oz	⅓ cup	92	0.6	0.12	19	0.9	66	83	high
Doongara Clever rice, Sunrice, Ricegrowers	2 oz	⅓ cup	82	0.1	0	18.2	0.3	90	54	low
Doongara rice, brown, Ricegrowers	2 oz	⅓ cup	92	0.6	0.1	19	0.9	66	66	med
Doongara rice, white, boiled, Ricegrowers	2 oz	⅓ cup	82	0.1	0	18.2	0.3	90	56	med
Glutinous rice, white, cooked in rice cooker	2 oz	⅓ cup	82	0.1	0	18.2	0.3	90	98	high
Instant rice, white, cooked 6 mins with water	2 oz	⅓ cup	82	0.1	0	18.2	0.3	90	87	high
Jasmine fragrant rice, Sunrice, Ricegrowers	2 oz	⅓ cup	82	0.1	0	18.2	0.3	90	89	high
Jasmine rice, white, long-grain, cooked in rice cooker	2 oz	⅓ cup	82	0.1	0	18.2	0.3	90	109	high
Long-grain rice, white, Mahatma, boiled 15 mins	2 oz	⅓ cup	82	0.1	0	18.2	0.3	90	50	low
Moolgiri rice	2 oz	⅓ cup	82	0.1	0	18.2	0.3	90	54	low
Pelde parboiled rice, Sungold	2 oz	⅓ cup	82	0.1	0	18.2	0.3	90	87	high
Sunbrown Quick® rice, Ricegrowers, boiled	2 oz	⅓ cup	92	0.6	0.1	19	0.9	66	80	high
Sunrice Koshihikari rice, Ricegrowers	2 oz	⅓ cup	82	0.1	0	18.2	0.3	90	73	high
Sunrice Medium Grain brown rice	2 oz	⅓ cup	92	0.6	0.1	19	0.9	66	59	med
Sunrice Premium White Long Grain rice	2 oz	⅓ cup	82	0.1	0	18.2	0.3	90	59	med
Uncle Ben's ® Ready Whole Grain Brown Rice (pouch)	5 oz	⅔ cup	220	4	0.5	39	2	5	48	low
Uncle Ben's ® Ready Whole Grain Chicken Flavored Brown Rice (pouch)	5¼ oz	⅔ cup	230	4.5	0.5	39	2	800	46	low
Uncle Ben's ® Ready Whole Grain Medley™ Brown & Wild (pouch)	5¼ oz	⅔ cup	240	3.5	0	38	1	500	45	low
Uncle Ben's ® Ready Rice ® Original Long Grain (pouch)	5 oz	⅔ cup	230	3.5	0	43	1	500	48	low
Uncle Ben's ® Ready Rice ® Long Grain & Wild (pouch)	5 oz	⅔ cup	240	3.5	0	43	1	500	49	low
Uncle Ben's ® Ready Rice ® Roasted Chicken Flavored (pouch)	5 oz	⅔ cup	230	4	0	43	1	960	51	low
Uncle Ben's ® Ready Rice ® Spanish Style (pouch)	5½ oz	⅔ cup	240	3.5	0	46	1	500	51	low
Wild rice, boiled	2½ oz	½ cup	70	0.2	0	13.3	1.2	2	57	med

Ⓖ program participant

SNACK FOODS

Food	Serve Size	Household Measure	Calories	Fat (g)	Saturated Fat (g)	Carbo-hydrate (g)	Fiber (g)	Sodium (mg)	GI	LOW MED HIGH
Cadbury's® milk chocolate, plain,	1 oz	1 row	147	8	5	16.4		36	49	low
Cashew nuts, salted	1¾ oz	⅓ cup	319	25.7	4.4	13.2	2.2	145	22	low
Chocolate, dark, plain, regular	1 oz	1 row family-sized block	144	8.5	7.8	16	1.3	13	41	low
Chocolate, milk, plain, Nestlé®	1 oz	1 row	145	7.7	4.7	17.3	0.2	25	42	low
Chocolate, milk, plain, reduced sugar	1 oz	1 row	108	7.8	4.7	17.3	0.2	25	35	low
Chocolate, milk, plain, regular	1 oz	1 row	145	7.7	4.7	17.3	0.2	25	41	low
Chocolate, milk, plain, with fructose instead of regular sugar	1 oz	1 row	145	7.7	4.7	17.3	0.2	25	20	low
Clif Bar, Chocolate Brownie	2¼ oz	1 bar	240	4.5	1.5	40	5	150	57	med
Clif Bar, Cookies n' Cream	2¼ oz	1 bar	240	4	1.5	42	5	180	101	high
CocoaVia Chocolate Almond Snack Bar	¾ oz	1 bar	80	2	1	12	1	60	63	med
CocoaVia Chocolate Covered Almonds	1 oz	1 pack	140	11	3.5	9	3	0	21	low
CocoaVia Crispy Chocolate Bar	¾ oz	1 bar	90	5	3	9	2	10	33	low
Combos Snacks Cheddar Cheese Crackers	1¾ oz	1 bag	240	11	5	30	1	490	54	low
Combos Snacks Cheddar Cheese Pretzels	1¾ oz	1 bag	240	8	5	33	1	790	52	low
Corn chips, plain, salted	1 oz	15 average chips	140	7.8	3.1	14	2.7	138	42	low
Dove®, milk chocolate	1 oz	½ bar	132	7.5	4.6	14.5	0	21	45	low
Gummi confectionary, based on glucose syrup	¾ oz	5 pieces	63	0.1	0.1	14.5		3	94	high
Jelly beans	¾ oz	6 pieces	62	0	0	14.6	0	25	78	high
K-Time® Just Right® breakfast cereal bar	½ oz	½ bar	62	0.5	0.1	12.9	0.9	4	72	high
Kudos Milk Chocolate Granola Bars, with M&M's	¾ oz	1 bar	100	3	1.5	16	1	80	52	low
Kudos Milk Chocolate Granola Bars, Peanut Butter Flavor	1 oz	1 bar	130	6	3	17	1	75	45	low
Licorice, soft	1 oz	2 pieces	61	0.2	0.2	13.5	0.8	31	78	high
Life Savers®, peppermint	½ oz	¾ roll	65	0.1	0.1	16	0	1	70	high
Mars Bar®, regular	1 oz	1 fun-size bar	114	4.4	2.6	17.9	0	37	62	med
Marshmallows, plain, pink and white	½ oz	4 round pieces	48	0	0	14.5	0	5	62	med
Milky Bar®, white, Nestlé®	1 oz	2 mini-bars	168	10.4	6.3	16.5	0	35	44	low
Milky Way Bar	2 oz	1 bar	260	10	7	40	1	95	62	med

Ⓖ program participant

Food	Serve Size	Household Measure	Calories	Fat (g)	Saturated Fat (g)	Carbo-hydrate (g)	Fiber (g)	Sodium (mg)	GI	LOW MED HIGH
M&M's®, peanut	1 oz	½ packet	142	7.5	3	16.5	0	15	33	low
Muesli bar, chewy, with choc chips or fruit	1 oz	¾ bar	98	3.1	1.1	15.1	0	60	54	low
Muesli bar, crunchy, with dried fruit	¾ oz	1 bar	85	2.2	0.3	14	0	64	61	med
NutriSystem, Apple Cinnamon Soy Chips	1 oz	1 container	110	3	0	10	2	135	36	low
NutriSystem, Blueberry Dessert Bar	1.5 oz	1 container	140	3.5	2.5	21	3	115	36	low
NutriSystem, Chocolate Crunch Bar	1 oz	1 container	130	6	5	15	0	130	41	low
NutriSystem, Chocolate Peanut Butter Dessert Bar	1.5 oz	1 container	180	8	2.5	18	2	170	48	low
NutriSystem, Honey Mustard Pretzels	1 oz	1 container	140	6	2	7	3	330	32	low
Nuts, mixed, roasted and salted	7 oz	1½ cup, chopped	1230	110	13.9	15.6	16.6	1180	24	low
Peanuts, roasted, salted	5½ oz	1 cup	871	72	8.1	13.7	12.5	900	14	low
Pecan nuts, raw	11 oz	2 ½ cups	2251	226	14.2	15.4	26.5	10	10	low
Popcorn, plain, cooked in microwave	1 oz	3 cups	89	1.1	0.2	13.9	5.5	1	72	high
Pop-Tarts!™, double chocolate	1 oz	½ tart	101	2.4	0.5	18.7	0.3	101	70	high
Potato chips, plain, salted	1 oz	1½ cups	86	9.6	4.2	14.2	3.6	192	54	low
Power Bar, Chocolate	2 oz	1 bar	230	1.5	0.5	40	4	200	53	low
President's Choice® Blue Menu™ Chewy Cranberry Apple Granola Bar	1 oz	1 bar	100	1.5	0	20	1	55	58	med
President's Choice® Blue Menu™ Chewy Chocolate Chip & Marshmallow	1 oz	1 bar	110	2	0.5	20	1	50	78	high
President's Choice® Blue Menu™ Flaxseed Tortilla Chips, Sea Salt	1¾ oz	17 chips	250	14	2	20	6	170	45	low
President's Choice® Blue Menu™ Flaxseed Tortilla Chips-Spicy	1¾ oz	17 chips	250	14	2	20	6	370	34	low
President's Choice® Blue Menu™ Fruit n' Nut Chewy Multi-Grain Bar, Cranberry & Almonds	1 oz	1 bar	140	4	0.4	24	5	105	75	high
President's Choice® Blue Menu™ Fruit n' Nut Bar, Apple & Almonds	1 oz	1 bar	130	2.5	0.3	20	5	90	65	med
President's Choice® Blue Menu™ Fruit & Yogurt Cranberry Blueberry Bars (Soy)	1½ oz	1 bar	170	5	1.5	21	2	130	33	low
President's Choice® Blue Menu™ Fruit & Yogurt Apple Cinnamon Chewy Bars (Soy)	1½ oz	1 bar	170	5	1.5	21	2	170	34	low

Ⓖ program participant

Food	Serve Size	Household Measure	Calories	Fat (g)	Saturated Fat (g)	Carbo-hydrate (g)	Fiber (g)	Sodium (mg)	GI	LOW MED HIGH
President's Choice® Blue Menu™ Rice & Corn Chips, Thai Curry	1¾ oz	30 chips	200	3	0.3	39	2	550	84	high
President's Choice® Blue Menu™ Rice & Corn Chips, Japanese Tamari	1¾ oz	30 chips	200	3	0.3	38	1	470	91	high
Pretzels, oven-baked, traditional wheat flavor	¾ oz	1 small packet	76	1.44	0.3	12.9	0.7	396	83	high
Rice Krispie Treat® bar, Kellogg's®	¾ oz	1 bar	91	2	1	17.2	0.2	81	63	med
Roll-Ups®, processed fruit snack	¾ oz	1	66	0.5	0.1	14.4	0.4	1	99	high
Shaklee weight management bars, Cinch, chocolate	1 oz	1 bar	120	2.5	1	12	3	170	29	low
Shaklee weight management bars, Cinch, lemon	1 oz	1 bar	120	2.5	0.5	12	3	150	23	low
Shaklee weight management bars, Cinch, peanut butter	1 oz	1 bar	120	3	0.5	12	3	190	22	low
Shaklee weight management powder, Cinch, prepared, chocolate	8 fl oz	1 cup	280	3	0.5	12	6	370	29	low
Shaklee weight management powder, Cinch, prepared, vanilla	8 fl oz	1 cup	280	3	0.5	12	6	370	29	low
Shaklee weight management powder, Cinch, prepared, café latte	8 fl oz	1 cup	290	3	0.5	12	6	370	29	low
Skittles®	¾ oz	5 pieces	82	0.9	0.5	18.1	0	9	70	high
Snickers Bar	2 oz	1 bar	280	14	5	34	1	140	43	low
Snickers, Marathon Energy Bar, Chewy Chocolate Peanut Flavor	2 oz	1 bar	210	8	3	21	5	250	36	low
Snickers, Marathon Energy Bar, Multi-Grain Crunch Flavor	2 oz	1 bar	220	7	2.5	25	3	220	50	low
Snickers, Marathon Low Carb Lifestyle Energy Bar, Chocolate Fudge Brownie Flavor	1¾ oz	1 bar	170	7	2.5	11	8	240	20	low
Snickers, Marathon Low Carb Lifestyle Energy Bar, Peanut Butter Flavor	1¾ oz	1 bar	160	6	2	11	7	260	21	low
Snickers, Marathon Protein Performance Bar, Caramel Nut Rush Flavor	2¾ oz	1 bar	290	8	3.5	33	8	180	26	low
Snickers, Marathon Protein Performance Bar, Chocolate Nut Burst Flavor	2¾ oz	1 bar	290	7	2.5	29	7	260	32	low
SoLo GI Nutrition Bar, Berry Bliss	1¾ oz	1 bar	200	6	2.5	22	3	125	28	low
SoLo GI Nutrition Bar, Mint Mania	1¾ oz	1 bar	200	7	3	22	4	120	23	low

Ⓖ program participant

Food	Serve Size	Household Measure	Calories	Fat (g)	Saturated Fat (g)	Carbo-hydrate (g)	Fiber (g)	Sodium (mg)	GI	LOW MED HIGH
SoLo GI Nutrition Bar, Chocolate Charger	1¾ oz	1 bar	200	7	3	22	4	120	28	low
SoLo GI Nutrition Bar, Peanut Power	1¾ oz	1 bar	200	8	3	20	3	125	27	low
SoLo GI Nutrition Bar, Lemon Lift	1¾ oz	1 bar	200	6	2.5	22	4	105	28	low
SoLo GI Snack Bar, Berry Bliss	1 oz	1 bar	100	3	1.5	11	2	60	28	low
SoLo GI Snack Bar, Mint Mania	1 oz	1 bar	100	3	1.5	10	2	60	23	low
SoLo GI Snack Bar, Chocolate Charger	1 oz	1 bar	100	3	1.5	10	2	60	28	low
SoLo GI Snack Bar, Peanut Power	1 oz	1 bar	100	3.5	1.5	10	2	60	27	low
SoLo GI Snack Bar, Lemon Lift	1 oz	1 bar	100	3	1.5	11	2	55	28	low
Ⓖ Sunripe School Straps Blackberry Sour Buzz	¾ oz	1 ½ bars	68	0	0	15.4	1.9	8	35	low
Ⓖ Sunripe School Straps, dried fruit snack	¾ oz	1 ½ bars	72	0	0	17.4	1.9	8	40	low
Twisties®, cheese-flavored snack	1 oz	½ 1¾ oz packet	108	7	3.5	15	0.5	278	74	high
Twix® bar	½ oz	1 fun-size bar	91	4.5	2.5	11.9		28	44	low
Zone Performance Bar, Double Chocolate	1¾ oz	1 bar	210	7	5	20	1	260	44	low

SOUPS

Food	Serve Size	Household Measure	Calories	Fat (g)	Saturated Fat (g)	Carbo-hydrate (g)	Fiber (g)	Sodium (mg)	GI	LOW MED HIGH
Black bean, canned	6½ oz	¾ cup	88	1.1	0.3	14.9	3.3	898	64	med
Green pea, canned	9 oz	½ can	180	6.8	4.3	19.3		613	66	med
Lentil, canned	9 oz	1 cup	98	1	0.3	12.9	4.6	867	44	low
Minestrone, Traditional, Campbell's® Country Ladle	9 oz	1 cup	140	3.6	1.3	13	9.6	520	39	low
President's Choice® Blue Menu™ Barley Vegetable Low Fat Instant Soup	1½ oz	1 container	160	1.5	0.3	28	5	430	41	low
President's Choice® Blue Menu™ Mushroom Barley, Ready-to-Serve	1 cup	1 container	80	2	0.4	9	3	480	45	low
President's Choice® Blue Menu™ Pasta e Fagioli Soup, Ready-to-Serve	1 cup	1 container	160	3	0.5	20	5	480	52	low
President's Choice® Blue Menu™ Spicy Black Bean Low Fat Instant Soup	1½ oz	1 container	240	1	0.2	32	13	680	57	med

Ⓖ program participant

Food	Serve Size	Household Measure	Calories	Fat (g)	Saturated Fat (g)	Carbo- hydrate (g)	Fiber (g)	Sodium (mg)	GI	LOW MED HIGH
President's Choice® Blue Menu™ Spicy Thai Instant Noodles with Vegetables Low Fat Instant Soup	2 oz	1 container	170	0.5	0.2	31	6	250	56	med
President's Choice® Blue Menu™ Vegetarian Chili Low Fat Instant Cup	2 oz	1 container	230	1.5	0.3	29	11	420	36	low
President's Choice® Blue Menu™ Vegetarian Chili, Ready-to-Serve	1 cup	1 container	200	3	0.5	29	5	480	39	low
President's Choice® Blue Menu™ Vegetable CousCous Low Fat Instant Soup Cup	2 oz	1 container	200	1	0.3	33	6	510	57	med
President's Choice® Blue Menu™ Indian Lentil Low Fat Instant Soup	2 oz	1 container	150	1.5	0.3	20	5	500	55	low
President's Choice® Blue Menu™ Lentil Soup	1 cup	1 container	140	3	0.5	19	4	480	56	med
President's Choice® Blue Menu™ Soupreme, Carrot Soup	1 cup	1 container	100	3	0.3	13	3	420	35	low
President's Choice® Blue Menu™ Soupreme, Tomato and Herb Soup	1 cup	1 container	80	0.5	0	14	2	340	47	low
President's Choice® Blue Menu™ Soupreme, Winter Squash Soup	1 cup	1 container	90	1.5	1	15	5	490	41	low
Pumpkin, Creamy, Heinz® Very Special!™	7 oz	½ can	106	2.1	0.4	15.5		672	76	high
Split pea, canned	4½ oz	½ cup	90	1.2	0.4	15	2.4	210	60	med
Tomato, canned	9 oz	1 cup	70	0.5	0	14.4	2.6	850	45	low

SOY PRODUCTS										
Ⓖ Bürgen® Soy-Lin Muesli	¾ oz	¼ cup	92	2.65	0.4	12.5	2.5	37	51	low
Ⓖ Bürgen® Soy-Lin, soy and flaxseed bread	1½ oz	1 slice	97	2.8	0.4	11.9	2.2	146	36	low
Ⓖ Country Life Rye Hi-soy and Flaxseed bread	1¾ oz	1½ slices	111	2	0.4	13.8	4.8	110	42	low
NutriSystem, Apple Cinnamon Soy Chips	1 oz	1 container	110	3	0	10	2	135	36	low
NutriSystem, Sour Cream and Onion Soy Chips	1 oz	1 container	110	3	0	10	2	320	41	low
President's Choice® Blue Menu™ Popcorn, Microwave, Natural Flavor	6 cups popped	½ bag	160	2.5	0.5	25	4	200	58	med

Ⓖ program participant

Food	Serve Size	Household Measure	Calories	Fat (g)	Saturated Fat (g)	Carbo-hydrate (g)	Fiber (g)	Sodium (mg)	GI	LOW MED HIGH
Ⓖ So Natural Calciforte, soy milk, calcium-enriched, full fat	8 fl oz	1 cup	172	7.3	0.75	18.7	1.3	233	40	low
So Natural Light, soy milk, reduced fat, calcium-fortified	8 fl oz	1 cup	105	1.2	0.25	14.2	1.2	98	44	low
So Natural Original, soy milk, full fat (3%)	8 fl oz	1 cup	158	7.3	0.7	18.5	1.3	225	44	low
Soy beans, canned, drained	15 oz	2½ cups	432	23.7	3.4	12.5	20.6	1590	14	low
Soy beans, dried, boiled	18 oz	3 cups	736	39.7	5.7	12.4	37.2	46	18	low
Vitasoy® Light Original, soy milk	12 fl oz	1½ cups	106	2.6	0.4	15	0	161	45	low
Vitasoy® Premium Calci Plus® High Fiber, soy milk, 98.5% fat free	8 fl oz	1 cup	121	3.8	0.8	13.8	3.8	110	16	low
Vitasoy® Premium Calci Plus®, soy milk	8 fl oz	1 cup	160	7.5	1.5	15	1.3	120	24	low

SPREADS & SWEETENERS

Food	Serve Size	Household Measure	Calories	Fat (g)	Saturated Fat (g)	Carbo-hydrate (g)	Fiber (g)	Sodium (mg)	GI	LOW MED HIGH
Cottee's 100% Fruit Jam Apricot	1 oz	1 tbsp	64	0.2	0.1	15		2.5	50	low
Cottee's 100% Fruit Jam Blackberry	1 oz	1 tbsp	66	0.2	0.1	15.3		2.5	46	low
Cottee's 100% Fruit Jam Breakfast Marmalade	1 oz	1 tbsp	68	0.2	0.1	16.7		2.5	55	low
Cottee's 100% Fruit Jam Raspberry	1 oz	1 tbsp	66	0.2	0.1	15.3		2.5	46	low
Cottee's 100% Fruit Jam Strawberry	1 oz	1 tbsp	65	0.2	0.1	15.2		2.5	46	low
Fructose, pure	½ oz	3 tsp	61	0	0	15	0	0	19	low
Ginger Marmalade, original	¾ oz	2 tsp	56	0.1	0.1	13.6		2	50	low
Glucose tablets or powder	½ oz	1 tbsp	59	0	0	15	0	2	100	high
Golden syrup	¾ oz	3 tsp	58	0	0	14.9	0	26	63	med
Hummus, regular	6 oz	⅔ cup	99	29	5.8	15.6	14.8	527	6	low
Honey, Capilano, blended	¾ oz	3 tsp	70	0	0	18	0	3	64	med
Honey, Ironbark	¾ oz	3 tsp	70	0	0	18	0	3	48	low
Honey, Red Gum	¾ oz	3 tsp	70	0	0	18	0	3	53	low
Honey, Salvation Jane	¾ oz	3 tsp	70	0	0	18	0	3	64	med
Honey, Stringybark	¾ oz	3 tsp	70	0	0	18	0	3	44	low
Honey, Yapunya	¾ oz	3 tsp	0	0	0	18	0	3	52	low
Honey, Yellow-box	¾ oz	3 tsp	0	0	0	18	0	3	35	low
Maple flavored syrup, Cottee's®	¾ oz	3 tsp	58	0	0	15.1	0	10	68	med
Maple syrup, pure, Canadian	¾ oz	3 tsp	52	0	0	13.4	0	2	54	low

Ⓖ program participant

Food	Serve Size	Household Measure	Calories	Fat (g)	Saturated Fat (g)	Carbo-hydrate (g)	Fiber (g)	Sodium (mg)	GI	LOW MED HIGH
Marmalade, orange	¾ oz	3 tsp	55	0.1	0.1	13.6	0.2	3	55	low
Nutella®, hazelnut spread	1 oz	1 ½ tbsp	157	9.6	2.9	16.6	0.4	15	33	low
Ⓖ Premium Agave Nectar, Sweet Cactus Farms	¾ oz	4 tsp	64	0	0	15.9	0	3	19	low
Strawberry jam, regular	¾ oz	3 tsp	53	0	0	13.4	0.3	3	51	low
Sugar	½ oz	6 tsp	65	0	0	16.9	0	2	60	med
Ⓖ Sweetaddin	½ oz	3 tsp	61	0	0	15	0	0	19	low

SUGARS

Food	Serve Size	Household Measure	Calories	Fat (g)	Saturated Fat (g)	Carbo-hydrate (g)	Fiber (g)	Sodium (mg)	GI	LOW MED HIGH
Glucose Syrup	¾ oz	3 tsp	65	0	0	16.3	0	29	100	high
Golden Syrup	¾ oz	3 tsp	58	0	0	14.9	0	26	68	med
Honey, general	¾ oz	3 tsp	70	0	0	18	0	3	52	low
Honey, Iron bark	¾ oz	3 tsp	70	0	0	18	0	3	48	low
Honey, Red gum	¾ oz	3 tsp	70	0	0	18	0	3	46	low
Honey, Stringy bark	¾ oz	3 tsp	70	0	0	18	0	3	44	low
Honey, Yellow-box	¾ oz	3 tsp	70	0	0	18	0	3	35	low
Maple-Flavored Syrup	¾ oz	3 tsp	58	0	0	15.1	0	10	68	med
Maple Syrup (100% Maple)	¾ oz	3 tsp	52	0	0	13.4	0	2	54	low
Sugar, brown	½ oz	6 tsp	65	0	0	16.9	0	2	61	med
Sugar, white	½ oz	6 tsp	65	0	0	16.9	0	2	61	med
Treacle	¾ oz	3 tsp	51	0	0	13	0.2	36	68	med

VEGETABLES

Food	Serve Size	Household Measure	Calories	Fat (g)	Saturated Fat (g)	Carbo-hydrate (g)	Fiber (g)	Sodium (mg)	GI	LOW MED HIGH
Baked potato, without skin	3½ oz	1 medium	72	0.2	0	13.7	1.2	8	85	high
Beets, canned	6 oz	1 cup sliced	82	0.2	0	16	4.5	540	64	med
Carrots, peeled, boiled	9 oz	1 ½ cups	84	0.3	0	14.4	7.7	106	41	low
Hash brown	2 oz	1 average	171	11.7	5.2	14.7	0.8	281	75	high
Kumara, boiled	3 oz	½ large	63	0.1	0	12.6	2.1	9	77	high
Mashed potato, made with milk	4 oz	½ cup	82	0.5	0.2	14.8	1.7	10	85	high
Parsnips, boiled	2¾ oz	½ cup	16	0	0	8	1	1	52	low
Peas, green	7 oz	1 ½ cups	128	0.2	0	14.6	12.7	2	45	low
Potato Chips, deep fried	1½ oz	10 average chips	126	7.0	3.2	13.5	1.4	72	75	high
Potatoes, Desiree, peeled, boiled 35 mins	4 oz	1 medium (2¾ inch diameter)	82	0.1	0	15.6	2.3	4	101	high

Ⓖ program participant

Food	Serve Size	Household Measure	Calories	Fat (g)	Saturated Fat (g)	Carbo-hydrate (g)	Fiber (g)	Sodium (mg)	GI	LOW MED HIGH
Potatoes, Nardine, peeled, boiled	4 oz	1 medium (2¾ inch diameter)	82	0.1	0	15.6	2.3	4	70	high
Potatoes, new, canned, microwaved 3 mins	5 oz	4 small (1 inch diameter)	84	0.1	0	16	2.2	470	65	med
Potatoes, new, unpeeled, boiled 20 mins	5 oz	4 small (1 inch diameter)	84	0.1	0	16	2.2	4	78	high
Potatoes, Pontiac, peeled, boiled 15 mins, mashed	4 oz	½ cup	74	0.1	0	14.2	2.2	4	91	high
Potatoes, Pontiac, peeled, boiled whole 30-35 mins	4 oz	1 medium (2¾ inch diameter)	82	0.1	0	15.6	2.3	4	72	high
Potatoes, Pontiac, peeled, microwaved 7 mins	4 oz	1 medium (2¾ inch diameter)	82	0.1	0	15.6	2.3	4	79	high
Potatoes, Sebago, peeled, boiled 35 mins	4 oz	1 medium (2¾ inch diameter)	82	0.1	0	15.6	2.3	4	87	high
Potato, instant, mashed, Idahoan	4 oz	½ cup, prepared	170	0	0	16	2	15	88	high
Potato salad, canned	4 oz	½ cup	147	8.3	1.6	15.8	1.2	408	63	med
Potato, wedge, with skin	1¼ oz	2 small	118	4.2	0.5	16.9	2.2	23	75	high
Pumpkin, boiled	7½ oz	1¼ cup	96	0.9	0.6	15	3	2	75	high
Squash, butternut, boiled	2¾ oz	½ cup	30	0	0	6	2	2	51	low
Sweet corn, honey and pearl variety, boiled	2¾ oz	1 medium (5 inches long)	84	0.8	0	15.3	2.4	6	37	low
Sweet corn, on the cob, boiled	2¾ oz	1 medium (5 inches long)	84	0.8	0	15.3	2.4	6	48	low
Sweet corn, whole kernel, canned, drained	3 oz	½ cup	90	0.9	0.1	16.3	2.7	238	46	low
Sweet potato, baked	3 oz	½ large	79	0.1	0	16.2	2.1	12	46	low
Taro, boiled	1½ oz	½ cup	63	0.1	0	15.2	2.2	7	54	low
Yam, peeled, boiled	2½ oz	½ cup	79	0.1	0	18.8	2.7	5	37	low

Ⓖ program participant

LOW- AND NO-CARBOHYDRATE FOODS

Food	Serve Size	Household Measure	Calories	Protein [g]	Fat [g]	Saturated Fat [g]	Carbo-hydrate [g]	Fiber [g]	Sodium [mg]
CHEESES									
Brie	1 oz	2 tbsp	102	5.8	8.7	5.6	0		182
Camembert	1 oz	2 tbsp	93	5.6	7.9	5.1	0		195
Cheddar	1 oz	1½ slices	122	7.6	10.1	6.5	0		197
Cheddar, 25% reduced fat	1 oz	1½ slices	99	8.6	7.1	4.5	0		216
Cheddar, 50% reduced fat	1 oz	1½ slices	80	9.4	4.7	3	0		207
Cheddar, low fat	1 oz	1½ slices	61	10.2	2.2	1.4	0		198
Cheddar, reduced salt	1 oz	1½ slices	123	7.3	11	6.7	0		111
Cheese spread, cheddar	1 oz	1½ tbsp	87	4.8	7.4	4.7	0.5		435
Cheese spread, cheddar, reduced fat	1 oz	1½ tbsp	72	5	5	3.3	1.9		480
Cottage cheese	1 oz	2 tbsp	37	5.3	1.7	1.1	0.7		95
Cottage cheese, low fat	1 oz	2 tbsp	27	4.6	0.4	0.2	0.5		39
Cream cheese	1 oz	1½ tbsp	102	2.6	9.9	6.4	0.7		126
Cream cheese dip	1 oz	1½ tbsp	76	1.4	6.5	4.1	3.2		204
Cream cheese, reduced fat	1 oz	1½ tbsp	58	2.5	5	3.3	0.9		102
Feta	1 oz	2 tbsp	84	5.3	7	4.6	0		321
Feta, low salt	1 oz	2 tbsp	113	5.7	10.1	6.5	0		66
Feta, reduced fat	1 oz	2 tbsp	70	7.7	4.4	2.8	0		330
Mozzarella	1 oz	1½ slices	91	7.8	6.6	4.2	0		113
Mozzarella, reduced fat	1 oz	1½ slices	86	9.5	5.4	3.5	0		174
Parmesan	1 oz	⅓ cup	133	11.4	9.7	6.2	0		432
Ricotta	1 oz	2 tbsp	44	3.2	3.4	2.2	0.3		59
Ricotta, reduced fat	1 oz	2 tbsp	38	3.1	2.6	1.7	0.6		56
Soy cheese	1 oz	1½ slices	95	5.5	8.2	0.6	0		180
DRESSINGS									
Caesar salad dressing	1 fl oz	1½ tbsp	149	0	16.5	2	0		6
Creamy mayonnaise 97% fat free	¾ fl oz	1 tbsp	24	0	0.5	0.2	4.8		152
French dressing	1 fl oz	1½ tbsp	82	0	7.4	0.9	3.6		567
French dressing, fat free, artificially sweetened	1 fl oz	1½ tbsp	3	0	0	0	0		514
Italian dressing	1 fl oz	1½ tbsp	95	0	9.4	1	2.1		399
Italian dressing ,fat free, artificially sweetened	1 fl oz	1½ tbsp	4	0	0	0	0.1		239
Mayonnaise	½ fl oz	1 tbsp	56	0	4.9	0.5	2.9		122

Ⓖ program participant

Food	Serve Size	Household Measure	Calories	Protein [g]	Fat [g]	Saturated Fat [g]	Carbo-hydrate [g]	Fiber [g]	Sodium (mg)
Salad dressing, homemade oil & vinegar	1 fl oz	1½ tbsp	178	0	19.8	2.4	0.1		7
Tartar Sauce	1 fl oz	1½ tbsp	71	0	6.9	1.1	1.6		157
Thousand island dressing	¾ fl oz	1 tbsp	56	0	4.5	0.5	3.7		210
Vinegar	½ fl oz	1 tbsp	2	0	0	0	0		1

EGGS

Food	Serve Size	Household Measure	Calories	Protein [g]	Fat [g]	Saturated Fat [g]	Carbo-hydrate [g]	Fiber [g]	Sodium (mg)
Egg white, raw	1 fl oz	1 average	15	3.5	0	0	0.1		54
Egg, whole raw	2 fl oz	1 average	77	2.7	5.5	1.7	0.1		72
Egg yolk, raw	½ fl oz	1 average	53	6.9	4.8	1.5	0		10

FATS AND OILS

Food	Serve Size	Household Measure	Calories	Protein [g]	Fat [g]	Saturated Fat [g]	Carbo-hydrate [g]	Fiber [g]	Sodium (mg)
Canola oil	⅓ fl oz	2 tsp	89	0	10	0.7	0		0
Copha	⅓ oz	2 tsp	83	0	9.3	8.6	0		0
Cream, pure, >35% fat	1 fl oz	1½ tbsp	120	0	12.8	8.5	0.8		6
Cream, sour, >35% fat	1 oz	1½ tbsp	120	0	12.7	8.4	0.9		9
Cream, thickened, >35% fat	¾ fl oz	1 tbsp	70	0	7.4	4.8	0.6		10
Dripping, pork	⅓ fl oz	2 tsp	83	0	9.3	3.8	0		0
Ghee	⅓ oz	2 tsp	97	0	10.9	7.2	0		0
Lard	⅓ oz	2 tsp	83	0	9.3	3.6	0		0
Margarine, cooking	⅓ oz	2 tsp	72	0	8	3.6	0		113
Safflower oil	⅓ fl oz	2 tsp	89	0	10	0.9	0		0
Sesame oil	⅓ fl oz	2 tsp	89	0	10	1.4	0		0
Soybean oil	⅓ fl oz	2 tsp	89	0	10	1.5	0		0
Suet	⅓ oz	2 tsp	76	0	8.1	4.6	1		0
Sunflower oil	⅓ fl oz	2 tsp	89	0	10	1.1	0		0

FRUITS

Food	Serve Size	Household Measure	Calories	Protein [g]	Fat [g]	Saturated Fat [g]	Carbo-hydrate [g]	Fiber [g]	Sodium (mg)
Avocado	2¾ oz	⅓ average	171	0	18.1	3.9	0.3	1.2	2
Kumquats	¾ oz	1 average	13	0	0.0	0	2.4	0.7	1
Loganberries	2½ oz	½ cup	51	0	0.2	0	3.5	5.8	1
Mulberries	2½ oz	½ cup	23	0	0.1	0	3	1.5	4
Raspberries	2 oz	½ cup	29	0	0.3	0	3.7	3.4	1
Rhubarb, stewed, unsweetened	3½ oz	⅓ cup	19	0	0.1	0	1.3	2.5	9
Strawberries	2½ oz	½ cup	17	0	0.1	0	1.9	1.6	4

Ⓖ program participant

Food	Serve Size	Household Measure	Calories	Protein [g]	Fat [g]	Saturated Fat [g]	Carbo-hydrate [g]	Fiber [g]	Sodium [mg]
MEAT AND ALTERNATIVES									
Bacon, fried	1 oz	1 small slice	38	5.5	1.5	0.5	0.7		500
Bacon, grilled	1 oz	1 slice	49	7.8	1.6	0.6	0.8		735
Beef									
Beef, corned silverside	¾ oz	1 slice	23	3.3	1.1	0.5	0		213
Beef, corned silverside, canned	1¾ oz	2 slices	96	11.3	5.6	2.4	0.1		570
Beef, roast	1 oz	2 slices	44	7.7	1.4	0.6	0		17
Beef steak, fat trimmed	6 oz	1 medium	356	50	17.1	7	0		119
Brains, cooked	2 oz	½ cup	89	8.4	6.2	1.7	0		73
Burger, fried	1¾ oz	1 average	101	17.7	5.5	1.3	2.7		241
Chicken									
Chicken breast, baked without skin	3 oz	⅓ small	140	21.2	6	1.7	0		65
Chicken breast, grilled without skin	3 oz	⅓ small	150	22.8	6.5	1.9	0		70
Chicken drumstick, grilled without skin	1½ oz	1 small	78	11.6	3.4	1	0		50
Chicken loaf	¾ oz	1 slice	42	3.1	2.3	0.7	2.2		172
Chicken chopped, cooked	3½ oz	½ cup	204	26.9	10.6	3	0		101
Chicken roll	¾ oz	1 slice	31	2.7	1.8	0.6	0.8		142
Chicken thigh fillet grilled, without skin	1¾ oz	½ large	113	13.2	6.7	2	0		55
Chicken wing grilled without skin	¾ oz	1 medium	37	5.3	1.8	0.5	0		19
Cold meats									
Pancetta	¾ oz	1 slice	40	3.8	2.7	1	0		275
Pepperoni	¾ oz	1 slice	106	5.7	9.3	4.1	0.8		365
Prosciutto	1½ oz	1 slice	51	7.3	2.3	0.8	0.1		753
Salami	¾ oz	1 slice	98	5.7	8.7	2.8	0.3		336
Duck and game									
Duck, roasted without skin	2 oz	½ breast	156	20.7	8.1	2.4	0		81
Quail	2¾ oz	1 average	151	21.1	7.3	1.9	0		
Hamburger pattie	2¾ oz	1 pattie	197	17.7	14	6.4	0		52
Lamb									
Lamb, ground, cooked	3½ oz	½ cup	218	24	13	6.8	0		80
Lamb, grilled chop, fat trimmed	1¾ oz	1 medium	108	15.3	5.2	2.7	0		36
Lamb, roasted loin, fat trimmed	2 oz	1 thick slice	141	12.9	9.9	5.3	0		34
Liver, cooked	2 oz	½ cup	158	18.3	8.4	3.1	2.1		53

Ⓖ program participant

Food	Serve Size	Household Measure	Calories	Protein [g]	Fat [g]	Saturated Fat [g]	Carbo-hydrate [g]	Fiber [g]	Sodium [mg]
Pork									
Frankfurter	2 oz	1 average	144	8.2	11.3	4.3	1.9		439
Ham, canned leg	1½ oz	1 thick slice	45	6.9	1.8	0.7	0.2		500
Pork, grilled chops, fat trimmed	3 oz	1 medium	171	27.2	6.8	2.6	0		71
Spam, lite	2 oz	2 slices	96	9	7.5	3	2		580
Spam, regular	1½ oz	2 slices	133	5	12.4	4.8	0.5		628
Speck	3½ oz	1 slice	212	22.1	13.7	5.4	0		1480
Turkey									
Turkey breast, deli-sliced	¾ oz	1 slice	34	6.5	0.9	0.2	0		46
Turkey breast, rolled roast	3 oz	2 thick slices	132	25	3.4	0.8	0		179
Turkey breast, smoked, without skin	3 oz	2 thick slices	132	25	3.4	0.8	0		179
Turkey leg, roasted without skin	3 oz	2 thick slices	146	22.8	5.6	1.9	0		145
Turkey, roasted breast without skin	2¾ oz	2 thick slices	117	22.1	3	0.7	0		158
Veal									
Veal, roasted, fat trimmed	3 oz	2 thick slices	122	26.9	1.4	0.4	0		43
Vegetarian									
Nutolene	3 oz	2 thick slices	214	9.3	17.6	2.7	3.9		281
Tofu, cooked	4½ oz	½ cup	96	10.5	5.5	0.8	0.7		5.2
Vegetarian sausages	3 oz	1 thick	109	13.8	4.3	0.8	2.7		381

SEAFOOD

Food	Serve Size	Household Measure	Calories	Protein [g]	Fat [g]	Saturated Fat [g]	Carbo-hydrate [g]	Fiber [g]	Sodium [mg]
Calamari, fried	2 oz	½ cup	70	10.5	3.1	0.9	0		192
Cod, fried	4 oz	1 fillet	192	22.8	9.7	2.5	3.4		163
Crab, cooked	2 oz	½ cup	34	24.5	0.3	0.1	0.6		218
Dory, fried	4 oz	1 fillet	203	27.4	10	2.7	3.4		181
Flounder, fried	4 oz	1 fillet	201	26.8	10.3	2.7	3.4		148
Kingfish, fried	4 oz	1 fillet	261	31.1	13.3	3.9	3.9		136
Ling, fried	4 oz	1 fillet	204	25.7	9.6	2.5	3.4		230
Lobster, cooked	2 oz	½ cup	53	11.9	0.5	0.1	0		213
Mullet, fried	4 oz	1 fillet	281	28	17	6.2	3.7		234
Mussels, cooked	2 oz	½ cup	76	10.8	1.6	0.5	4.3		562
Ocean perch, fried	4 oz	1 fillet	210	25.1	10.3	2.7	3.8		147
Octopus, cooked	2 oz	½ cup	69	14.2	1	0.2	0.5		204

Ⓖ program participant

Food	Serve Size	Household Measure	Calories	Protein [g]	Fat [g]	Saturated Fat [g]	Carbo-hydrate [g]	Fiber [g]	Sodium [mg]
Salmon, pink, no added salt, drained	2 oz	⅔ small can	90	13.4	4	1.2	0		67
Salmon, red, no added salt, drained	2 oz	⅔ small can	119	13.4	7.3	2	0		67
Sardines, canned in oil, drained	2 oz	⅔ small can	137	13.4	9.6	3.1	0		372
Scallops, cooked	2 oz	½ cup	56	13.3	0.8	0.2	0.3		91
Seafood marinara, canned	2 oz	⅔ small can	67	11.7	1	0.3	2.9		367
Shark, fried	4 oz	1 fillet	231	11.5	8.9	2.4	3.4		164
Snapper, fried	4 oz	1 fillet	251	33.9	12.3	3.5	3.9		181
Sole, fried	4 oz	1 fillet	206	30.7	10.5	2.9	3.4		186
Seafood									
Shrimp, cooked	2 oz	½ cup	55	12	0.7	0.2	0		228
Trevally, fried	4 oz	1 fillet	234	26.6	12.3	3.4	3.4		131
Trout, cooked	4 oz	1 fillet	164	27.2	5.6	1.3	0		70
Trout, fried	4 oz	1 fillet	200	7.1	8.7	2.5	3.5		129
Tuna, cooked	4 oz	1 fillet	213	28	8	3.2	0		57
Tuna in brine, drained	2 oz	⅔ small can	76	15.1	1.6	0.6	0		253
Tuna in oil	2 oz	⅔ small can	177	12.7	14.2	2.1	0		253

SPREADS

Food	Serve Size	Household Measure	Calories	Protein [g]	Fat [g]	Saturated Fat [g]	Carbo-hydrate [g]	Fiber [g]	Sodium [mg]
Anchovette fish spread	¾ oz	1 tbsp	37	4.35	1.7	0.6	0.9		240
Butter	⅓ oz	2 tsp	80	0.07	8.9	5.9	0		78
Cashew spread	⅓ oz	2 tsp	58	1.8	4.7	0.9	2.7		2
Dairy blend, with canola oil	⅓ oz	2 tsp	67	0.05	7.5	3.9	0		52
Extra virgin olive oil spread	¼ oz	1 tsp	31	0.05	3.5	0.9	0		18
Jam, sweetened with aspartame	⅓ oz	2 tsp	3	0.12	0	0	0.4		8
Jam, sweetened with sucralose	⅓ oz	2 tsp	2	0.03	0	0	0.4		8
Lemon butter, homemade	⅓ oz	2 tsp	32	0.49	2.1	1.2	2.8		18
Margarine, canola	⅓ oz	2 tsp	62	0.03	7	1.2	0		79
Marmalade, sweetened with aspartame	⅓ oz	2 tsp	2	0.12	0	0	0.2		3
Marmalade, sweetened with sucralose	⅓ oz	2 tsp	1	0.01	0	0	0.2		3
Tahini	¾ oz	1 tbsp	131	4.08	12.1	1.5	0.2		16

VEGETABLES

Canned vegetables

Food	Serve Size	Household Measure	Calories	Protein [g]	Fat [g]	Saturated Fat [g]	Carbo-hydrate [g]	Fiber [g]	Sodium [mg]
Artichoke hearts in brine, drained	3 oz	2 hearts	19		0.3	0	1	2.49	249
Artichoke hearts, whole	1½ oz	1 heart	14		0.2	0.1	0.5		80

Ⓖ program participant

Food	Serve Size	Household Measure	Calories	Protein [g]	Fat [g]	Saturated Fat [g]	Carbo-hydrate [g]	Fiber [g]	Sodium [mg]
Artichokes in brine	1½ oz	1 heart	12	0	0		2		130
Asparagus, drained	3 oz	¾ cup	22	0.1	0		1.3	3.5	216
Asparagus green/white spears	2 oz	½ cup	12	0.1	0		1.3		104
Asparagus in springwater	2 oz	½ cup	8	0.1	0		0.6		110
Baby corn, cut	1¾ oz	⅓ cup	13	0.2	0.1		1.8		135
Baby corn spears, whole	1¾ oz	⅓ cup	13	0.2	0.1		1.9		105
Bamboo shoots	1 oz	¼ cup	4	0	0		0.3	0.6	3
Champignons, whole	2 oz	⅓ cup	18	0.3	0.2		1.1		179
Green beans, sliced	3 oz	⅓ cup	30	0.1	0		4.5	2.6	281
Mixed vegetables, Chinese	3 oz	⅓ cup	26	0.3	0		4.5	1.4	68
Mushrooms	1 oz	3 small	11	0.5	0.1		0.5	0.8	5
Mushrooms, shiitake	1 oz	3 small	8	0.3	0.3		1.3		96
Onions, sautéed and diced	1¾ oz	1 medium	26	1.1	0.2		3.2		215
Pepper, green	1½ oz	¼ cup	8	0	0		0.9	0.4	1
Pepper, red	1½ oz	¼ cup	12	0.1	0		1.6	0.5	0
Sauerkraut	2½ oz	½ cup	12	0.4	0.2		0.7	3	322
Tomatoes, in tomato juice	3 oz	⅓ cup	19	0.2	0		2.8	1.1	56
Tomatoes, Italian diced	4½ oz	½ cup	28	1.3	1.3		4.5		125
Tomatoes, Italian whole peeled roma	4½ oz	½ cup	30	1.3	1.3		4.5		125
Tomatoes, whole peeled; no added salt	4½ oz	½ cup	25	0.1	0		4	0.6	6
Tomato, onion, pepper, celery	3 oz	⅓ cup	19	0.2	0		2.8	1.2	60
Tomato puree	2 oz	¼ cup	20	0.1	0		3.2	1.2	221
Water chestnuts, drained	¾ oz	2 tbsp	11	0.2	0		1.8	0.5	2
Cooked vegetables									
Artichoke, globe	4 oz	1 medium	28	0.2	0		1.6	1.1	7
Asparagus	3 oz	8 small spears	20	0.1	0		1.4	1.4	2
Bean sprouts	2 oz	½ cup	16	0.1	0		0.9	1.9	1
Beans, snake	2½ oz	½ cup	21	0.2	0		1.1	2.7	1
Bok choy	3 oz	½ cup	30	2.4	0.6		0.8	1	21
Broccoflower	1½ oz	½ cup	13	0.1	0		0.6	1.4	8
Broccoli	3½ oz	1 cup	34	0.3	0		0.6	4.2	20
Brussels sprouts	2¾ oz	4 sprouts	25	0.2	0		1.6	2.7	23
Cabbage, Chinese	3 oz	½ cup	29	2.3	0.6		0.7	1	18
Cabbage, green	3 oz	½ cup	20	0.1	0		2.1	3	15
Cabbage, red	3 oz	½ cup	26	0.3	0		2.5	3.2	14
Cauliflower	3 oz	¾ cup	21	0.2	0		1.9	1.7	13
Celery	2½ oz	2 medium stalks	13	0.1	0		1.8	1.7	63

Ⓖ program participant

Food	Serve Size	Household Measure	Calories	Protein [g]	Fat [g]	Saturated Fat [g]	Carbo-hydrate [g]	Fiber [g]	Sodium [mg]
Chilli, banana	1¾ oz	1 average	10	0.1	0		1.2	0.9	2.2
Chilli, hot thin	¾ oz	1 average	6	0.1	0		0.6	0.6	0.6
Choko	1½ oz	¼ average	9	0.1	0		1.5	0.7	3
Eggplant	1¾ oz	1 slice	12	0.1	0		1.3	1.2	2
Endive	3 oz	½ cup	16	0.2	0		0.4	2.4	81
Fennel	2½ oz	½ cup	20	0.1	0		2.6	2.9	26
Kohlrabi	3 oz	½ cup	36	0.1	0		3.9	3.1	12
Leeks	3 oz	1 average	27	0.3	0		3.1	2.4	13
Okra	3 oz	½ cup	29	0.2	0		1.4	4.1	2
Onion	1 oz	½ medium	13	0	0		2.1	0.6	4
Parsley	1½ oz	½ cup	10	0.1	0		0.1	2.1	21
Shallots	1 oz	3 medium	9	0.1	0		1.3	0.4	33
Snowpeas	2¾ oz	20 average	39	1.2	0.1		3.6	1.8	1
Spinach, English	3 oz	⅔ cup	28	0.4	0		0.7	5.7	18
Squash	2½ oz	2 average	22	0.1	0		2.3	1.8	1
Swiss Chard	4 oz	1 cup	24	0.4	0		1.5	3.8	213
Turnips	1¾ oz	⅓ cup	14	0	0		1.9	1.6	12
Zucchini	3 oz	1 medium	17	0.3	0		1.6	1.5	1
Raw vegetables									
Alfalfa sprouts	½ oz	6 tbs	4	0.1	0		0	0.4	7
Beans, green	1¾ oz	10 average	14	0.1	0		1.3	1.5	2
Bean sprouts	1 oz	⅓ cup	6	0.1	0		0.2		69
Cabbage, green	3 oz	1 cup	23	0.1	0		2.4	3.4	17
Cabbage, red	3 oz	1 cup	30	0.3	0		2.9	3.7	15
Celery	1 oz	2 small stalks	5	0	0		0.7	0.6	28
Chilli, banana	2 oz	1 average	10	0.1	0		1.2	0.9	2
Chilli, hot thin	1 oz	1 average	9	0.1	0		0.8	0.8	1
Chives	¼ oz	1 tbsp	1	0	0		0.1	0.1	0
Choko	2¾ oz	½ average	17	0.2	0		2.8	1.3	6
Cucumber	1 oz	3 slices	3	0	0		0.4	0.1	5
Cucumber, Lebanese	1 oz	3 slices	4	0	0		0.5	0.3	5
Eggplant	1½ oz	½ cup	9	0.1	0		1	0.9	2
Fennel	1¾ oz	½ cup	12	0.1	0		1.6	1.4	19
Garlic	¼ oz	1 clove	4	0.1	0		0.3	0.5	0
Horseradish	¼ oz	1 average	4	0	0		0.5	0.4	0
Leeks	3 oz	1 average	28	0.3	0		3.4	2.6	14
Lettuce, cos	¾ oz	3 medium leafs	5	0.1	0		0.4	0.5	4
Lettuce, iceberg	¾ oz	3 medium leafs	2	0	0		0	0.4	5

Ⓖ program participant

Food	Serve Size	Household Measure	Calories	Protein (g)	Fat (g)	Saturated Fat (g)	Carbo-hydrate (g)	Fiber (g)	Sodium (mg)
Lettuce, mignonette	¾ oz	3 medium leafs	4	0.1	0	0.2	0.5	4	
Mushrooms	1¼ oz	½ cup	11	0.1	0	0.5	0.9	3	
Onions, sautèed and diced	½ oz	1 medium slice	6	0	0	0.9	0.2	2	
Parsley	¼ oz	1 tbsp	1	0	0	0	0.2	2	
Pepper, green	1½ oz	4 rings	7	0	0	0.8	0.3	1	
Pepper, red	1½ oz	4 rings	11	0.1	0	1.6	0.5	0	
Radishes, red	2 oz	6 large	9	0.1	0	1.1	0.6	12	
Arugula	¾ oz	3 medium leaves	6	0.2	0	0.5	0.4	6	
Seaweed	1½ oz	½ cup	13	0.2	0	0	5	60	
Shallots	½ oz	2 average	4	0	0	0.5	0.2	16	
Snowpeas	1 oz	10 average	12	0.1	0	1.5	0.7	0	
Spinach, English	1 oz	1 cup	6	0.1	0	0.1	0.8	6	
Tomatoes	1¾ oz	½ small	9	0.1	0	1	0.7	3	
Zucchini	2 oz	½ medium	10	0.2	0	0.9	0.9	1	

Ⓖ program participant

What Sweetener Is That?

Nutritive Sweeteners

Fructose

GI 19

4 cal (16 kJ) per gram

11 cal (46 kJ) per teaspoon table sugar equivalent*

Fructose or fruit sugar has a relatively small effect on blood glucose levels. It is sweeter than table sugar, but has the same number of calories per gram.

Sweetness relative to table sugar = up to 70% more, depending on the temperature of the food

Glucose

GI 100

4 cal (16 kJ) per gram

26 cal (108 kJ) per teaspoon table sugar equivalent*

Brand name: Lucozade

Glucose is the sugar found in blood. When eaten, it causes blood glucose levels to rise rapidly. It is not as sweet as table sugar, but has the same number of calories per gram.

Sweetness relative to table sugar = 25% less

Golden syrup

GI 63

3 cal (12 kJ) per gram

11 cal (45 kJ) per teaspoon table sugar equivalent*

Golden syrup has a moderate effect on blood glucose levels, very similar to table sugar. It is sweeter than table sugar, and has fewer calories per gram.

Sweetness relative to table sugar = 33% more

Grape syrup

GI 52

4 cal (16 kJ) per gram

16 cal (68 kJ) per teaspoon table sugar equivalent*

Grape syrup or nectar has a moderate effect on blood glucose levels. It is a little sweeter than table sugar, but has the same number of calories.

Sweetness relative to table sugar = 20% more

Honey

GI 35–64

4 cal (16 kJ) per gram

20 cal (83 kJ) per teaspoon table sugar equivalent*

Honey has a variable effect on blood glucose levels depending on whether it is a blend or a pure floral honey. The pure floral honeys appear to have lower GIs. On average, honey is slightly less sweet than table sugar, but has about the same number of calories per teaspoon.

Sweetness relative to table sugar = about the same

*The number of calories in the volume of alternative sweetener that provides the equivalent sweetness to 1 teaspoon of table sugar.

Isomalt

GI 60

3 cal (11 kJ) per gram

26 cal (110 kJ) per teaspoon table sugar equivalent*

Isomalt has a moderate effect on blood glucose levels similar to table sugar. It is only half as sweet as table sugar, but has fewer calories, and may have a laxative effect if eaten in large quantities.

Sweetness relative to table sugar = half as sweet

Lactose

GI 46

4 cal (16 kJ) per gram

120 cal (500 kJ) per teaspoon table sugar equivalent*

Lactose is the sugar found in milk. It causes blood glucose levels to rise slowly. It is not very sweet at all, but has the same number of calories as table sugar.

Sweetness relative to table sugar = 85% less

Maltitol

GI 69

3 cal (13 kJ) per gram

21 cal (87 kJ) per teaspoon table sugar equivalent*

Maltitol has a moderate to high effect on blood glucose levels greater than that of table sugar. It is only three-quarters as sweet as table sugar, and has the same number of calories, and may have a laxative effect and cause wind and diarrhea if eaten in large quantities.

Sweetness relative to table sugar = 25% less sweet

Maltodextrin

GI not known

4 cal (16 kJ) per gram

35 cal (146 kJ) per teaspoon table sugar equivalent*

The effect of maltodextrin on blood glucose levels is not exactly known, though it is likely to be similar to that of glucose. It is only half as sweet as table sugar, and has the same number of calories.

Sweetness relative to table sugar = half as sweet

Maltose

GI 105

4 cal (16 kJ) per gram

60 cal (250 kJ) per teaspoon table sugar equivalent*

Maltose or malt causes blood glucose levels to rise rapidly. It is only one-third as sweet as table sugar, and has the same number of calories.

Sweetness relative to table sugar = 67% less sweet

*The number of calories in the volume of alternative sweetener that provides the equivalent sweetness to 1 teaspoon of table sugar.

Mannitol

GI n/a	Mannitol has essentially no effect on blood glucose levels. It is only three-quarters as sweet as table sugar, but has only half the amount of calories, and may have a laxative effect and cause gas and diarrhea if eaten in large quantities.
2 cal (9 kJ) per gram	
15 cal (64 kJ) per teaspoon table sugar equivalent*	
	Sweetness relative to table sugar = 25% less

Maple syrup

GI 54	Real maple syrup has a moderate effect on blood glucose levels. It is a little sweeter than table sugar, but has fewer calories.
3 cal (11 kJ) per gram	
15 cal (61 kJ) per teaspoon table sugar equivalent*	
	Sweetness relative to table sugar = 10% more

Polydextrose

GI 7	Polydextrose has very little effect on blood glucose levels. It is not sweet, but is used as a bulking agent with nonnutritive sweeteners. It has only one-third the amount of calories as table sugar, but may have a laxative effect if eaten in large quantities.
1 cal (5 kJ) per gram	
6 cal (25 kJ) per teaspoon table sugar equivalent*	
Brand name: Litesse	
	Sweetness relative to table sugar = not sweet

Table sugar (sucrose)

GI 60 (average)	Sucrose or table sugar is the most common sweetener eaten in North America. Despite popular misconceptions, it causes blood glucose levels to rise only moderately (less than white bread).
4 cal (16 kJ) per gram	
16 cal (67 kJ) per teaspoon	
	Sweetness = 100%
	Castor sugar, brown sugar, raw sugar, confectioners' sugar are all forms of sugar.

Xylitol

GI 21	Xylitol is a sugar alcohol that has little effect on blood glucose levels. It is as sweet as sugar and has fewer calories, but may have a laxative effect and cause gas and diarrhea if consumed in large quantities.
3 cal (12 kJ) per gram	
14 cal (60 kJ) per teaspoon table sugar equivalent*	
	Sweetness relative to table sugar = 100%

*The number of calories in the volume of alternative sweetener that provides the equivalent sweetness to 1 teaspoon of table sugar.

Nonnutritive Sweeteners

Acesulphame potassium or Acesulphame K	
GI 0	Acesulphame K is much sweeter than sugar, has no effect on blood glucose levels, and doesn't provide any calories because it is not absorbed into the body.
0 cal (0 kJ) per gram	
0 cal (0 kJ) per teaspoon table sugar equivalent*	
Food additive code 950	Sweetness relative to table sugar = 200 times more
Brand names: Sweet One, Sunett	

Alitame	
GI 0	Alitame is two thousand times sweeter than sugar, and has essentially no effect on blood glucose levels. Because it is a protein. it does provide some calories, but because it is so sweet, you only use it in tiny amounts.
4 cal (17 kJ) per gram	
0 cal (0 kJ) per teaspoon table sugar equivalent*	
	Sweetness relative to table sugar = 2,000 times more

Aspartame	
GI 0	Aspartame is a couple of hundred times sweeter than sugar, and has essentially no effect on blood glucose levels. Because it is a protein it does provide some calories, but because it is very sweet, you only use it in small amounts.
4 cal (17 kJ) per gram	
0.3 cal (1.4 kJ) per teaspoon table sugar equivalent*	
Brand names: Nutrasweet, Equal, Equal Spoonful	
	Sweetness relative to table sugar = 150–250 times more
	Warning: Aspartame should not be used by people with phenylketonuria.

Cyclamate	
GI 0	Cyclamate is considerably sweeter than sugar, has essentially no effect on blood glucose levels and is not metabolized by most people.
0 cal (0 kJ) per gram	
0 cal (0 kJ) per teaspoon table sugar equivalent*	
	Sweetness relative to table sugar = 15–50 times more

*The number of calories in the volume of alternative sweetener that provides the equivalent sweetness to 1 teaspoon of table sugar.

Neotame

GI 0	Neotame is many thousands of times sweeter than sugar, and has essentially no effect on blood glucose levels. Because it is a protein it does provide some calories, but because it is extremely sweet, it is only used in tiny amounts.
4 cal (17 kJ) per gram	
0 cal (0 kJ) per teaspoon table sugar equivalent*	
	Sweetness relative to table sugar = 7,000–13,000 times more
	While neotame is approved by the Food and Drug Administration (FDA), it is not currently found in many foods or beverages.

Saccharin

GI 0	Saccharin is hundreds of times sweeter than sugar, has no effect on blood glucose levels and is not metabolized by the human body.
0 cal (0 kJ) per gram	
0 cal (0 kJ) per teaspoon table sugar equivalent*	
Brand names: Sweet 'n Low, Sugar Twin	Sweetness relative to table sugar = 300–500 times more

Stevia

GI 0	Sweetness relative to table sugar = 30 times more
2.7 cal (11 kJ) per gram	
0.7 cal (3 kJ) per teaspoon table sugar equivalent*	Currently stevia is not approved as a food additive by the FDA and Health Canada, but it is available in health food stores as a dietary supplement.
Stevia is considerably sweeter than sugar and has essentially no effect on blood glucose levels.	

Sucralose

GI 0	Sucralose is hundreds of times sweeter than sugar, has no effect on blood glucose levels, and does not provide any calories because it is not absorbed into the body.
0 cal (0 kJ) per gram	
0 cal (0 kJ) per teaspoon table sugar equivalent*	
Brand name: Splenda	Sweetness relative to table sugar = 400–600 times more

*The number of calories in the volume of alternative sweetener that provides the equivalent sweetness to 1 teaspoon of table sugar.

Further Resources
and Key Contacts

*F*or **further information** and advice, we recommend that you contact the following organizations.

American Diabetes Association (ADA)

ADA is the nation's leading nonprofit health organization for people with diabetes in the United States, providing information on diabetes and diabetes prevention, as well as tips and resources for living well with diabetes. ADA has offices nationwide; to find the office closest to you, call 800-DIABETES (800-342-2383).

www.diabetes.org

American Heart Association

The American Heart Association has offices all around the country. Contact the Heartline at 800-AHA-USA-1 (800-242-8721) for information, or go to their Web site

www.americanheart.org

Canadian Diabetes Association

The Canadian Diabetes Association is the primary consumer health organization for people with diabetes in Canada. The aim of the organization is to promote the health of Canadians through diabetes research, education, service and advocacy.

www.diabetes.ca

Crisis Services Kids Helpline (United States)

877-KIDS-400 (877-543-1400)

www.kidscrisis.com

Diabetes Educators

In the United States

American Association of Diabetes Educators (AADE)

100 West Monroe, Suite 400

Chicago, IL 60603

800-338-3633

www.aadenet.org

In Canada

Canadian Diabetes Educator Certification Board

2878 King Street

Caledon, ON L7C 0R3

905-838-4898

www.cdecb.ca

Dietitians

In the United States

American Dietetic Association

120 South Riverside Plaza, Suite 2000

Chicago, Illinois 60606

800-877-1600

www.eatright.org

In Canada

Dietitians of Canada
480 University Avenue, Suite 604
Toronto, ON M5G 1V2
416-596-0857
www.dieticians.ca

Exercise Specialists

Personal Trainers' Network
An international database for locating personal trainers.
www.personaltrainers.net

In the United States

American Physical Therapy Association
800-999-APTA (800-999-2782)
www.apta.org and click on "Find a PT"

American Society of Exercise Physiologists
www.asep.org

In Canada

Canadian Physiotherapy Association
800-387-8679
www.physiotherapy.ca and click on "Find a Physiotherapist"

Canadian Society for Exercise Physiology
877-651-3755
www.csep.ca

Glycemic Index

For the latest information on the glycemic index (GI)
www.glycemicindex.com

www.ginews.blogspot.com
www.gisymbol.com

Glycemic Index Laboratories

www.gilabs.com

Heart and Stroke Foundation (Canada)

Call 613-569-4361 to find the Heart and Stroke Foundation office nearest you.
www.heartandstroke.ca

HopeLine (United States)

800-394-HOPE (800-394-4673)
www.thehopeline.com

Juvenile Diabetes Research Foundation International

www.jdrf.org and click on "Locations"

Kids Help Phone (Canada)

800-668-6868
www.kidshelpphone.ca

Mood Disorder Society of Canada

For anyone suffering from depression and all other mood disorders, including depression, bipolar disorders and anxiety, Mood Disorder Society provides resources to find help.
www.mooddisordersofcanada.ca

National Alliance on Mental Illness (NAMI) (United States)

NAMI provides information and support for people living with mental illnesses and their friends and family.
Info helpline: 800-950-NAMI (800-950-6264)
www.nami.org

Podiatrists

In the United States

American Podiatric Medical Association
www.apma.org

In Canada

Podiatrists in Canada
www.footdoctors.ca

Quit Line

If you need help to stop smoking, call
United States: 800-QUIT-NOW (800-784-8669)
Canada: 877-513-5333

Acknowledgments

*A*s we say in our dedication, this book is for all the people who live with diabetes and have so openly shared their experience with us over the years. We could not have written it without you. In particular, we would like to thank those who allowed us to publish their "success stories" here.

We would also like to thank our numerous colleagues who generously provided us with indispensable feedback as we were working on this book.

To publish GI tables that include all the latest foods that have been tested, we need the help of the team at the University of Sydney who keep the GI database up to date: Fiona Atkinson, manager of the Sydney University Glycemic Index Research Service, and Associate Professor Gareth Denyer—thank you both. And we greatly appreciation the contributions of Katherine Corbett and all those at GI Labs in Toronto.

Our thanks also to Peter Howard for the recipes he created for us and for giving us permission to reproduce three recipes from his cookbook, *Delicious Living* (New Holland, 2006), and to Diane

Temple for testing and developing recipes to meet our nutritional guidelines.

As ever, we are indebted to our tireless publisher, Matthew Lore, for his passion and commitment to publishing this book on diabetes. Of course we know he has the backing of a great team at Marlowe & Company and we would especially like to thank Courtney Napoles and Kathleen Hanuschak for their attention to every detail.

From the start, two people held on to the vision for this book and helped us make it a reality: our editor Vanessa Radnidge and our agent Philippa Sandall. Thank you both, we couldn't have done it without you.

Lastly, we thank our wonderful, encouraging and supportive families—John Miller; Jonathan Powell; Ruth Colagiuri; Sharon, Marcus and Michael Barclay; and especially Kaye's young children, Rowan and April, for all the times when "mommy" was working!

Index

About the Authors

MEET THE MEDICAL DOCTORS, SCIENTISTS AND CLINICIANS BEHIND *THE NEW GLUCOSE REVOLUTION FOR DIABETES*

Jennie Brand-Miller, PhD, is one of the world's foremost authorities on carbohydrates and the glycemic index and has championed the GI approach to nutrition for more than twenty-five years. Professor of Human Nutrition at the University of Sydney and the immediate past president of the Nutrition Society of Australia, Dr. Brand-Miller is also chair of the board of directors of the not-for-profit Glycemic Index Ltd., which administers a GI food-labeling program in collaboration with the Juvenile Diabetes Research Foundation and Diabetes Australia, to ensure that claims about the GI are scientifically correct and applied only to nutritious foods. Winner of Australia's prestigious ATSE Clunies Ross Award in 2003 for her commitment to advancing science and technology and coauthor of the entire *New York Times*–best-selling New Glucose Revolution series of books, Dr. Brand-Miller is an in-demand speaker, and her laboratory at the

University of Sydney is recognized worldwide for cutting-edge research on carbohydrates and health.

Kaye Foster-Powell, M Nutr & Diet, an accredited dietitian-nutritionist with extensive experience in diabetes management, counsels hundreds of people a year on how to improve their health and well-being and reduce their risk of diabetic complications through a low-GI diet. Foster-Powell is the coauthor with Dr. Jennie Brand-Miller of the New Glucose Revolution series of books, as well as of the authoritative international tables of GI values published in the *American Journal of Clinical Nutrition*.

Stephen Colagiuri, MD, is Professor of Metabolic Health at the University of Sydney and a fellow of the Royal Australasian College of Physicians. A coauthor of many books in the New Glucose Revolution series, Dr. Colagiuri has more than 100 scientific papers to his name, many concerned with the importance of carbohydrates in the diet of people with diabetes.

Alan W. Barclay, APD, B Sci, Grad Dip Dietetics, PhD Candidate, is an accredited practicing dietitian who has worked for Diabetes Australia since 1998, most recently as Research and Development Manager in New South Wales. He is a member of the editorial boards of Diabetes Australia's consumer magazine, *Conquest*, and *Diabetes Management Journal*. Barclay is currently acting CEO of Glycemic Index Ltd.

The Marlowe Diabetes Library

Good control is in your hands.

MARLOWE DIABETES LIBRARY titles are available from on-line and bricks-and-mortar retailers nationally. For more information about the Marlowe Diabetes Library or any of our books or authors, visit www.marlowepub.com/diabetes library or e-mail us at goodcontrol@avalonpub.com

TYPE 1 DIABETES
A Guide for Children, Adolescents, Young Adults—and Their Caregivers
Ragnar Hanas, MD, PhD | Forewords by Stuart Brink, MD,
and Jeff Hitchcock ■ $24.95

KNOW YOUR NUMBERS, OUTLIVE YOUR DIABETES
Five Essential Health Factors You Can Master to Enjoy a Long and Healthy Life
Richard A. Jackson, MD, and Amy Tenderich ■ $14.95

INSULIN PUMP THERAPY DEMYSTIFIED
An Essential Guide for Everyone Pumping Insulin
Gabrielle Kaplan-Mayer | Foreword by Gary Scheiner, MS, CDE ■ $15.95

LOSING WEIGHT WITH YOUR DIABETES MEDICATION
How Byetta and Other Drugs Can Help You Lose More Weight
than You Ever Thought Possible
David Mendosa | Foreword by Joe Prendergast, MD ■ $14.99

1,001 TIPS FOR LIVING WELL WITH DIABETES
Firsthand Advice that Really Works
Judith H. McQuown | Foreword by Harry Gruenspan, MD, PhD ■ $16.95

DIABETES ON YOUR OWN TERMS
Janis Roszler, RD, CDE, LD/N ■ $14.95

THINK LIKE A PANCREAS
A Practical Guide to Managing Diabetes with Insulin
Gary Scheiner, MS, CDE | Foreword by Barry Goldstein, MD ■ $15.95

THE ULTIMATE GUIDE TO ACCURATE CARB COUNTING
Gary Scheiner, MS, CDE ■ $9.95

THE MIND-BODY DIABETES REVOLUTION
A Proven New Program for Better Blood Sugar Control
Richard S. Surwit, PhD, with Alisa Bauman ■ $14.95